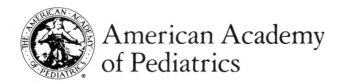

American Academy
of Pediatrics

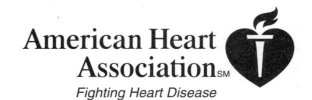

American Heart
Association℠

*Fighting Heart Disease
and Stroke*

Textbook of
Pediatric
Advanced Life Support

Editors

Leon Chameides, MD
Mary Fran Hazinski, MSN, RN

Subcommittee on Pediatric Resuscitation, 1991-1994

Mary Fran Hazinski, MSN, RN, Cochair
Linda Quan, MD, Cochair
Leon Chameides, MD, Cochair,
   1991-1993
James S. Seidel, MD, PhD, Chair,
   1987-1991
David J. Burchfield, MD

Arthur Cooper, MD
Charles J. Coté, MD
J. Michael Dean, MD
Mary E. Fallat, MD
Wayne H. Franklin, MD
Mark G. Goetting, MD
Harriet Hawkins, RNC, CCRN

Karin A. McCloskey, MD
Lyle F. McGonigle, MD
Olga E. Mohan, MD
Vinay M. Nadkarni, MD
John R. Raye, MD
Kathryn A. Taubert, PhD
Timothy S. Yeh, MD

Contributors and Reviewers

Julius Landwirth, MD, JD
Joseph J. Tepas, MD

I. David Todres, MD
Arno L. Zaritsky, MD

James A. Glenski, MD

Neonatal Resuscitation Program Steering Committee, 1991-1994

David J. Burchfield, MD, Cochair
William J. Keenan, MD, Cochair
John R. Raye, MD, Immediate Past Chair

Ronald S. Bloom, MD
Catherine Cropley, MN, RN
Susan E. Denson, MD

Allen Erenberg, MD
John Kattwinkel, MD
Martha D. Mullett, MD

Committee on Emergency Cardiac Care, 1991-1994

Joseph P. Ornato, MD, Chair
Richard E. Kerber, MD, Immediate Past Chair
Richard O. Cummins, MD, MPH, MSc,
   Vice-Chair

Richard K. Albert, MD
Donald D. Brown, MD
Nisha Chibber Chandra, MD
Mary Fran Hazinski, MSN, RN

Richard J. Melker, MD, PhD
Linda Quan, MD
W. Douglas Weaver, MD

ISBN 0-87493-635-7

Credit Listing of 1988 Edition

Editor

Leon Chameides, MD, FAAP

Contributing Editors

Ronald S. Bloom, MD, FAAP
Deborah L. Burkett, EdD
Frederick W. Campbell, MD
Peter R. Holbrook, MD, FAAP
Julius Landwirth, MD, JD, FAAP

Robert C. Luten, MD, FAAP
James H. McCrory, MD
Richard J. Melker, MD, PhD, FAAP
Richard A. Schieber, MD, FAAP
Alan Jay Schwartz, MD, MSEd

James S. Seidel, MD, PhD, FAAP
Ann E. Thompson, MD, FAAP
Robert E. Wood, MD, PhD, FAAP
Arno L. Zaritsky, MD, FAAP

Prepared under the direction of the
Subcommittee on Pediatric Resuscitation

James S. Seidel, MD, PhD, Chair
Robert C. Luten, MD

James H. McCrory, MD
John R. Raye, MD

Arno L. Zaritsky, MD

Of the American Heart Association
Committee on Emergency Cardiac Care

Judith H. Donegan, MD, PhD, Chair
Ramiro Albarran-Sotelo, MD

Allan S. Jaffe, MD
Joseph Ornato, MD

John A. Paraskos, MD

Special Acknowledgment

Many AHA staff members have contributed in numerous ways to the development of this text. In particular, we would like to acknowledge the invaluable assistance of F.G. Stoddard, PhD, AHA copy editor.

Contents

Preface

Five years have passed since the first edition of this textbook was published as a companion to the Pediatric Advanced Life Support Course. The course and text have been widely accepted. It is difficult to gauge the full impact of the Pediatric Advanced Life Support program on the acute care of critically ill children. Nevertheless, we believe that the clinical approach to assessment, intervention, and reassessment emphasized in the course has had a salutary effect on outcome.

Changes in resuscitation guidelines made as a result of the 1992 National Conference on Cardiopulmonary Resuscitation and Emergency Cardiac Care* have necessitated a revision of the textbook. This has given us an opportunity to critically review its content, update it, and to add several important chapters. These include chapters on trauma, the most common cause of cardiopulmonary collapse in infants and children, and the Emergency Medical Services system, which emphasizes the importance of appropriate prehospital care for a good outcome.

We are grateful to the many contributors, without whose patience and work this textbook would have been impossible. Because this revised textbook is built on the firm foundation of the contributors to the first edition, we have included their names with our thanks. Finally, we are indebted to the many correspondents who have written us with suggestions, many of which have been incorporated in this revision.

Leon Chameides, MD, FAAP
Mary Fran Hazinski, MSN, RN, FAAN
Coeditors

*Emergency Cardiac Care Committee and Subcommittees. American Heart Association. Guidelines for cardiopulmonary resuscitation and emergency cardiac care, V, VI, VII. *JAMA*. 1992;268:2251-2281.

He who has saved one life has saved the whole world.
—*Mishnah Sanhedrin*

Introduction

And it came to pass after these things, that the son of the woman, the mistress of the house, fell sick; and his sickness was so sore, that there was no breath left in him ... And [Elijah] said unto her, Give me thy son. And he took him out of her bosom, and carried him up into a loft, where he abode, and laid him upon his own bed. And he cried unto the Lord, and said, O Lord my God, hast thou also brought evil upon the widow with whom I sojourn, by slaying her son? And he stretched himself upon the child three times, and cried unto the Lord, and said, O Lord my God, I pray thee, let this child's soul come into him again. And the Lord heard the voice of Elijah; and the soul of the child came into him again, and he revived.

—I Kings 17:17-22
King James Version

Some of the modern concepts of cardiopulmonary resuscitation (CPR) are already evident in this first "case report" of a pediatric resuscitation. There is a victim (the child) and a bystander (the mother), who correctly assesses the problem and seeks a rescuer (Elijah), who lies down on the victim (mouth-to-mouth ventilation?), and the victim recovers.

Reanimation, however, remained only a dream for many centuries until Kouwenhoven and associates[1] demonstrated that chest compressions in victims of cardiac arrest can provide sufficient blood flow to maintain life until definitive treatment is provided.

Historical Setting

Although there have been periodic national conferences on basic and advanced life support (BLS and ALS) for adults, pediatricians were not involved in the 1966 or 1973 national conferences, and the only reference to infants and children in the resulting standards was a drug dosage chart. To correct this omission, a working group on pediatric resuscitation chaired by Dr Leon Chameides was formed in 1978 under the auspices of the American Heart Association (AHA) Subcommittee on Emergency Cardiac Care. This group developed standards in pediatric BLS and guidelines for neonatal resuscitation that were accepted by the 1979 national conference.[2] The 1985 national conference included three speakers on various aspects of pediatric resuscitation. Three panels—Pediatric BLS, Pediatric ALS, and Neonatal Resuscitation—revised the standards for pediatric BLS and the guidelines in neonatal resuscitation and devel-

oped pediatric ALS guidelines.[3] These were subsequently endorsed by the American Academy of Pediatrics (AAP). A large number of pediatricians representing the full range of subspecialties and personnel caring for critically ill children participated in the 1992 national conference.[4] Among the new features were a state-of-the-art presentation and a panel discussion on injury prevention.

In December 1983 a national conference on pediatric resuscitation was convened under the auspices of the AHA and the chairmanship of Dr Leon Chameides. Experts in the field were joined by representatives of the Section of Pediatric Emergency Medicine and the Committee on the Fetus and Newborn of the AAP, the American Academy of Family Physicians, the American College of Cardiology, the American College of Surgeons, the American Medical Association, the American Society of Anesthesiology, the Canadian Heart Foundation, the National Perinatal Association, and the Nurses Association of the American College of Obstetricians and Gynecologists. The conference concluded that courses in pediatric and neonatal ALS were urgently needed and defined their general content.

Three pediatric resuscitation courses were introduced in the fall of 1988. The Neonatal Resuscitation Program (NRP) was offered for the first time at the annual AAP meeting in New Orleans, and the Pediatric BLS and ALS courses were introduced to a select group of instructors at meetings in Jacksonville, Fla, Los Angeles, Calif, and Kansas City, Mo.

Administration of the pediatric BLS and ALS courses is the responsibility of the AHA and its affiliates. The neonatal resuscitation course is administered by the AAP and a steering committee composed of representatives of both organizations.

Since their introduction, the three courses have enjoyed wide popularity in this country and internationally. To date, over 500 000 healthcare providers have taken the neonatal resuscitation course, over 50 000 have taken the pediatric ALS course, and an untold number have taken the pediatric BLS course.

Overview

This textbook, which provides the student with a reference on various aspects of ALS for infants and children, is a companion to the Pediatric Advanced Life Support Course. The course includes lectures, skill stations, and interactive sessions that integrate knowledge and skills into a clinically useful discipline.

The structure of the text makes the contents of the chapters appear isolated from each other, although they, like resuscitation itself, must be viewed as a continuum in *time:*

Preresuscitation ⇒ Resuscitation ⇒ Postresuscitation

and in *activity:*

Assessment ⇒ Action ⇒ Reassessment

The resuscitative process involves information presented in many chapters. The relation of text to steps of the resuscitative process (Figure) begins with assessment of the cardiovascular and respiratory systems.

The conclusion of the assessment may be that

- The systems are stable, in which case no further action is necessary
- The systems are unstable, in which case the action depends on the nature and degree of instability
- The assessment is inconclusive, in which case the child needs careful observation and repeated assessments.

This text concentrates on assessment, signs that indicate a need for intervention, and the nature of the intervention.

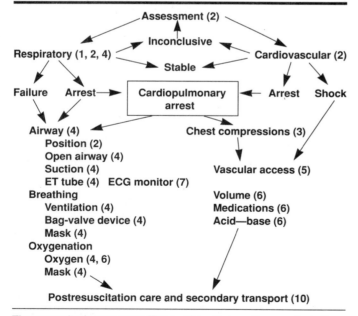

The resuscitation process. The numbers in parentheses refer to the chapters in which the information is located.

References

1. Kouwenhoven WB, Jude JR, Knickerbocker GG. Closed-chest cardiac massage. *JAMA.* 1960;173:1064-1067.
2. Standards and guidelines for cardiopulmonary resuscitation (CPR) and emergency cardiac care (ECC). *JAMA.* 1980;244:453-509.
3. Standards and guidelines for cardiopulmonary resuscitation (CPR) and emergency cardiac care (ECC). *JAMA.* 1986;255:2905-2984.
4. Emergency Cardiac Care Committee and Subcommittees. American Heart Association. Guidelines for cardiopulmonary resuscitation and emergency cardiac care, V, VI, VII. *JAMA.* 1992;268: 2251-2281.

Emergency Medical Services for Children

Chapter 1

The functional survival of critically ill and injured children is influenced by the provision of timely and appropriate pediatric emergency care. This care includes a broad spectrum of services, from early identification of problems through prehospital, hospital, and rehabilitative care. Emergency Medical Services for Children (EMS-C) must therefore be integrated into emergency medical services (EMS) systems at state, regional, and local levels. The specific needs of pediatric patients within the EMS system are now appreciated as a result of efforts by the pediatric and emergency medicine communities and projects funded through the US Department of Health and Human Services, Health Services and Resources Administration, Maternal and Child Health Branch, in collaboration with the National Highway Traffic Safety Commission.[1,2]

The first links in the "chain of survival" for pediatric emergencies involve identification of problems and early intervention. Parents, caretakers, and school personnel must be trained to (1) recognize ill and injured children, (2) provide first aid, (3) activate the EMS system, and (4) be familiar with the resources for emergency care in their communities. Although courses in BLS[3] are available in most communities, even parents of children at high risk may not be adequately trained in CPR. Caretakers of children must be able to recognize an emergency, initiate emergency care (particularly rescue breathing), and call EMS *fast*.

Access to EMS Services

Entry into the EMS system occurs when the rescuer or bystander calls the local emergency telephone number and speaks with a dispatcher. The accessibility of this critical contact and the speed and quality of the dispatcher response vary widely throughout the United States.

While the universal emergency access number 911 is an excellent concept, 911 access is not universal and is determined entirely by local (community) jurisdiction and funding. In 1991 only 60% of the population and 42% of the US could access emergency services by dialing 911.[4] "Enhanced 911" services are available to even fewer communities. An enhanced service enables immediate computerized identification of the telephone number and location of the caller so that the dispatcher can send appropriate help regardless of the quality of the information provided by the caller. Such an enhanced system would particularly benefit children as well as callers who may be distraught or disoriented or have trouble speaking.

Although all dispatchers must complete an approved training course, the information dispatchers give callers varies widely and is controlled by local jurisdiction. Use of dispatcher protocols would reduce the variability of information provided by dispatchers and ensure that succinct, accurate emergency information is provided to every caller. Currently such protocols are used by less than 20% of EMS dispatchers.[5] Even fewer have pediatric protocols. Protocols must be developed and implemented so that dispatchers can properly instruct callers in pediatric CPR, relief of foreign-body airway obstruction, and essential first aid until EMS personnel arrive.[6,7]

The first link in the chain of survival is the general public. For children this link includes parents, caretakers, older siblings, and school personnel, who must be educated about the appropriate use of the EMS system. Too often EMS services are inappropriately used to provide basic health care or transportation.[8] For example, a study in King County, Wash, revealed that 25% of children admitted to a hospital with a diagnosis of epiglottitis were inappropriately transported in private automobiles.[9] Physicians must be taught how to evaluate critically ill or injured children and determine the optimal mode of transport.

EMS services are sometimes underused in emergencies.[10,11] A recent survey of health maintenance organizations (HMOs) in Chicago revealed that most instructed their subscribers to call the HMO first in an emergency, and many did not provide any information to subscribers about activation of emergency services.[12] Increased implementation of managed care may further impede access to emergency care.[13]

EMS Prehospital Care: Preparation and Education

The outcome of pediatric out-of-hospital asystolic cardiopulmonary arrest is dismal.[14-16] It is not known, however, if improved critical prehospital care can improve this outcome.[17] Paramedics and emergency medical technicians (EMTs) provide the initial care for the most seriously ill or injured children. In Los Angeles County, for example, all pediatric cases referred to the coroner's office for autopsy involved contact with the EMS system.[18] In general, however, the average EMS provider receives little education about the care of a seriously ill or injured child, has little experience in pediatric care, and is therefore poorly equipped to provide such care.

Basic EMTs are required to complete 100 hours of education, but only a few of these hours are devoted to pediatric assessment or care. Although paramedics generally complete 1000 hours of education, most programs devote only a small number of these hours to pediatric care. If the pediatric experience of EMS personnel is only classroom-based or if their clinical experience consists

Table 1. Prehospital Pediatric Equipment for Basic Life Support Units

Rigid cervical collars — infant, child, adult*
Oropharyngeal airways — infant, child, adult (0-5)
Resuscitator — child and adult reservoir†
Masks for resuscitator — infant, child, adult
Blood pressure cuffs — infant, child, adult
Oxygen delivery devices
    Masks — infant, child, adult
    Nasal cannulas — infant, child, adult
Portable suction device
Suction catheters, tonsil tip and 6F-14F
Bulb suction device
Backboard
Cervical immobilization device††
Extremity splints
Burn dressings⌐
Sterile scissors∥

*Cervical immobilization of small infants may be better achieved by the use of towels and tape rather than a rigid collar, which may not fit properly.

†Ventilation bags used for resuscitation should be self-refilling. The child and adult bags are suitable for supporting adequate tidal volumes for the entire pediatric age range. A child-sized bag has a reservoir of at least 450 mL but no more than 750 mL. An adult-sized bag has a reservoir of at least 1000 mL. Bags without pop-off valves are preferred.

††A cervical immobilization device can immobilize the neck of an infant, child, or adult. This device may consist of towel rolls or may be a commercially available device specifically for cradling the neck.

⌐Burn dressings may include commercially available packs or clean sheets and dressings.

∥Sterile scissors are used to cut the umbilical cord and may be stocked separately from the obstetrical pack to ensure sterility. Commercially available cord-clamp cutting devices may be substituted for the scissors.

only of the care of a few children in stable condition, they may be unable to recognize a distressed infant or child and perform such critical pediatric procedures as endotracheal intubation or establishing vascular access.

Approximately 10% of EMS contacts in both rural and urban areas are for children under 14 years of age,[19,20] with trauma being the most frequent reason between the ages of 5 and 14 years. For children younger than 5 years of age, the EMS system is most frequently activated in response to medical illness. Serious illness, including cardiorespiratory arrest, is most common in children under 2 years of age.[19] Thus it is mandatory that EMS personnel develop and maintain expertise in the assessment and stabilization of infants and young children. If such experience cannot be maintained in the field, EMS personnel must be able to arrange practicum experiences in local pediatric critical care units, emergency departments, and operating rooms. Such pediatric-focused educational experience is mandatory for EMS pediatric providers and must be extended to prehospital providers who may not be employees of the EMS system.[1,21,22]

The optimal type of training required to ensure skilled field performance is unclear. A recent nationwide survey of training programs documented that 97% of the programs include pediatric intubation in the curricula.[23] The method of teaching intubation, however, varies widely. Paramedics can learn to intubate children proficiently in the operating room, but field intubation may require unique modification of these skills.[24] Many programs use only manikins for training; some use animal models. Further study of intubation and other interventions is necessary to determine the optimal method of teaching field procedures.

The effects of critical prehospital procedures on the outcome of seriously ill or injured children have not been determined and require study.[17] A study of submersion injuries in King County, Wash, suggested improved outcomes in pediatric patients with cardiac arrest who received advanced prehospital airway management,[25] but several other studies on prehospital intubation failed to demonstrate any significant difference in survival from those receiving bag-valve–mask ventilation.[26-28] The success rate in one study of prehospital intubation was only 64%.[26] Many of the pediatric field intubation studies are not well controlled and not prospective in design. The high complication rate reported in several studies of pediatric prehospital intubation is worrisome.[27,28]

Prehospital Equipment

If prehospital providers are expected to assess and stabilize children with critical illnesses and injuries, they must have the proper equipment.[21] All emergency vehicles must contain specific equipment and supplies that will enable EMTs and paramedics to provide efficient and appropriate pediatric emergency care. Examples of minimal and enhanced lists of supplies and equipment are shown in Tables 1 and 2. Too often pediatric intubation equipment, blood pressure cuffs, or intravenous catheters are missing from emergency vehicles.[29]

Prehospital Protocols and Communication

Protocols for field management of pediatric illness and injury should be part of the training, systems development, and quality assurance programs for all EMS agencies.[6]

Communication between the EMS provider and the hospital must be formalized so that critical information is not omitted. Currently, vital signs and other parameters of circulatory status are often not assessed, and neurological evaluations often are not completed for pediatric patients.[19,29] The younger the patient, the less likely that complete vital signs are obtained.[29] If the prehospital provider fails to obtain crucial information, the base station physician must request it.

Table 2. Prehospital Pediatric Equipment for Advanced Life Support Units

Advanced life support units should have all the equipment in the BLS list plus the following items:

Monitor defibrillator[†]
*Laryngoscope with straight blades 1-2, curved blades 2-4
*Pediatric and adult size stylets for endotracheal tubes
*Pediatric and adult Magill forceps
*Endotracheal tubes, uncuffed sizes 2.5-6.0 and cuffed 6.0-8.0
Arm boards — infant, child, and adult sizes
Intravenous catheters, 14-24 gauge
Microdrip IV devices[††]
*Intraosseous needles
Drug dose chart or tape[ε]
Intravenous fluids that meet the local standard of practice
Resuscitation drugs that meet the local standard of practice

*These items are required only if the skill is part of the local scope of practice of EMS providers.

[†]The defibrillator should be able to deliver 5 to 400 J. The addition of pediatric paddles may give the responding unit enhanced capabilities. Units carrying only adult paddles/pads should ensure that providers are trained in the proper use of these paddles in infants and children.
[††]Burettes, microdrip tubing, or in-line volume controllers.
[ε]This may include charts listing the drug doses in milliliters or milligrams per kilogram, precalculated doses based on weight, or a tape that generates the drug dose based on the patient's height or length.

Physician and Hospital Care

The professional community, a key link in the chain of survival, must learn to use the EMS system appropriately and to manage pediatric emergencies.[30-32] Pediatric physician offices and ambulatory and urgent care centers in which acutely ill and injured children are treated may not have the necessary equipment for pediatric emergency care[33] (Table 3). To assist pediatricians in the development of community (and office) readiness for emergency care, the American Academy of Pediatrics has published guidelines for the role of the primary provider in EMS for children.[34]

The next link in the chain of survival that requires strengthening is pediatric care in emergency departments. The American Hospital Association estimates that 92 million visits were made to emergency departments in the United States in 1990. In some areas as many as 30% of these visits were by patients in the pediatric age group. Many hospital emergency departments are neither staffed nor equipped to manage pediatric emergencies.[35] Education of physicians and nurses in pediatric emergency care and the development of pediatric guidelines for emergency departments are important. Implementation of an EMS-C component within the EMS system may improve outcome.[34]

An estimated 240 children per 100 000 pediatric population require intensive care services annually. Many of these children currently receive care in community hospital adult intensive care units (ICUs).[36] Studies have

demonstrated differences in outcome for patients kept in adult ICUs compared with pediatric intensive care units (PICUs).[37] Access to specialized pediatric critical care services, such as pediatric trauma centers and PICUs, directly from the prehospital scene or by secondary transport from an emergency department improves outcome of critically ill or injured children in a limited number of studies.[38,39] Interfacility transfer agreements, provision of PICU transport team services, and educational outreach by PICUs to community hospitals may also improve outcome (see also chapter 10).[40] Optimal EMS-C services thus include integration of PICU, burn, reimplantation, and hyperbaric oxygen centers into the EMS-C component of EMS.

Table 3. Suggested Emergency Equipment for Physician Offices

<u>Airway Management</u>
Oxygen source with flowmeter (to deliver $\geq$ 15 mL/min)
Oxygen masks — infant, child, adult
Self-inflating bag-valve–mask resuscitators, including reservoir — infant, child, adult
Suction — wall or machine
Suction catheters — Yankauer, 8F, 10F, 14F
Oral airways — 0-5
Nasal cannulas — infant, child, and adult sizes 1-3
Optional for intubation
— Laryngoscope handle with Miller or Wishipple blades — 0, 1, 2, 3
— Laryngoscope batteries and bulbs
— Endotracheal tubes, uncuffed — 3.0, 3.5, 4.0, 4.5, 5.0, 6.0, 7.0, 8.0
— Stylets — small, large
— Magill forceps

<u>Fluid Management</u>
Intraosseous needles — 15 and 18 gauge
IV catheters, short, over-the-needle — 20, 22, 24 gauge
Butterfly needles — 21, 23, 25 gauge
IV boards, tape, alcohol swabs, tourniquet
Pediatric drip chambers and tubing
D_5/0.45% normal saline
Isotonic fluids (normal saline or lactated Ringer's solution)
Optional: over-guidewire catheters — 3F, 4F, 5F

<u>Miscellaneous Equipment</u>
Blood pressure cuffs — infant, child, adult
Nasogastric tubes — 10F, 14F
Feeding tubes — 3F, 5F
Foley urine catheters — 8F, 10F
Sphygmomanometer
Cardiac arrest board
Medication table or tape

Optional Equipment
Portable ECG monitor/defibrillator
Noninvasive blood pressure monitor
Pulse oximeter

Each year the pediatric population spends more than 10 million days in bed because of injuries. Brain injuries in children are common and result in tremendous disability.[40-42] A conservative estimate is that 29 000 persons aged 0 to 19 years have permanent disabilities from traumatic brain injuries. Even children with relatively minor brain trauma may have residual damage.[1] Rehabilitation should begin at the time the child enters the EMS system and continue until the child has reached full potential. The goal of rehabilitation is to achieve an optimal level of function by restoring or enhancing impaired or residual biologic function. These services are not available to most injured or ill children despite legislation that promotes their implementation.[1,2]

If outcome for critically ill and injured infants, children, and young adults is to improve, all EMS-C components must be integrated into existing EMS systems, and the public must be educated to activate EMS appropriately and provide first aid and CPR until help arrives.[2,3]

References

1. Seidel JS, Henderson DP, eds. *Emergency Medical Services for Children: A Report to the Nation.* Washington, DC: National Center for Education in Maternal and Child Health; 1991.
2. Durch JS, Lohr KN, eds. *Emergency Medical Services for Children.* Washington, DC: National Academy Press; 1993.
3. Guidelines for cardiopulmonary resuscitation and emergency cardiac care, V: pediatric basic life support. *JAMA.* 1992;268: 2251-2261.
4. Emergency medical services: sixteenth annual EMS state and province survey. *Emerg Med Serv.* 1992;21:202-226.
5. Montgomery WH, Brown DD, Hazinski MF, et al. Citizen response to cardiopulmonary emergencies. *Ann Emerg Med.* 1993;22: 428-434.
6. Dieckmann RA. Pediatrics in EMS: the effect of dispatch center and base hospitals on the quality of field care. *Pediatr Emerg Care.* 1990;6:76-77.
7. Clawson JJ. Telephone treatment protocols: reach out and help someone. *J Emerg Med Serv.* 1986;11:43-46.
8. Chi PS. Medical utilization patterns of migrant farm workers in Wayne County, New York. *Public Health Rep.* 1985;100:480-490.
9. DiGuiseppi C, Quan L. Acute epiglottitis: diagnosis and transport. *Pediatr Emerg Care.* 1989;5:286. Abstract.
10. Knolle LL, McDermott RJ, Ritzel DO. Knowledge of access to and use of the emergency medical services system in a rural Illinois county. *Am J Prev Med.* 1989;5:164-169.
11. White-Means SI, Thornton MC, Yeo JS. Sociodemographic and health factors influencing black and Hispanic use of the hospital emergency room. *J Natl Med Assoc.* 1989;81:72-80.
12. Hossfeld G, Ryan M. HMOs and utilization of emergency medical services: a metropolitan survey. *Ann Emerg Med.* 1989;18: 374-377.
13. Shaw KN, Selbst SM, Gill FM. Indigent children who are denied care in the emergency department. *Ann Emerg Med.* 1990;19: 59-62.
14. Eisenberg M, Bergner L, Hallstrom A. Epidemiology of cardiac arrest and resuscitation in children. *Ann Emerg Med.* 1983;12: 672-674.
15. Freisen RM, Duncan P, Tweed WA, Bristow G. Appraisal of pediatric cardiopulmonary resuscitation. *Can Med Assoc J.* 1982;126:1055-1058.
16. O'Rourke PP. Outcome of children who are apneic and pulseless in the emergency room. *Crit Care Med.* 1986;14:466-468.
17. Losek JD, Hennes H, Glaeser P, Hendley G, Nelson DB. Prehospital care of the pulseless, nonbreathing pediatric patient. *Am J Emerg Med.* 1987;5:370-374.
18. Gausche M, Seidel JS, Henderson DP, et al. Pediatric deaths and emergency medical services (EMS) in urban and rural areas. *Pediatr Emerg Care.* 1989;5:158-162.
19. Seidel JS, Henderson DP, Ward P, Wayland BW, Ness B. Pediatric prehospital care in urban and rural areas. *Pediatrics.* 1991;88: 681-690.
20. Tsai A, Kallsen G. Epidemiology of pediatric prehospital care. *Ann Emerg Med.* 1987;16:284-292.
21. Seidel JS. Emergency medical services and the pediatric patient: are the needs being met? II: training and equipping emergency service providers for pediatric emergencies. *Pediatrics.* 1986;78: 808-812.
22. Sinclair LM, Baker MD. Police involvement in pediatric prehospital care. *Pediatrics.* 1991;87:636-641.
23. Stratton SJ, Underwood LA, Whalen SM, Gunter CS. Prehospital pediatric endotracheal intubation: a survey of the United States. *Prehosp Disaster Med.* 1993;8:323-326.
24. Brownstein DR, Quan L, Orr R, Wentz KR, Copass MK. Paramedic intubation training in a pediatric operating room. *Am J Emerg Med.* 1992;10:418-420.
25. Quan L, Wentz KR, Gore EJ, Copass MK. Outcome and predictors of outcome in pediatric submersion victims receiving prehospital care in King County, Washington. *Pediatrics.* 1990;86:586-593.
26. Aijian P, Tsai A, Knopp R, Kallsen GW. Endotracheal intubation of pediatric patients by paramedics. *Ann Emerg Med.* 1989;18: 489-494.
27. Pointer JE. Clinical characteristics of paramedics' performance of pediatric endotracheal intubation. *Am J Emerg Med.* 1989;7: 364-366.
28. Nakayama DK, Gardner MJ, Rowe MI. Emergency endotracheal intubation in pediatric trauma. *Ann Surg.* 1990;211:218-223.
29. Gausche M, Henderson DP, Seidel JS. Vital signs as part of the prehospital assessment of the pediatric patient: a survey of paramedics. *Ann Emerg Med.* 1990;19:173-178.
30. Fuchs S, Jaffe DM, Cristoffel KK. Pediatric emergencies in office practices: prevalence and office preparedness. *Pediatrics.* 1989;83:931-939.
31. Hodge D III. Pediatric emergency office equipment. *Pediatr Emerg Care.* 1988;4:212-214.
32. Altieri M, Bellet J, Scott H. Preparedness for pediatric emergencies encountered in the practitioner's office. *Pediatrics.* 1990;85: 710-714.
33. Seidel JS, Henderson DP, Lewis JB. Emergency medical services and the pediatric patient, part III: resources of ambulatory care centers. *Pediatrics.* 1991;88:230-235.
34. Singer J, Ludwig S, eds. *Emergency Medical Services for Children: the Role of the Primary Care Provider.* Elk Grove Village, Ill: American Academy of Pediatrics; 1992.
35. Seidel JS, Gausche M. Standards for emergency departments. In: Dieckmann RA, ed. *Pediatric Emergency Care Systems: Planning and Management.* Baltimore, Md: Williams & Wilkins; 1992.
36. Pettigrew AH. Pediatric intensive care systems in northern and central California. In: Haller JA, ed. *Emergency Medical Services for Children: Report of the 97th Ross Conference on Pediatric Research.* Columbus, Ohio: Ross Laboratories; 1989.
37. Pollack MM, Alexander SR, Clarke N, Ruttimann UE, Tesselaar HM, Bachulis AC. Improved outcomes from tertiary center pediatric intensive care: a statewide comparison of tertiary and nontertiary care facilities. *Crit Care Med.* 1991;19:150-159.
38. Haller JA, Beaver B. A model: systems management of life threatening injuries in children for the state of Maryland, USA. *Intensive Care Med.* 1989;15(suppl 1):S53-S56.
39. Haller JA Jr, Shorter N, Miller D, Colombani P, Hall J, Buck J. Organization and function of a regional pediatric trauma center: does a system of management improve outcome? *J Trauma.* 1983;23:691-696.
40. Rivara FP, Thompson RS, Thompson DC, Calonge N. Injuries to children and adolescents: impact on physical health. *Pediatrics.* 1991;88:783-788.
41. Kraus JF, Rock A, Hemyari P. Brain injuries among infants, children, adolescents, and young adults. *Am J Dis Child.* 1990;144:684-691.
42. Guyer B, Ellers B. Childhood injuries in the United States: mortality, morbidity, and cost. *Am J Dis Child.* 1990;144:649-652.

Recognition of Respiratory Failure and Shock

Anticipating Cardiopulmonary Arrest

Cardiopulmonary arrest in infants and children is rarely a sudden event. Instead, it is often the end result of progressive deterioration in respiratory and circulatory function. Regardless of the initiating event or disease process, the final common pathway in this deterioration is the development of cardiopulmonary failure (Fig 1) and possible cardiopulmonary arrest. If pulseless cardiac arrest ensues, the outcome is dismal.[1-4] Cardiopulmonary arrest can often be prevented if the clinician recognizes symptoms of respiratory failure or shock and promptly initiates therapy. This chapter presents guidelines for anticipating cardiopulmonary arrest in infants and children and for establishing priorities in care.

Respiratory failure is clinically characterized by inadequate ventilation or oxygenation. It may be caused by intrinsic lung or airway disease, airway obstruction, or inadequate respiratory effort (eg, apnea or shallow respirations).

A compensated state may precede respiratory failure. The patient is able to maintain adequate gas exchange by increasing breathing rate (tachypnea) or depth (hyperpnea). This compensation, which occurs at the expense of increased work of breathing, is characterized by signs of respiratory distress (tachypnea, nasal flaring, the use of accessory muscles of respiration, inspiratory retractions) and tachycardia.

The definition of respiratory failure has traditionally placed a heavy emphasis on arterial blood gas analysis, including criteria such as hypoxemia (fall in PaO_2), hypercarbia (rise in $PaCO_2$), acidosis (pH <7.4), and evidence of significant intrapulmonary shunt.[5] However, this approach is problematic for several reasons. Most important, arterial blood gas analysis may not be available (eg, during transport) or may delay the initiation of therapy. Second, a single blood gas analysis often is not helpful, since evaluation of patient trends and response to therapy is necessary. Third, interpretation of the results requires consideration of the patient's clinical appearance and must be modified based on the patient's underlying condition. For example, the infant with bronchopulmonary dysplasia may always demonstrate hypoxemia and hypercarbia, so diagnosis of acute respiratory failure relies heavily on clinical examination and evaluation of the pH (acidosis will be apparent if respiratory failure is significantly worse than the child's baseline status).

This chapter emphasizes the recognition of *potential* respiratory failure, based on *clinical* evaluation of the child. If any child with potential respiratory failure fails to improve after initial therapy such as oxygen administra-

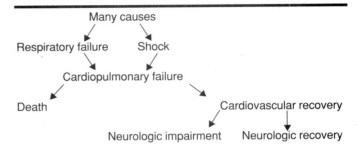

Fig 1. Path of various disease states leading to cardiopulmonary failure in infants and children.

tion or if further deterioration is observed, more aggressive therapy is clearly indicated and actual respiratory failure is likely to be present. Arterial blood gas analysis may be used to confirm the clinical impression or evaluate the child's response to therapy but is not necessary to detect potential respiratory failure.

Shock is a clinical state characterized by inadequate delivery of oxygen and metabolic substrates to meet the metabolic demands of tissues. It produces signs of inadequate organ and tissue perfusion and function, such as oliguria and lactic acidosis. Shock may occur with a normal, increased, or decreased cardiac output and normal, increased, or decreased blood pressure.[6,7] Shock may also be classified as compensated or decompensated. In compensated shock the blood pressure is normal. Decompensated shock is characterized by hypotension and often by a low cardiac output.

Respiratory failure and shock may begin as clinically distinct problems, but these often progress to a state of cardiopulmonary failure in the final moments preceding cardiopulmonary arrest. Cardiopulmonary failure is characterized by insufficient oxygen delivery to the tissues and inadequate clearance of metabolites.

Oxygen delivery is determined by arterial oxygen content and cardiac output:

| Oxygen delivery (DO_2) | = | Arterial oxygen content | × | Cardiac output | × | 10 |

Arterial oxygen content is determined by the hemoglobin concentration and its saturation with oxygen in the following formula:

$$\text{Arterial oxygen content (mL } O_2\text{/dL blood)} =$$

| Hemoglobin concentration (g/dL) | × | 1.34 mL oxygen/g | × | Oxyhemoglobin saturation |

The normal arterial oxygen content is approximately 18 to 20 mL O_2/dL blood. The cardiac output is a product of heart rate and ventricular stroke volume:

$$Cardiac\ output = Heart\ rate \times Stroke\ volume$$

If either arterial oxygen content or cardiac output falls without a commensurate and compensatory increase in the other component, oxygen delivery to the tissues will fall. When decompensated respiratory failure is present, the arterial oxygen content is reduced. If cardiac output can increase sufficiently, oxygen delivery to the tissues may be maintained at normal or near-normal levels. However, if cardiac output cannot increase sufficiently, oxygen delivery to tissues will fall. Additional deleterious effects of respiratory failure include the development of hypercarbia with resultant respiratory acidosis.

Oxygen content cannot increase in response to changes in cardiac output, so any fall in cardiac output (such as occurs in some forms of shock or with some arrhythmias) is likely to result in a decrease in oxygen delivery. Cardiac output and oxygen delivery must be evaluated in terms of tissue requirements (demands) rather than compared with normative data. When tissue oxygen requirements exceed oxygen delivery, anaerobic metabolism leads to lactic acid accumulation.

Potential cardiopulmonary failure is present in any infant or child who demonstrates respiratory distress, a reduced level of consciousness, cyanosis or pallor, or who has suffered severe trauma (Table 1). Clinical signs of shock and respiratory failure result from end-organ dysfunction caused by tissue hypoxia and acidosis. These signs include tachycardia, altered levels of consciousness (irritability or lethargy), oliguria, hypotonia, weak central (proximal) pulses with weak or absent peripheral pulses, and prolonged capillary refill despite a warm ambient temperature. Bradycardia, hypotension, and irregular respirations are late, ominous signs.

Evaluation of Respiratory Performance

Normal spontaneous ventilation is accomplished with minimal work and is quiet. The normal respiratory rate is inversely related to age; it is rapid in the neonate, then decreases in older infants and children. The neonatal respiratory rate is typically 40 to 60 breaths per minute or less, the respiratory rate of a 1-year-old is approximately 24 breaths per minute, and the normal respiratory rate in the 18-year-old is approximately 12 breaths per minute during quiet breathing. These rates would be expected to increase in the presence of excitement, anxiety, exercise, pain, or fever. Tidal volume, the volume of each breath per kilogram of body weight, remains fairly constant throughout life. Adequacy of tidal volume is assessed clinically by observation of chest wall excursion and auscultation of the lungs, noting the quality of air movement.

Table 1. Conditions Requiring Rapid Cardiopulmonary Assessment and Potential Cardiopulmonary Support

Respiratory rate >60
Heart rate
    Child ≤5 yr old: <80 bpm or >180 bpm
    Child >5 yr old: <60 bpm or >160 bpm
Increased work of breathing (retractions, nasal flaring, grunting)
Cyanosis or a decrease in oxyhemoglobin saturation
Altered level of consciousness (unusual irritability or lethargy or failure to respond to parents)
Seizures
Fever with petechiae
Trauma
Burns totaling >10% of body surface area

bpm indicates beats per minute.

When respiratory distress or failure is present, minute ventilation (Minute ventilation = Tidal volume × Respiratory rate) may be inadequate (hypoventilation) because each breath is shallow or because too few breaths are taken each minute. Abnormal respirations can be classified as too fast (tachypnea), too slow (bradypnea), absent (apnea), or associated with increased work of breathing.

Acute respiratory failure can result from any airway, pulmonary, or neuromuscular disease that impairs oxygen exchange (oxygenation) or elimination of carbon dioxide (ventilation).[5] The resultant hypoxemia, hypercapnia, and respiratory acidosis reflect the severity of respiratory failure.

Infants and children at risk for respiratory arrest may initially demonstrate

- Increased respiratory rate, increased respiratory effort, or diminished breath sounds
- Diminished level of consciousness or response to parents or pain
- Poor skeletal muscle tone
- Cyanosis

The assessment of respiratory function requires careful evaluation of

- Respiratory rate
- Respiratory mechanics
- Color of the skin and mucous membranes
- Temperature of the skin

Pulse oximetry is a useful noninvasive adjunct to clinical assessment of oxygen saturation; it gives no information about the adequacy of ventilation.

Respiratory Rate

Tachypnea is often the first manifestation of respiratory distress in infants. Tachypnea without other signs of respiratory distress ("quiet tachypnea") is often an attempt to maintain a normal pH by increasing minute ventilation, thereby causing a compensatory respiratory alkalosis. It commonly results from nonpulmonary diseases such as metabolic acidosis associated with shock, diabetic ketoacidosis, some congenital heart abnormalities, inborn errors of metabolism, salicylism, severe diarrhea, and chronic renal insufficiency.

A slow or irregular respiratory rate in an acutely ill infant or child is ominous. Possible causes include hypothermia, fatigue, and central nervous system depression. Fatigue is a common cause of slowing of the respiratory rate — an infant breathing at a rate of 80 breaths per minute will eventually tire. For this reason, *a decreasing respiratory rate or irregular respiratory rhythm may indicate deterioration rather than improvement in the child's clinical condition.*

Respiratory Mechanics

Increased work of breathing often produces nasal flaring and intercostal, subcostal, and suprasternal inspiratory retractions. These signs may be observed in children with airway obstruction or alveolar disease. As work of breathing increases, a greater proportion of the cardiac output must be delivered to the respiratory muscles, which in turn produce more carbon dioxide.

Head bobbing, grunting, stridor, and prolonged expiration are signs of significant alteration in respiratory mechanics. Bobbing of the head with each breath is often a sign of increased respiratory effort. Severe chest retractions accompanied by abdominal distention cause "seesaw" or "rocky" respirations and are usually indicative of upper airway obstruction. Seesaw respirations may also be called *abdominal breathing* because the chest wall retracts and the abdomen expands when the diaphragm contracts. This is a very inefficient form of ventilation because the tidal volume is reduced and fatigue may develop in a short time.

Grunting is produced by premature glottic closure accompanying late expiratory contraction of the diaphragm. Infants and children grunt to increase airway pressure, thereby preserving or increasing functional residual capacity. Grunting is demonstrated by patients who have experienced alveolar collapse and loss of lung volume associated with pulmonary edema, pneumonia, or atelectasis.

Stridor (an inspiratory, high-pitched sound) is a sign of upper airway (extrathoracic) obstruction. Causes of upper airway obstruction include congenital abnormalities (eg, a large tongue, laryngomalacia, vocal cord paralysis, hemangioma, airway tumor, or cyst), infections (eg, epiglottitis or croup), upper airway edema (eg, allergic reaction, following intubation or with gastroesophageal reflux), and aspiration of a foreign body.

Prolonged expiration, usually accompanied by wheezing, is a sign of intrathoracic airway obstruction, most often at the bronchial or bronchiolar level. Causes of prolonged expiration include bronchiolitis, asthma, pulmonary edema, or intrathoracic foreign body.

Air Entry

Tidal volume and effectiveness of ventilation are clinically assessed by evaluation of chest expansion and auscultation of breath sounds. The chest should expand bilaterally during inspiration. The expansion may be subtle during spontaneous quiet breathing but should be readily observed during positive-pressure ventilation (such as during bag-valve–mask ventilation or mechanical ventilation). Decreased chest expansion may result from hypoventilation, airway obstruction, atelectasis, pneumothorax, hemothorax, pleural effusion, mucous plug, or foreign-body aspiration.

Breath sounds should be equal and easily heard bilaterally. The child's chest wall is thin, so breath sounds are readily transmitted and readily heard. In fact, a decrease in intensity of breath sounds may be difficult to appreciate when listening over an area of atelectasis, pneumothorax, or pleural fluid because referred breath sounds are transmitted from other areas of the lung. Therefore, the intensity and the pitch of breath sounds must be evaluated; both should be equal over all lung fields. Breath sounds should be auscultated over the anterior and posterior chest as well as in the axillary areas.

Skin Color and Temperature

The child's skin color and skin temperature should be consistent over the trunk and extremities if the child is in a warm environment. Mucous membranes, nail beds, and the palms of the hands and soles of the feet will be pink in the presence of normal cardiorespiratory function. The skin over the trunk or extremities, however, may become mottled if hypoxemia or poor perfusion develops. In addition, hands and feet may become pale or dusky and cool.

Central cyanosis may be apparent in a child with hypoxemia. For central cyanosis to be clinically apparent, however, approximately 5 g desaturated hemoglobin must be present per deciliter of blood. Thus, a polycythemic child (eg, one with uncorrected cyanotic heart disease) is more likely to demonstrate cyanosis in the presence of hypoxemia than is the child with a normal or low hemoglobin concentration. Cyanosis may not be apparent in an anemic child despite the presence of profound hypoxemia. For this reason, the appearance of central cyanosis is not a reliable or an early indicator of hypoxemia.

The ambient temperature should be considered when the child's skin color and temperature are evaluated. If the child is exposed to a cold environmental temperature, peripheral vasoconstriction may produce mottling or pallor with cool skin and delayed capillary refill (particularly in the extremities).[8] When the child is warmed, however, the color should improve, and the extremities should again feel warm with brisk capillary refill. The capillary refill is only one clinical parameter and must be evaluated in light of ambient temperature and other clinical findings.[9]

Pulse oximetry should be used to monitor hemoglobin oxygen saturation if a child is at risk for developing hypoxemia. Arterial blood gases should be evaluated if respiratory impairment (particularly hypercarbia or acidosis) is suspected.

Evaluation of Cardiovascular Performance

Shock is present when cardiovascular dysfunction results in inadequate perfusion of vital organs.[6,7,10] Failure to deliver adequate metabolic substrate and remove metabolites leads to anaerobic metabolism, accumulation of lactic acid, and cellular damage. Death may then rapidly result from cardiovascular collapse or later from multiple organ system dysfunction.

Cardiac output is the volume of blood ejected by the heart each minute (heart rate × stroke volume). Stroke volume is the volume of blood ejected by the ventricles with each contraction. Arterial blood pressure is the product of flow (cardiac output) and resistance (systemic vascular resistance) (Fig 2). Organ perfusion depends on both cardiac output and perfusion pressure. Of the variables affecting and affected by cardiac output, only the heart rate and blood pressure can be easily measured (see Fig 2). Stroke volume and systemic vascular resistance must be indirectly assessed by examining the quality of pulses and evaluating tissue perfusion.

Shock may be classified according to etiology or by its effect on blood pressure or cardiac output. Any method of classification represents an oversimplification since most children in shock have cardiovascular dysfunction requiring more than a single therapy. When shock is classified by etiology, the terms *hypovolemic, cardiogenic,* and *distributive* shock are used. Hypovolemic shock is characterized by inadequate intravascular volume relative to the vascular space. Hypovolemic shock is the leading form of shock in children worldwide. It often results from dehydration or hemorrhage but may also be caused by "third-spacing" of fluids (extravascular fluid shifts) such as may be observed in children with burns or with systemic vasodilation (as in sepsis). Cardiogenic shock is characterized by myocardial dysfunction; typically, intravascular volume is adequate or even increased, but cardiac dysfunction limits cardiac output. Distributive shock is characterized by inappropriate distribution of blood volume. This form of shock may be caused by sepsis or anaphylaxis. This etiologic classification of shock is useful because the diagnosis clarifies the focus of therapy. However, any child with severe or sustained shock has some degree of myocardial dysfunction. In addition, most children with shock will require careful titration of fluid administration, and many will require pharmacologic therapy to increase or redistribute cardiac output.

Shock may also be characterized as *compensated* or *decompensated.* When compensated shock is present,

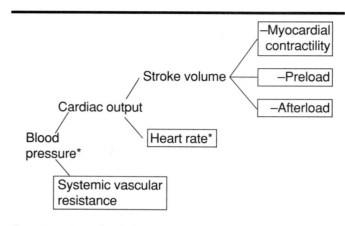

Fig 2. Hemodynamic relations.

*Measurable. Box indicates variables manipulated by therapy.

the child's blood pressure is normal, although signs of inadequate tissue and organ perfusion (eg, lactic acidosis, oliguria, altered level of consciousness) are observed. Decompensated shock is present when hypotension develops.

Finally, shock may be characterized by the patient's cardiac output. Although shock is often associated with low cardiac output, septic and anaphylactic shock may be characterized by high cardiac output.[10-12] For this reason the cardiac output should not simply be evaluated as normal, low, or high but should also be determined to be either *adequate* or *inadequate* to meet tissue metabolic requirements. Virtually any child in shock will require support of cardiovascular function and cardiac output.

When shock is associated with a low flow state, such as occurs with hypovolemic or cardiogenic shock, sympathetic nervous system compensatory mechanisms may be activated to divert blood flow from the skin, mesenteric, and renal circulations. The skin becomes cool, and systemic vascular resistance is high. Initially, arterial blood pressure may be maintained by redistribution of cardiac output and increased systemic vascular resistance.

Septic or anaphylactic shock is characteristically associated with high cardiac output. However, the cardiac output is unevenly distributed, so some tissue beds remain inadequately perfused. Low systemic vascular resistance results in increased skin blood flow and bounding peripheral pulses. However, there is a mismatch between tissue blood flow and tissue requirements. Some tissue beds receive excessive blood flow while other tissue beds receive inadequate flow. The ischemic tissue beds generate lactic acid, leading to acidosis. Therefore, despite the presence of a high cardiac output, shock and metabolic acidosis develop because blood flow is inappropriately distributed.

Early signs of sepsis are often subtle and thus may be difficult to recognize. Sepsis is diagnosed when the child develops fever or hypothermia, tachycardia, tachypnea with respiratory alkalosis, and a change in white blood cell count (leukocytosis, leukopenia, or an increase in immature or band forms of white blood cells) in the presence of suspected infection.[11,13] This diagnosis requires a high index of suspicion. Severe sepsis is present when signs of sepsis are observed in association with evidence of inadequate organ perfusion and function (eg, altered mental status, oliguria, or lactic acidosis).[13] Thus, evaluation of systemic perfusion and analysis of blood gases should allow the identification of sepsis before decompensated shock develops. Septic shock is often present when the patient with severe sepsis develops hypotension despite fluid administration or when normotension is maintained only with vasoactive drug support.[13]

Heart Rate

Normal heart rates in infants and children are provided in chapter 7. Sinus tachycardia is a common response to many types of stress (eg, anxiety, pain, fever, hypoxia, hypercapnia, hypovolemia, or cardiac impairment). The presence of tachycardia therefore mandates further evaluation (see chapter 7).

The cardiac output of neonates, infants, and children is influenced more by heart rate than by stroke volume. In children cardiac output is increased primarily by increasing the heart rate. Although neonates often demonstrate bradycardia in response to hypoxemia, older children will initially demonstrate tachycardia. When the tachycardia fails to maintain adequate tissue oxygenation, tissue hypoxia and hypercapnia produce acidosis, and bradycardia ensues. The development of bradycardia in a child with cardiorespiratory distress is an ominous sign, usually indicating that cardiopulmonary arrest is imminent.

Blood Pressure

Blood pressure is determined by cardiac output (flow) and systemic vascular resistance. Normal blood pressure can be maintained despite a fall in cardiac output only if compensatory vasoconstriction occurs. Tachycardia and increased cardiac contractility will also attempt to restore cardiac output. When these compensatory mechanisms fail, hypotension develops and decompensated shock is present.

Tachycardia persists until cardiac reserve is depleted. A model of the cardiovascular response to hemorrhagic shock (based on normative data) is depicted in Fig 3. Although cardiac output falls as blood volume is depleted, blood pressure is initially maintained by an increase in systemic vascular resistance. Hypotension is a late and often sudden sign of cardiovascular decompensation. Therefore, even mild hypotension must be treated quickly and vigorously because it signals decompensation, and cardiopulmonary arrest may be imminent.

Normal blood pressure values according to age are provided in Table 2. The median (50th percentile) systolic blood pressure for children older than 1 year may be approximated by the following formula:

$$90 \text{ mm Hg} + (2 \times \text{age in years})$$

The *lower limit* (5th percentile) of systolic blood pressure can be estimated with this formula:

$$70 \text{ mm Hg} + (2 \times \text{age in years})$$

An observed fall of 10 mm Hg in systolic blood pressure should prompt careful serial evaluations for additional signs of shock.

Hemodynamic Response to Hemorrhage

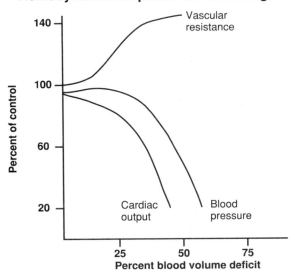

Fig 3. Model for cardiovascular response to hypovolemia from hemorrhage (based on normative data).[16]

Table 2. Normal Blood Pressures in Children*

Age	Systolic Pressure (mm Hg)	Diastolic Pressure (mm Hg)
Birth (12 hr, <1000 g)	39-59	16-36
Birth (12 hr, 3 kg)	50-70	25-45
Neonate (96 hr)	60-90	20-60
Infant (6 mo)	87-105	53-66
Toddler (2 yr)	95-105	53-66
School age (7 yr)	97-112	57-71
Adolescent (15 yr)	112-128	66-80

*Blood pressure ranges taken from the following sources: **Neonate:** Versmold H and others: Aortic blood pressure during the first 12 hours of life in infants with birth weight 610-4220 gms. *Pediatrics.* 1981;67:107. Tenth to 90th percentile ranges used. **Children:** Horan MJ, chairman: Task Force on Blood Pressure Control in Children, report of the Second Task Force on Blood Pressure in Children. *Pediatrics.* 1987;79:1. Fiftieth to 90th percentile ranges indicated.

Reproduced from Hazinski MF. Children are different. In: Hazinski MF, ed. *Nursing Care of the Critically Ill Child*, 2nd ed. St Louis, Mo: Mosby Year Book; 1992.

The child's circulating blood volume can be estimated if the body weight is known. The circulating blood volume in neonates is approximately 85 mL/kg, in infants approximately 80 mL/kg, and in children approximately 75 mL/kg. The circulating blood volume should be calculated, and all blood lost or drawn for laboratory analysis should be totaled and evaluated in light of the estimated circulating blood volume. An acute blood loss of 5% to 10% of circulating blood volume may be significant. Hypotension is usually not observed unless the child loses approximately 25% of circulating blood volume acutely.[14-16]

Systemic Perfusion

Because tachycardia is a nonspecific sign of distress and hypotension is a late sign of shock, recognition of early compensated shock requires evaluation of indirect signs of blood flow and systemic vascular resistance. This is best accomplished by evaluating the presence and volume of peripheral pulses and evidence of end-organ perfusion and function.

Evaluation of Pulses

The carotid, axillary, brachial, radial, femoral, dorsalis pedis, and posterior tibial pulses are readily palpable in healthy infants and children. A discrepancy in volume between central and peripheral pulses may be caused by vasoconstriction associated with a cold ambient temperature or may be an early sign of decreased cardiac output. Pulse volume is related to pulse pressure (difference between systolic and diastolic pressures). When cardiac output decreases (low cardiac output shock), the pulse pressure narrows, making the pulse "thready" and finally impossible to feel. In contrast, early septic shock is a high-output state and is often characterized by a wide pulse pressure with bounding pulses. Loss of *central* pulses is a premorbid sign and should be treated as cardiac arrest.

Skin

Decreased perfusion of the skin can be an early sign of shock. When the child is well perfused and the ambient temperature is warm, the hands and feet should be warm and dry and the palms pink to the distal phalanx. When cardiac output decreases, cooling of the skin begins peripherally (in the fingers and toes) and extends proximally (toward the trunk).[17] Sluggish (delayed) capillary refill (more than 2 seconds) after blanching is caused by shock, fever, or a cold ambient temperature.[8,9,17] When capillary refill is evaluated, the extremity should be lifted slightly above the level of the heart to ensure assessment of arteriolar capillary (and not venous stasis) refill.

Mottling, pallor, delayed capillary refill, and peripheral cyanosis often indicate poor skin perfusion. Acrocyanosis, however, may be normal in newborn or polycythemic patients. Severe vasoconstriction produces a gray or ashen color in newborns and pallor in older children.

Brain

The clinical signs of brain hypoperfusion are determined by the severity and duration of the ischemia.[18] When the ischemic insult is sudden, few signs of neurologic compromise precede loss of consciousness. Muscular tone is lost, and generalized seizures and pupillary dilation may be observed.

When the onset of the ischemic insult is more gradual, neurological symptoms are typically more insidious. Alteration of consciousness occurs, with confusion, irritability, and lethargy. Agitation may alternate with lethargy. After 2 months of age an infant should normally be able to focus on his or her parents' faces. Failure to recognize parents and failure to make eye contact with parents may be early, ominous signs of cortical hypoperfusion or cerebral dysfunction. Failure to respond to a painful stimulus is also an ominous sign in a previously normal child. Parents may be the first to recognize these signs but may be unable to describe them other than to say something is wrong.

More profound degrees of hypoperfusion produce greater changes in the level of consciousness. In decreasing levels of consciousness, the child may be

- Awake
- Responsive to voice
- Responsive to pain
- Unresponsive

Deep tendon reflexes may be depressed, pupils may be small but reactive, and breathing patterns may be altered.

Hypotonia and intermittent flexor or extensor posturing may occur with prolonged cerebral hypoperfusion or extreme hypoxemia (PaO_2 <30 mm Hg).

Kidneys

Urine output is directly proportional to glomerular filtration rate and renal blood flow. Although the urine output is a good indicator of renal function, it is not very helpful in the initial evaluation of renal perfusion, because it is often difficult for parents to estimate recent urine production. Normal urine output averages 1 to 2 mL/kg per hour. Urine flow of less than 1 mL/kg per hour in the absence of known renal disease is often a sign of poor renal perfusion or hypovolemia. An indwelling urinary catheter facilitates accurate and continuous determination of urine flow.

Rapid Cardiopulmonary Assessment

Recognition of cardiorespiratory deterioration in the infant or child requires skilled physical examination. Laboratory tests are useful adjuncts in determining the severity of physiologic derangements but are not essential to the initial evaluation. Every clinician who works with children should be able to recognize potential pulmonary and circulatory failure and impending cardiopulmonary arrest based on a rapid cardiopulmonary assessment (Table 3). The assessment requires less than 30 seconds to complete and, by integrating important physical findings, is designed to evaluate pulmonary and cardiovascular function and their effects on end-organ perfusion and function.

Table 3. Rapid Cardiopulmonary Assessment

Respiratory Assessment	Cardiovascular Assessment

A. **A**irway patency
• Able to maintain independently
• Requires adjuncts/assistance to maintain
 	
B. **B**reathing
Rate
Mechanics
  Retractions
  Grunting
  Accessory muscles
  Nasal flaring
Air entry
  Chest expansion
  Breath sounds
  Stridor
  Wheezing
  Paradoxical chest movement
Color
	C. **C**irculation
	Heart rate
	Blood pressure
	  Volume/strength of central pulses
	Peripheral pulses
	  Present/absent
	  Volume/strength
	Skin perfusion
	  Capillary refill time (consider ambient temperature)
	  Temperature
	  Color
	  Mottling
	CNS perfusion
	  Responsiveness
	    Awake
	    Responds to voice
	    Responds to pain
	    Unresponsive
	  Recognizes parents
	  Muscle tone
	  Pupil size
	  Posturing

CNS indicates central nervous system.

The assessment uses the ABC approach used in CPR:

Airway: The airway is determined to be (1) patent; (2) maintainable with head positioning, suctioning, or adjuncts; or (3) unmaintainable and requiring interventions, such as intubation, removal of a foreign body, or cricothyrotomy. Inspiratory sounds (eg, stridor) and work of breathing should also be evaluated.

Breathing: Evaluation of breathing focuses on determination of the respiratory rate and assessment of inspiratory breath sounds, work of breathing, adequacy of tidal volume, and resultant chest expansion. The minute ventilation must be determined to be adequate or inadequate to sustain heart rate, oxygenation, and circulation.

Circulation: Qualitative examination of the systemic circulation provides indirect evidence of the efficacy/ effectiveness of cardiac output. The presence and quality of peripheral pulses, capillary refill time (consider ambient temperature), and skin perfusion as well as end-organ function are assessed using criteria discussed previously.

Examination of the ill infant or child does not end when the rapid cardiopulmonary assessment is completed. Often the condition of these patients is dynamic, and repeated assessments are necessary to evaluate trends in the patient's condition and the patient's response to therapy.

Priorities in Management

On the basis of the rapid cardiopulmonary assessment, the child is categorized as

• Stable
• In potential respiratory failure or shock
• In definite respiratory failure or shock
• In cardiopulmonary failure

When clinical signs of distress are subtle and potential respiratory or circulatory failure is suspected, frequent sequential assessments must be made. Supplemental laboratory studies, especially pulse oximetry, arterial blood gas analysis, and chest x-ray, may be useful. When inadequate ventilation, oxygenation, or perfusion threatens cardiopulmonary stability, interventions and reassessments should be performed promptly and continued until the child is stable, before definitive diagnostic testing is attempted.

A child with potential respiratory failure or compensated shock should be approached promptly and efficiently yet thoughtfully and gently to minimize fear and oxygen demand. Supplemental oxygen should be administered in a nonthreatening manner whenever possible. Infants should be supported with the head in a neutral position. Older patients should be allowed to assume a position of maximal comfort to minimize the work of breathing and to optimize airway patency. Normal ambient and body temperature should be maintained and feeding withheld.

If signs of actual respiratory failure are present, a patent airway must be established and adequate ventilation ensured with maximum supplemental oxygen provided (see chapter 4). When signs of shock are present, vascular access should be established rapidly (see chapter 5) and volume expansion and medications administered as needed (see chapter 6).

When cardiopulmonary failure is detected, initial priority is given to ventilation and oxygenation. If circulation and perfusion fail to improve rapidly, therapy for shock is provided (see chapter 6).

Special Conditions Predisposing an Infant or Child to Cardiopulmonary Arrest

Certain conditions place infants and children at high risk for development of cardiopulmonary failure. More comprehensive information about the pathophysiology and management of these conditions can be found in texts on pediatric trauma, pediatric emergency care, and critical care medicine and nursing.

Trauma (see also chapter 8)

Respiratory failure in children who have suffered trauma may occur as a result of central nervous system injury or depression, upper airway obstruction, pneumothorax or hemothorax, pulmonary contusion, or flail chest. Cervical spinal injury should be suspected whenever head injury or multisystem trauma has occurred, and neck immobilization should be maintained until that diagnosis has been excluded. Hemorrhagic shock usually is caused by hepatic or splenic injury, but hemothorax, a fractured femur with vascular laceration, multiple extremity fractures or pelvic fractures, scalp lacerations, and intracranial hemorrhage may be other sources of major blood loss.[14]

Burns

Children with major burns (≥10% to 15% of total body surface area) require significant fluid administration during the initial 24 to 48 hours following the burn to replace fluid lost through the burn surface and into extravascular tissue.[19] In addition, inhalation injury should be suspected and careful and frequent assessments required to detect the development of shock or respiratory failure. Patients with severe burns of the head and neck and those burned in a closed space (eg, house or automobile) may require prompt endotracheal intubation to protect the airway before edema caused by inhalation injury distorts the anatomy. Prophylactic tracheostomy is *not* recommended. Carbon monoxide (CO) poisoning should be suspected and immediately treated with maximal supplemental oxygen. Carboxyhemoglobin (COHb) levels should also be evaluated through blood sampling,[20] since the pulse oximeter will not accurately reflect oxyhemoglobin saturation in the presence of carbon monoxide poisoning. Burned children 2 years old or younger are particularly likely to develop complications of fluid resuscitation, so transfer of these children to a pediatric intensive care unit (or intensive care unit with pediatric expertise) should be considered.

Gastroenteritis

Gastrointestinal infection and diarrhea may cause dehydration, and severe fluid loss may result in hypovolemic shock. Gastroenteritis with dehydration is the leading cause of shock in children worldwide. Signs of dehydration include weight loss, irritability, absence of tearing, dry mucous membranes, a sunken fontanelle in infants, and dry, sometimes doughy or tenting skin. Signs of shock include tachycardia, diminished peripheral pulses, oliguria, irritability or lethargy, and acidosis. Rapid volume replacement is indicated to prevent cardiovascular collapse.

Epiglottitis

Epiglottitis is an acute respiratory emergency characterized by inflammation and edema of the epiglottis, false cords, and aryepiglottic folds, which can result in severe upper airway obstruction. Since most epiglottitis in children is caused by *Haemophilus influenzae B*, the *H influenzae* vaccine has almost eradicated this disease in children. Healthcare providers may, however, encounter epiglottitis in the occasional patient who has not been immunized.

Acute epiglottitis is characterized by abrupt onset of fever, sore throat, drooling, muffled voice, and inspiratory stridor. The child often attempts to maintain a patent airway by leaning forward while sitting and holding his or her head in a sniffing position. This position should be supported, and the child should be disturbed as little as possible. Supplemental oxygen can be administered while the child is sitting in a parent's lap. Respiratory arrest can result from total airway obstruction or from a combination of partial airway obstruction and fatigue. If epiglottitis is strongly suspected, the patient should be taken *directly* to the operating room for intubation. These patients require definitive airway management under optimal conditions by the staff physician most skilled in pediatric intubation and airway management because the inflamed, swollen supraglottis makes intubation difficult. If respiratory arrest occurs, bag-mask ventilation with 100% oxygen should precede any attempt to intubate the patient.

Deterioration During Positive-Pressure Ventilation

Cardiovascular collapse caused by hypoxemia may occur despite tracheal intubation and positive-pressure ventilation. The most likely causes of *acute* deterioration include endotracheal tube obstruction, displacement, or migration; development of tension pneumothorax; or failure of the mechanical ventilation device. See chapter 4 for recognition and management of these problems.

Tracheostomy

An infant with a tracheostomy is at high risk for respiratory arrest because mucous plugs frequently develop and may obstruct the artificial airway (see chapter 4). The risk of obstruction is particularly high in infants with small tracheal tube diameter. The obstruction may remain undetected because infants with tracheostomies are unable to speak or cry for help. Tracheal obstruction should be considered as a cause of an arrest in any patient with a tracheostomy until tube patency is verified. If a brief attempt at suctioning fails to relieve the obstruction or if a catheter cannot be passed through the tube, the tracheostomy tube should be removed immediately. The infant often has enough reserve to breathe spontaneously before the stoma is suctioned and a new tube is inserted. If ventilation through the stoma is unsuccessful and the upper airway is patent, the stoma can be manually occluded and ventilation or oxygenation provided with a bag and face mask until orotracheal intubation is accomplished or the tracheostomy tube is replaced. Alternatively, a standard endotracheal tube may be passed through the tracheostomy site if no replacement tracheostomy tube is readily available.

Seizures

Respiratory distress may develop during seizures as the result of respiratory depression, upper airway obstruction by secretions, or prolapse of soft tissue into the hypopharynx. In addition, some medications used to treat the seizures may cause apnea. For these reasons the child's respiratory status must be closely monitored and supported as needed.

Coma

When an infant or child is comatose, intubation may be required to treat hypoventilation and provide airway protection. Intracranial hypertension, which may be present in some comatose patients, may be aggravated if hypoxemia or hypercarbia develop during prolonged attempts at intubation. Bag-mask hyperventilation and oxygenation should be provided in such situations, and tracheal intubation should be performed by a skilled clinician using muscle relaxants and an anesthetic regimen for neuroinduction. The patient should be observed closely for signs of increased intracranial pressure. Cushing's triad (bradycardia, hypertension, and irregular respiration or apnea) is typically a very late manifestation of increased intracranial pressure. Increased intracranial pressure may be present despite the absence of these signs. Early signs of increased intracranial pressure may include change in responsiveness, inability to follow commands, pupil dilation with sluggish response to light, unequal pupils, and any development of or change in posturing or response to painful stimuli.

Critically Ill Patients

All infants and children who require intensive care, including those in an intensive care unit or an operating room or emergency department or in transit within or between hospitals, should be considered at high risk for the development of cardiopulmonary arrest. Cardiopulmonary arrest may result from

- The natural history of a life-threatening disease
- A complication of therapy
- Premature withdrawal of support, including mechanical ventilation, supplemental oxygen, or vasoactive drugs
- The unintentional withdrawal of such support (eg, spontaneous extubation)

Immediately following any resuscitation, cardiovascular instability and arrest may recur because

- Catecholamines administered during resuscitation have been metabolized and not replaced by a continuous infusion
- The inciting event recurs
- Hypoxic-ischemic myocardial, pulmonary, or cerebral damage has occurred
- Iatrogenic complications arise

References

1. Zaritsky A, Nadkarni V, Getson P, Kuehl K. CPR in children. *Ann Emerg Med.* 1987;16:1107-1111.
2. Eisenberg M, Bergner L, Hallstrom A. Epidemiology of cardiac arrest and resuscitation in children. *Ann Emerg Med.* 1983; 12:672-674.
3. Lewis JK, Minter MG, Eshelman SJ, Witte MK. Outcome of pediatric resuscitation. *Ann Emerg Med.* 1983;12:297-299.
4. O'Rourke PP. Outcome of children who are apneic and pulseless in the emergency room. *Crit Care Med.* 1986;14:466-468.
5. Downes JJ, Fulgencio T, Raphaely RC. Acute respiratory failure in infants and children. *Pediatr Clin North Am.* 1972;19:423-445.
6. Perkin RM, Levin DL. Shock in the pediatric patient, part I. *J Pediatr.* 1982;101:163-169.
7. Perkin RM, Levin DL. Shock in the pediatric patient, part II: therapy. *J Pediatr.* 1982;101:332.
8. Gorelick MH, Shaw KN, Baker MD. Effect of ambient temperature on capillary refill in healthy children. *Pediatrics.* 1993;92:699-702.
9. Baraff LJ. Capillary refill: is it a useful clinical sign? *Pediatrics.* 1993;92:723-724. Editorial.
10. Hazinski MF, Barkin RM. Shock. In: Barkin RM, ed. *Pediatric Emergency Medicine: Concepts and Clinical Practice.* St Louis, Mo: Mosby Year Book Inc; 1992.
11. Hazinski MF, Iberti TJ, MacIntyre NR, Parker MM, Tribett D, Prion S, Chmel H. Epidemiology, pathophysiology and clinical presentation of gram-negative sepsis. *Am J Crit Care.* 1993;2: 224-335.
12. Parker MM, McCarthy KE, Ognibene FP, Parrillo JE. Right ventricular dysfunction and dilatation, similar to left ventricular changes, characterize the cardiac depression of septic shock in humans. *Chest.* 1990;97:126-131.
13. Bone RC, Balk RA, Cerra FB, Dellinger RP, Fein AM, Knaus WA, Schein RM, Sibbald WJ. American College of Chest Physicians/Society of Critical Care Medicine Consensus Conference: definitions for sepsis and organ failure and guidelines for the use of innovative therapies in sepsis. *Crit Care Med.* 1992;20:864-874. Also *Chest.* 1992;101:1644-1655.
14. *Advanced Trauma Life Support Course.* Chicago, Ill: American College of Surgeons; 1993.

15. Fleisher GR, Ludwig S. *Textbook of Pediatric Emergency Medicine.* 2nd ed. Baltimore, Md: Williams and Wilkins; 1988.
16. Schwaitzberg SD, Bergman KS, Harris BH. A pediatric trauma model of continuous hemorrhage. *J Pediatr Surg.* 1988;23: 605-609.
17. Joly HR, Weil MH. Temperature of the great toe as an indication of the severity of shock. *Circulation.* 1969;39:131-138.
18. Plum F, Posner JB. *The Diagnosis of Stupor and Coma.* 3rd ed. Philadelphia, Pa: FA Davis Co; 1980.
19. Carvajal HF. Resuscitation of the burned child. In: Carvajal HF, Parks DH, eds. Burns in children: pediatric burn management. Chicago, Ill: Year Book Medical Publishers; 1988.
20. Herndon DN, Thompson PB, Linares HA, Traber DL. Postgraduate course: respiratory injury, part I: incidence, mortality, pathogenesis and treatment of pulmonary injury. *J Burn Care Rehabil.* 1986; 7:184-191.

Pediatric Basic Life Support

Chapter 3

Cardiopulmonary resuscitation (CPR) and life support for infants and children should be part of a community-wide effort that integrates

- Education about injury prevention
- Pediatric basic life support (PBLS)
- Easy access to an EMS system sensitive to and prepared for the needs of children
- Pediatric advanced life support (ALS)
- Pediatric postresuscitation care

Out-of-hospital cardiopulmonary arrest is most likely to occur while children are under the supervision of parents or their surrogates.[1-5] BLS courses should therefore be offered to expectant parents, parents of young children, and others into whose care children are entrusted, such as day-care personnel, teachers, and sports supervisors. Many children who require resuscitation suffer from underlying conditions that predispose them to development of cardiopulmonary failure.[2] Parents of children at high risk — those with chronic diseases — should be particularly targeted for these courses. The content of BLS courses should emphasize preventive strategies, training in BLS techniques, and access to the EMS system. Although BLS requires no adjuncts, the healthcare provider should use adjuncts that are readily available, such as a barrier device and ventilation bag and mask, if the provider is trained in their use. Pediatric ALS courses should be mandatory for all prehospital and hospital personnel who care for infants and children.

Epidemiology

The epidemiology of pediatric cardiopulmonary arrest is different from that of adults. Sudden, primary cardiac arrest in young children is uncommon. Ventricular fibrillation has been reported in only 10% to 15% of children younger than 10 years who experience pulseless arrest outside of the hospital.[1,6-8] Ventricular tachycardia or fibrillation is more likely to be observed in older children (10 years or older), submersion victims, children with complex congenital heart disease, and children who arrest in the hospital.[7,8] More commonly, injury or disease causes respiratory or circulatory failure, which progresses to cardiopulmonary failure with hypoxemia and acidosis, culminating in asystolic or pulseless cardiac arrest.

Intact survival from prehospital normothermic *asystolic* or *pulseless* cardiac arrest in infants and children is uncommon. Survival averages 10% in most reports, and many of those who are resuscitated suffer permanent neurological damage.[2,6,7,9-12] The survival rate is slightly higher if ventricular fibrillation is present on the initial electrocardiogram.[7,8] In contrast, respiratory arrest alone is associated with a survival rate exceeding 50% when prompt resuscitation is provided, and most patients survive neurologically intact.[2,9,11] Aggressive prehospital BLS and ALS have also improved the outcome of drowning victims in pulseless cardiac arrest.[13,14] To improve the outcome of resuscitation in all children, vigorous prehospital resuscitation should be encouraged, with particular emphasis on providing effective ventilation and oxygenation and preventing cardiac arrest.

Pediatric cardiopulmonary arrest occurs most commonly at either end of the age spectrum — in children younger than 1 year and in adolescence. During infancy the most common causes of arrest are intentional and unintentional injury, apparent life-threatening events (including the condition formerly referred to as "near-miss" sudden infant death syndrome), respiratory diseases, airway obstruction (including foreign-body aspiration), submersion, sepsis, and neurological diseases.[2-6] Beyond infancy, injuries are the leading cause of pediatric prehospital cardiopulmonary arrest.[5,6,10,11]

Injury Prevention

Incidence

Injury is a leading cause of death in children and young adults and is responsible for more childhood deaths than all other causes combined.[15] Annually, pediatric injuries account for approximately 25 000 deaths, 600 000 hospital admissions, and 16 million emergency department visits, with direct costs exceeding $7.5 billion.[15-17] Injuries should be viewed as preventable.

The Science of Injury Control

Injury control attempts to prevent injury or to minimize its effects on the child and family. Injury control addresses preinjury, injury, and care of the injured patient. Examples of preinjury intervention include prevention of drunk driving and construction of barriers surrounding swimming pools. An intervention that may alter the consequence of injury is the use of restraining devices for children traveling in motor vehicles. Postinjury care of children must focus on public and professional education to ensure performance of optimal bystander CPR, skilled prehospital and hospital care, and effective rehabilitation.

In planning injury prevention strategies, three principles (based on the work of Haddon and others[18]) should be emphasized:

1. Passive injury prevention strategies, such as air bags or automatic seat and shoulder belts in cars,

are generally more effective than active strategies that require repeated and conscious efforts.

2. Specific instructions are more likely to be followed than general advice.

3. Individual education, reinforced by communitywide educational programs, is more effective than isolated educational sessions.[18-20]

Epidemiology and Prevention of Common Childhood Injuries

Injury prevention programs will be most effective if they focus on injuries that are frequent and severe and for which proven prevention strategies are available. The six most common types of severe childhood injuries nationwide are motor vehicle passenger injuries, pedestrian injuries, bicycle injuries, submersion, burns, and firearm injuries.[15,19,21] Prevention of these would substantially reduce childhood deaths and disability.

Motor Vehicle Injuries

Motor vehicle–related trauma accounts for nearly half of all pediatric injuries and deaths.[15,21] Contributing factors include failure to use proper passenger restraints, inexperienced adolescent drivers, and alcohol abuse. Each of these factors should be addressed by injury prevention programs.

Proper use of child seat restraints and lap-shoulder harnesses can prevent an estimated 65% to 75% of serious injuries and fatalities to passengers under 4 years of age and 45% to 55% of all pediatric motor vehicle passenger injuries and deaths.[22] Use of proper seat restraints should be required and enforced by law in every state and taught to parents of infants as well as to children during their early primary school education. A 19-city National Highway Traffic Safety Administration (NHTSA) study documented that 20% of all child safety seats examined were seriously misused, and 1989-1990 estimates from voluntary screening programs have indicated that as many as 80% to 92% of child restraint devices in use are improperly installed.[23] Correct use of child restraint devices and safety belts must be taught and verified. Passive restraint devices, including adjustable shoulder harnesses and automatic lap and shoulder belts and air bags, should be further developed and implemented.

Adolescent drivers are responsible for a disproportionate number of motor vehicle–related injuries. Adolescent driver education classes *do not* reduce the incidence of collisions involving adolescent drivers. They have resulted in an increased number of licensed adolescent drivers without an improvement in safety.[24]

Adolescent drivers are inexperienced, and this inexperience, especially if coupled with alcohol, increases the risk of collision. Approximately 50% of adolescent motor vehicle fatalities involve alcohol.[22] In fact, a large proportion of all pediatric motor vehicle occupant deaths occur in vehicles operated by inebriated drivers.[25] Legislative and educational efforts must focus on elimination of drunk driving.

Pedestrian Injuries

Pedestrian injuries are a leading cause of death among children aged 5 to 9 years.[15,19] Injuries typically occur when a child darts out into the street and is struck by an automobile. Although promising educational programs attempt to improve the street-related behavior of children, roadway interventions such as adequate lighting, construction of sidewalks, and roadway barriers must also be pursued.

Bicycle Injuries

Every year approximately 200 000 children and adolescents are injured and more than 600 die from bicycle-related trauma.[15,16,21] Head injuries cause most bicycle-related morbidity and mortality, and bicycle-related trauma is a leading cause of severe pediatric closed-head injuries.[26] Use of bicycle helmets can prevent an estimated 85% of head injuries and 88% of brain injuries,[26] but many parents are unaware of the need for helmets, and children may be reluctant to wear them.[27] A successful bicycle helmet education program includes an ongoing communitywide multidisciplinary approach that provides focused information about the need for and effectiveness of helmets. To be successful, such programs must ensure the acceptability, accessibility, and affordability of helmets.[16,27]

Submersion

Drowning is a significant cause of death and disability in children younger than 4 years and is the leading cause of death in this age group in several states.[15,19] For every death due to submersion, six children are hospitalized, and approximately 20% of hospitalized survivors suffer severe neurological sequelae.[15]

Parents should be aware of the dangers to children posed by any body of water. Young children and children with seizure disorders should never be left unattended in bathtubs or near swimming pools, ponds, or beaches. Drownings in swimming pools may be prevented if the pool is completely surrounded by a 5-foot fence with a self-closing, self-latching gate. The house *cannot* serve as a barrier to the pool if one of the house doors opens onto the pool area. Older children and adults who reside in homes with swimming pools should learn CPR, since prompt provision of BLS contributes to improved survival after submersion.[13,14] Children aged 5 years and older should know how to swim. No one should ever swim alone, and even supervised children should wear personal flotation devices when playing in rivers, streams, or lakes. Alcohol appears to be a significant risk factor in adolescent drowning. Hence control of alcohol and the use of personal flotation devices on waterways should be encouraged.

Burns

Approximately 80% of fire- and burn-related deaths result from house fires.[15,17] Most fire-related deaths occur in private residences,[28] usually in homes without working smoke detectors.[29] Smoke inhalation, scalds, and contact and electric burns are especially likely to affect children younger than 4 years. Socioeconomic factors such as overcrowding, single-parent families, scarce financial resources, inadequate child care/supervision, and distance from a fire department contribute to increased risk for burn injury.

Smoke detectors are one of the most effective interventions for prevention of deaths from burns and smoke inhalation. When used correctly, they can reduce the potential for death and severe injury by nearly 90%.[29] Parents should be aware of the effectiveness of these devices and the need to change smoke detector batteries twice every year.

Continued improvements in flammability standards for furniture, bedding, and home builders' materials should reduce the incidence of fire-related injuries and deaths. Child-resistant ignition products should also be explored. School-based fire-safety programs should be continued and evaluated.

Firearm Injuries

Firearms, particularly handguns, are responsible for an increasing number of unintentional pediatric injuries and an increasing number of pediatric homicides and suicides.[30] Annually more than 4500 children under 20 years of age die from firearm injuries, and thousands more are injured.[31] Firearm homicide is the leading cause of death among African-American adolescents and young adults and the second leading cause of death in all adolescent males.[31,32] The United States has the highest firearm-related homicide rate among young males of any industrialized nation, more than four times that of any other country.[31] The rising incidence of firearm injuries has paralleled the increased availability of handguns.[33] More than 66% of all homes in the United States contain firearms, and at least one home in every two contains handguns.[34] Thirty-four percent of surveyed high school students report easy access to guns, and an increasing number of children are carrying guns to school.[35-37] Most guns used in unintentional shootings are found in the home and are typically found loaded in readily accessible places.[34,38-41] The presence of a gun in the home has also been linked to an increased likelihood of adolescent suicide.[42]

Reduction in the incidence of firearm injuries requires removal of guns from each child's environment.[43] Every gun owner, potential gun purchaser, and parent must be made aware of the risks of firearms and the need to ensure that weapons are inaccessible to children.[43-45] Guns must be stored *only* in areas inaccessible to children. They should be stored unloaded, and ammunition should be stored in an area apart from the guns. The use of trigger locks should be encouraged and their efficacy determined. Owner liability laws and controlled distribution of handguns should be monitored for effectiveness. If such laws are found to be effective, their extension should be considered.

Prehospital Care

EMS systems were developed primarily for adults, and the requirements of pediatric victims have only recently been considered. Prehospital equipment is often inadequate to meet the needs of critically ill or injured infants and children, and prehospital personnel receive little pediatric emergency education. In EMS systems death rates are higher among children than adults, especially in areas where tertiary pediatric care is unavailable.[46-50] To overcome these deficiencies, communities should ensure that EMS personnel are trained and equipped to care for pediatric emergencies, that medical dispatchers have emergency protocols appropriate for children, and that emergency departments caring for children are appropriately staffed and equipped.[48-50] Emergency departments caring for acutely ill or injured children should have formal agreements with a pediatric tertiary service so that postresuscitation care for infants and children can be provided in a pediatric intensive care unit under the supervision of trained personnel (see chapter 1).

The Sequence of Pediatric BLS: The ABCs of CPR and EMS Activation

Pediatric BLS includes sequential assessments and motor skills designed to support or restore effective ventilation and circulation to the child in respiratory or cardiorespiratory arrest. BLS can be performed by any trained bystander and is essential for the victim's eventual recovery. When cardiorespiratory arrest is present or impending, prompt access to advanced life support is also required.

Determine Responsiveness

The rescuer must quickly assess the presence or extent of injury and determine whether the child is conscious. The level of responsiveness is determined by tapping the child and speaking loudly to elicit a response. The victim should not be moved unnecessarily or shaken if spinal cord injury is suspected because such handling may aggravate the injury. If the child is unresponsive but breathing or struggling to breathe, the EMS system must be accessed so that the child can be rapidly transported to an advanced life support facility. Children with respiratory distress will often position themselves to maintain patency of a partially obstructed airway, and they should be allowed to remain in the position that is most comfortable for them.

Once unresponsiveness has been determined, the lone rescuer should shout for help and then provide BLS to the child, if necessary, for approximately 1 minute before the EMS system is activated. Since cardiac and cardiopulmonary arrest in children is most commonly associated with the development of hypoxemia rather than with ventricular arrhythmias, approximately 1 minute of rescue support may restore oxygenation and effective ventilation or may prevent the child with respiratory arrest from developing cardiac arrest. If trauma has not occurred, the single rescuer may consider moving a small child close to a telephone so that the EMS system may be more easily called. The EMS medical dispatcher may then guide the rescuer through CPR. Movement of the child is mandatory if the child is found in a dangerous location (eg, in a burning building) or if CPR cannot be performed where the child is found (see also "Coordination of Compressions and Rescue Breathing" below). If a second rescuer is present during the initial assessment of the child, that rescuer should activate the EMS system as soon as the presence of cardiorespiratory distress is recognized.

A child should always be moved carefully, particularly if there is evidence of trauma. The likelihood of neck, spine, or bone injuries may be evident from the child's location and position. For example, traumatic injuries should be expected if a child is found unconscious at the side of the road or the base of a tree but will be unlikely if an unconscious infant is found in bed. If trauma is suspected, the cervical spine must be completely immobilized, and neck extension, flexion, and rotation must be prevented. When the child is moved, the head and body must be held and turned as a unit and the head and neck firmly supported so that the head does not roll, twist, or tilt.

Airway

Hypoxemia and respiratory arrest may cause or contribute to acute deterioration and cardiopulmonary arrest during childhood. Thus, establishment and maintenance of a patent airway and support of adequate ventilation are the most important components of BLS.

Assessment of Airway

Relaxation of muscles and passive posterior displacement of the tongue may lead to airway obstruction in the unconscious victim.[51] Whenever an unconscious, non-breathing victim is found, the airway should be opened immediately. This is usually accomplished by the head tilt–chin lift maneuver. If neck injury is suspected, head tilt should be avoided and the airway opened by a jaw thrust while the cervical spine is completely immobilized. If the child is conscious and demonstrates spontaneous but labored respiratory efforts, time should not be wasted on an attempt to open the airway further. The child should instead be transported to an advanced life support facility as rapidly as possible.

Opening of Airway

Head Tilt–Chin Lift (Fig 1). To perform this technique:
- Place one hand on the child's forehead and tilt the head gently back into a neutral position. The neck is slightly extended.
- Place fingers, but not the thumb, of the other hand under the bony part of the lower jaw at the chin, and lift the mandible upward and outward.
- Be careful not to close the mouth or push on the soft tissues under the chin, because such maneuvers may obstruct rather than open the airway.
- If a foreign body or vomitus is visible, remove it.

Jaw Thrust. The jaw-thrust technique without head tilt is the safest method of opening the airway of the victim with suspected neck or cervical spine injury because it can be accomplished without extension of the neck.
- Place two or three fingers under each side of the lower jaw at its angle and lift the jaw upward and outward (Fig 2).
- If jaw thrust alone does not open the airway, slight head tilt may be added in patients with no evidence of cervical spine injury.

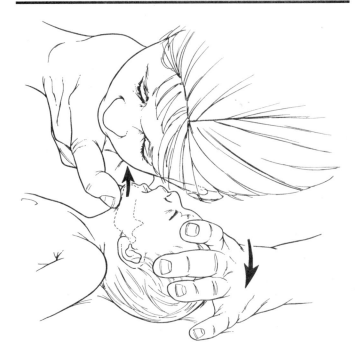

Fig 1. Opening the airway with the head tilt–chin lift maneuver. One hand is used to tilt the head, extending the neck. The index finger of the rescuer's other hand lifts the mandible outward by lifting on the chin. Head tilt should not be performed if cervical spine injury is suspected.

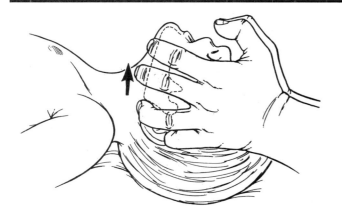

Fig 2. Opening the airway with the jaw-thrust maneuver. The airway is opened by lifting the angle of the mandible. The rescuer uses two or three fingers of each hand to lift the jaw while the remaining fingers guide the jaw upward and outward.

- If trauma is suspected and a second rescuer is present, that rescuer should immobilize the cervical spine (see "BLS in Trauma" below).

Breathing

Assessment of Breathing

After the airway is opened, the rescuer must determine if the child is breathing. The rescuer **looks** for a rise and fall of the chest and abdomen, **listens** for exhaled air, and **feels** for exhaled air flow at the mouth. If spontaneous breathing is present, a patent airway must be maintained. If the infant or child is unresponsive, has no evidence of trauma, and is obviously breathing effectively, the rescuer should place the victim in the **recovery position** and activate the EMS system. If the victim is breathing effectively and is small enough and is without evidence of trauma, the rescuer may carry the victim to the telephone to enable rapid activation of the EMS system.

To place the victim in the **recovery position**:

- Move the victim's head, shoulders, and torso simultaneously.
- Turn the victim onto his or her side.
- The leg not in contact with the ground may be bent and the knee moved forward to stabilize the victim.
- Note that the victim should *not* be moved in any way if trauma is suspected and should not be placed in the recovery position if rescue breathing or CPR is required.

Rescue Breathing

If no spontaneous breathing is detected, rescue breathing must be provided while a patent airway is maintained by a chin lift or jaw thrust. If a mask with one-way valve or other infection control barrier is readily available, it should be used during rescue breathing. However,

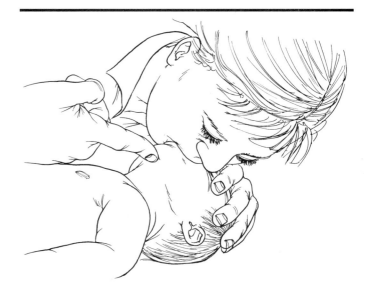

Fig 3. Rescue breathing in an infant. The rescuer's mouth covers the infant's nose and mouth, creating a seal. One hand performs head tilt while the other hand lifts the infant's jaw. Avoid head tilt if the infant has sustained head or neck trauma.

ventilation should not be delayed while such a device is located.

- First inhale deeply.
- *If the victim is an infant (under 1 year old)*, place your mouth over the infant's nose and mouth, creating a seal (Fig 3).
- *If the victim is a large infant or a child (1 to 8 years old)*, make a mouth-to-mouth seal and pinch the victim's nose tightly with the thumb and forefinger of the hand maintaining head tilt (Fig 4).
- Give two slow breaths (1 to 1½ seconds per breath) to the victim, pausing after the first breath to take a breath.

Pausing to take a breath maximizes oxygen content and minimizes carbon dioxide concentration in the delivered breaths.[52] If the rescuer fails to take this replenishing breath, the rescue breath will be low in oxygen and high in carbon dioxide.

Rescue breaths are the most important support for a nonbreathing infant or child. There is wide variation in the size of pediatric victims, so it is impossible to make precise recommendations about optimal pressure or volume of ventilations. The volume and pressure should be sufficient to cause the chest to rise. *If the child's chest does not rise during rescue breathing, ventilation is not effective.* The small airways of infants and children provide high resistance to airflow. To minimize the pressure required for ventilation and to prevent the development of gastric distention, breaths should be delivered slowly.[53] Slow delivery of breaths will allow delivery of an adequate volume of air and ensure effective lung and chest expansion. *The correct volume for each breath is the volume that causes the chest to rise.*

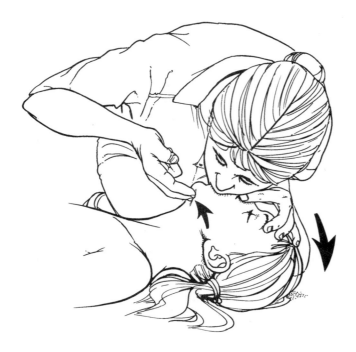

Fig 4. Rescue breathing in a child. The rescuer's mouth covers the mouth of the child, creating a mouth-to-mouth seal. One hand maintains head tilt; the thumb and forefinger of the same hand are used to pinch the child's nose. If head or neck trauma is suspected, immobilize the head in neutral position and *do not* perform head tilt.

If air enters freely and the chest rises, the airway is clear. If air does not enter freely (if the chest does not rise), either the airway is obstructed or more breath volume or pressure is necessary. Since improper opening of the airway is the most common cause of airway obstruction, the rescuer should be prepared to reattempt opening of the airway and reattempt ventilation if initial ventilation attempts are unsuccessful (ie, the chest does not rise). The victim's head will be placed in the neutral or sniffing position for the first attempt at ventilation. If ventilation is unsuccessful, the rescuer should move the victim's head into several positions of progressive neck extension, until a position of optimal airway patency results in effective rescue breathing (Fig 5). Such manipulation, however, should not be performed if neck or cervical spine trauma is suspected. Under these conditions airway opening should be provided by the jaw lift. If rescue breathing fails to produce chest expansion despite attempts at opening the airway, a foreign-body airway obstruction must be suspected (see "Foreign-Body Airway Obstruction" below).

Rescue breathing, especially if performed rapidly, may cause gastric distention.[54,55] Excessive gastric distention can, in turn, interfere with rescue breathing by elevating the diaphragm and thus compromise lung volume. Gastric distention may be minimized if rescue breaths are delivered slowly, since slow breaths will enable delivery of effective tidal volume at low inspiratory pressure. If two

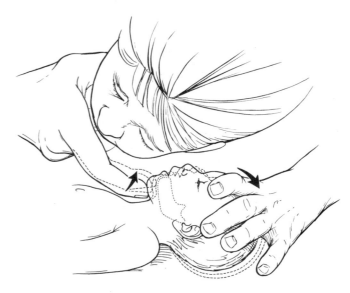

Fig 5. Movement of victim's head into positions of progressive neck extension until position of optimum airway patency (and effective ventilation) is achieved. Such manipulation of the head should *not* be performed if head, neck, or cervical spine injury is suspected.

rescuers are present, the second rescuer may provide cricoid pressure to displace the trachea posteriorly, compressing the esophagus against the vertebral column. This maneuver may prevent gastric distention and reduce the likelihood of regurgitation. It cannot be performed by a single rescuer.

Tracheostomy

Some pediatric victims, particularly those with chronic respiratory disease, may have a temporary tracheostomy tube in the trachea. Ventilation is provided through this tube. To prevent leakage of air when the rescuer blows into the tracheostomy tube, the victim's mouth and nose usually must be sealed by the rescuer's hand or by a tightly fitting face mask.

Mouth to Barrier Device

Some rescuers may prefer to use a barrier device during mouth-to-mouth ventilation. Many devices have been introduced, but few have been adequately studied. Two broad categories of devices are available: masks and face shields. Most masks have a one-way valve so that exhaled air does not enter the rescuer's mouth. Many face shields have no exhalation valve, and often air leaks around the shield. Barrier devices should ideally have a low resistance to gas flow to prevent rescuer fatigue. If rescue breathing is deemed necessary:

- Position the barrier device (face mask or face shield) over the victim's mouth and nose.
- Ensure an adequate air seal.

- Give slow inspiratory breaths (1 to 1½ seconds) as described above. Further evaluation of the effectiveness of these devices is warranted.

Circulation

Once the airway is opened and two rescue breaths have been provided, the rescuer determines the need for chest compression. The rescuer should be positioned beside the victim.

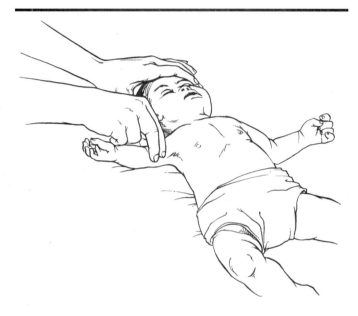

Fig 6. Palpating the brachial artery pulse in an infant.

Assessment of Circulation: Pulse Check

If cardiac contractions are ineffective or absent, there will not be a palpable pulse in the central arteries. Two studies have documented the difficulty that laypersons have in locating peripheral pulses and counting the pulse rate in children.[56,57] If the child is not breathing spontaneously, heart rate and stroke volume are probably inadequate, so chest compressions are usually required. Complications associated with CPR (including cardiac compression) are uncommon in infants and children. Although rib fractures and injuries to the bony thorax have been observed following CPR in adults,[58] they have not been reported in infants[59] or children.[60] Thus the need for and validity of a pulse check by prehospital providers is questionable. Landmarks for locating pulses are provided here, but the lay rescuer should spend only a few seconds attempting to locate a pulse in a nonbreathing infant or child before providing chest compressions.

It is important to note that precordial activity represents an *impulse* rather than a pulse. The child's precordium may be quiet, and a precordial impulse may not be palpated despite the presence of satisfactory cardiac function and strong central pulse.[56] For this reason the apical impulse is not used in the pulse check.

Pulse Check in Infants. The short, chubby neck of infants under 1 year of age makes rapid location of the carotid artery difficult, so palpation of the *brachial artery* is recommended.[56] The femoral pulse is often palpated by healthcare professionals in a hospital setting. The brachial pulse is on the inside of the upper arm, between the infant's elbow and shoulder.

- With your thumb on the outside of the arm, gently press your index and middle fingers until you feel the pulse (Fig 6).

Pulse Check in Children. In children older than 1 year, the *carotid artery,* on the side of the neck, is the most accessible central artery to palpate. The carotid artery lies on the side of the neck between the trachea and the sternocleidomastoid muscles. To feel the artery:

- Locate the victim's thyroid cartilage (Adam's apple) with two or three fingers of one hand while maintaining head tilt with the other hand.
- Slide your fingers into the groove on the side of the neck closer to you, between the trachea and the sternocleidomastoid muscles.
- Gently palpate the artery (Fig 7).

If a pulse is present but spontaneous breathing is absent:

- Provide rescue breathing alone at a rate of 20 breaths per minute (once every 3 seconds) for the infant or the child until spontaneous breathing resumes.
- After giving approximately 20 breaths, activate the EMS system (see "Activation of the EMS System" below).

If a pulse is not palpable or heart rate is less than 60 *and* signs of poor systemic perfusion are present:

- Begin chest compressions.
- Coordinate compressions and ventilation.
- After providing approximately 20 cycles of compressions and ventilations, activate the EMS system.

Chest Compressions

Chest compressions are serial, rhythmic compressions of the chest that circulate oxygen-containing blood to the vital organs (heart, lungs, and brain) until advanced life support can be provided. Chest compressions must always be accompanied by ventilations.

The mechanism by which blood flow is circulated during chest compressions in pediatric victims remains controversial.[61-66] The thoracic pump theory suggests that blood circulates as a result of a change in intrathoracic versus extrathoracic pressures. According to the cardiac pump theory, circulation results from direct compression of the heart. In infants and perhaps in children, because

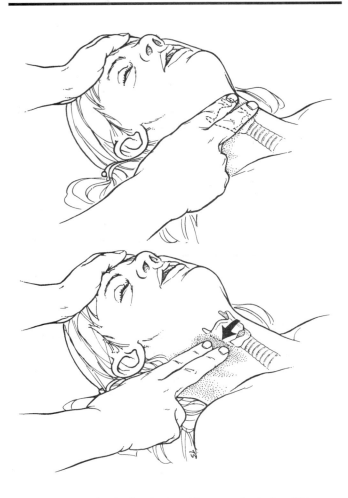

Fig 7. Locating and palpating the carotid artery pulse in the child.

of the greater mobility of the thoracic cage, direct heart compression may be an important mechanism of blood flow during compressions.[64]

To achieve optimal compressions:

• The child should be supine on a hard, flat surface.

For an infant the hard surface may be the rescuer's hand or forearm, with the palm supporting the infant's back (Fig 8, top). This maneuver effectively raises the infant's shoulders, allowing the head to tilt back slightly, into a position of airway patency.

If the infant is carried during CPR, the hard surface is created by the rescuer's forearm, which supports the length of the infant's torso, while the infant's head and neck are supported by the rescuer's hand. Care should be taken to keep the infant's head no higher than the rest of the body. The rescuer's other hand performs chest compression. The rescuer can lift the child to provide ventilation (Fig 8, bottom).

Chest Compression in the Infant. In infants the area of compression is the lower half of the sternum[67-69] (Fig 9). The technique for chest compression is as follows:

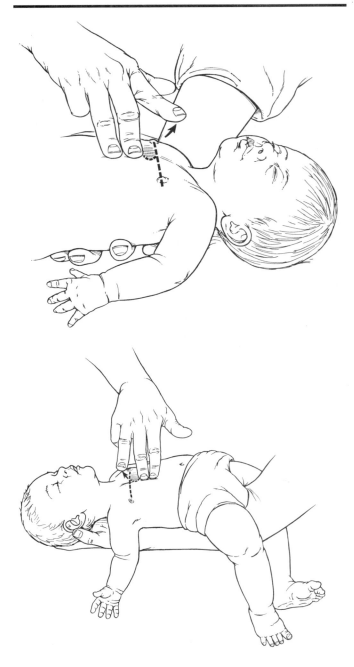

Fig 8. Cardiac compressions. Top, Infant supine on palm of the rescuer's hand. Bottom, Performing CPR while carrying the infant or small child. Note that the head is kept level with the torso. (Compare Fig 9.)

1. Use one hand to maintain the infant's head position (unless your hand is under the child's back). This may make it possible to ventilate without delaying to reposition the head.
2. Use your other hand to compress the chest. Place the index finger of that hand on the sternum just below the level of the infant's nipples. Place the middle fingers on the sternum, adjacent to the index finger. Sternal compression is performed approximately the width of one finger below the level of the

nipples. Avoid compression of the xiphoid process, which is at the lowermost portion of the sternum, because such compression may injure the liver, stomach, or spleen.[70]

3. Using two or three fingers, compress the sternum approximately one third to one half the depth of the chest. This will correspond to a depth of about ½ to 1 inch, although these measurements are not precise.

   • The compression rate should be *at least* 100 times per minute.
   • Compressions must be coordinated with ventilations in a 5:1 ratio.

   With pauses for ventilation, the number of compressions will actually be at least 80 per minute.

4. At the end of each compression, release pressure without removing the fingers from the chest. Allow the sternum to return briefly to its normal position. A smooth compression-relaxation rhythm without jerky movements should be developed, with equal time for compression and relaxation.

5. Activate the EMS system after you have provided approximately 1 minute of CPR (20 cycles).

6. If the victim resumes effective breathing, place the victim in the recovery position.

Chest Compression in the Child. Any child older than approximately 1 year up to 8 years is considered a child for the purposes of BLS. If the child is large or older than approximately 8 years, chest compression should be provided as described for adults.

1. Use one hand to maintain the child's head position so that it may be possible to ventilate without repositioning the head.

2. Using two fingers of the other hand, trace the lower margin of the victim's rib cage, on the side of the chest nearer you, to the notch where the ribs and sternum meet.

3. Note the location of the notch (where the ribs and stenum meet) and avoid compression over that notch, which includes the xiphoid.

4. Place the heel of your hand over the lower half of the sternum (between the nipple line and the notch), avoiding the xiphoid process. The long axis of the heel is over the long axis of the sternum (Fig 10).

5. Compress the chest to approximately one third to one half its total depth. This corresponds to a compression depth of about 1 to 1½ inches, but these measurements are not precise.

   • The compression rate is 100 times per minute.
   • Compressions must be coordinated with ventilation in a 5:1 compression-to-ventilation ratio.

   With pauses for ventilation, the number of compressions will actually be approximately 80 compressions per minute.

6. The compressions should be smooth. Hold your fingers up off the ribs while the heel of your hand remains on the sternum. Allow the chest to return to its resting position after each compression, but do not lift your hand off the chest. Compression and relaxation should be of approximately equal duration.

7. Activate the EMS system after you have provided approximately 1 minute of CPR (20 cycles).

8. If the victim resumes effective breathing, place the victim in the recovery position.

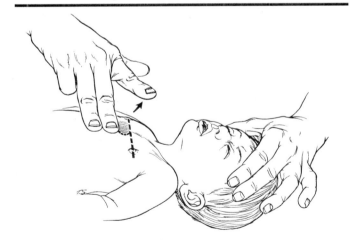

Fig 9. Locating proper finger position for chest compression in infant. Note that the rescuer's other hand is used to maintain head position to facilitate ventilation.

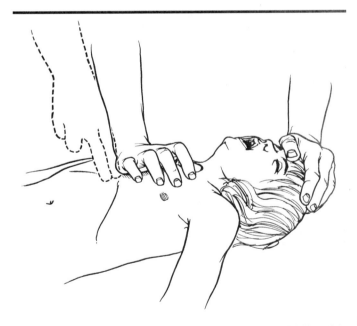

Fig 10. Locating hand position for chest compression in child. Note that the rescuer's other hand is used to maintain head position to facilitate ventilation.

Coordination of Compressions and Rescue Breathing

Chest compressions must always be accompanied by rescue breathing. At the end of every fifth compression, a pause of 1 to 1½ seconds should be allowed for a ventilation. The 5:1 compression-ventilation ratio for infants and children is used for both one and two rescuers. (The two-rescuer technique should be used only by healthcare providers.) The infant and child should be reassessed after 20 cycles of compressions and ventilations (approximately 1 minute, although this measurement is not precise) and every few minutes thereafter for any sign of resumption of spontaneous breathing or pulses.

Coordination of such rapid compressions and ventilations by a single rescuer may be difficult. Therefore, during cardiac compressions and between breaths for the infant, airway patency is maintained by head tilt using the hand that is not performing compression (Fig 9). Maintenance of head tilt in this way may reduce the time required to provide ventilation, enabling provision of an adequate number of compressions and ventilations every minute. Ventilation is adequate if effective chest expansion is observed with each breath provided by the rescuer. If the chest does not rise, the hand performing chest compressions should perform a chin lift to open the airway while ventilation is provided. That hand then returns to the compression position after ventilation.

In children, head tilt alone is often inadequate to maintain airway patency. Typically both hands are needed to perform the head tilt–chin lift maneuver with each ventilation. The time needed to position the hands for each breath, to locate landmarks, and to reposition the hand to perform compressions will reduce the total number of compressions provided. Therefore, when positioning the hand to perform chest compressions after ventilation, the rescuer should visualize the chest and return the hand to the approximate location used for the previous sequence of compressions. The full procedure to relocate the landmarks should not be performed each time a cycle of 5 compressions is begun.

A summary of BLS maneuvers in infants and children is presented in the Table. Note: Two-person CPR can be performed in children in a fashion similar to that for adults with appropriate changes in chest compressions and ventilations.

Activation of the EMS System

If the rescuer is alone, the EMS system should be activated after approximately 1 minute of rescue support (20 breaths including chest compressions, if necessary). If head and neck trauma are not present and the victim resumes spontaneous breathing, the rescuer should turn the unconscious victim to the side (recovery position) before leaving the victim to activate the EMS system. If head or neck trauma is suspected, the victim *should not* be turned.

Summary of BLS Maneuvers in Infants and Children

Maneuver	Infant (<1 y)	Child (1 to 8 y)
Airway	Head tilt–chin lift (if trauma is present, use jaw thrust)	Head tilt–chin lift (if trauma is present, use jaw thrust)
Breathing		
Initial	Two breaths at 1 to 1½ s/breath	Two breaths at 1 to 1½ s/breath
Subsequent	20 breaths/min (approximate)	20 breaths/min (approximate)
Circulation		
Pulse check	Brachial/femoral	Carotid
Compression area	Lower half of sternum	Lower half of sternum
Compression width	2 or 3 fingers	Heel of 1 hand
Depth	Approximately one third to one half the depth of the chest	Approximately one third to one half the depth of the chest
Rate	At least 100/min	100/min
Compression-ventilation ratio	5:1 (pause for ventilation)	5:1 (pause for ventilation)
Foreign-body airway obstruction	Back blows/chest thrusts	Heimlich maneuver

If the victim is small and trauma is not suspected, it may be possible to carry the child (supporting the head and neck carefully) to a telephone while CPR is provided so that the EMS system can be activated. If the rescuer is unable to activate the EMS system, CPR should continue until help arrives or the rescuer becomes too exhausted to continue.

The rescuer calling the EMS system should be prepared to give the following information:

- The location of the emergency, including address and names of streets or landmarks
- The telephone number from which the call is being made
- What happened, eg, auto accident, drowning
- The number of victims
- The condition of the victim(s)
- The nature of the aid being given
- Any other information requested

The caller should hang up only after the dispatcher breaks the connection or if specifically instructed to do so by the dispatcher.

Foreign-Body Airway Obstruction

More than 90% of deaths from foreign-body aspiration in the pediatric age group occur in children younger than 5 years; 65% of the victims are infants.[71] With the development of consumer product safety standards regulating the minimum size of toys and toy parts for young children, the incidence of foreign-body aspiration has decreased.

However, toys, balloons, or small objects and especially foods (eg, hot dogs, round candies, nuts, and grapes) may still be aspirated.[72,73] Foreign-body airway obstruction should be suspected in infants and children who demonstrate the *sudden* onset of respiratory distress associated with coughing, gagging, stridor (a high-pitched, noisy sound), or wheezing.

Signs and symptoms of airway obstruction may also be caused by infections such as epiglottitis and croup, which produce airway edema. Infection should be suspected as the cause of airway obstruction if the child has a fever, particularly if accompanied by congestion, hoarseness, drooling, lethargy, or limpness. Children with an *infectious* cause of airway obstruction must be taken immediately to an emergency facility. Time should not be wasted in a futile and probably dangerous attempt to relieve this form of obstruction.

Attempts to clear the airway should be considered when foreign-body aspiration is witnessed or strongly suspected or when the airway remains obstructed (no chest expansion) during attempts to provide rescue breathing to the unconscious, nonbreathing infant or child. If foreign-body aspiration is witnessed or strongly suspected, the rescuer should encourage the child to continue spontaneous coughing and breathing efforts as long as the cough is forceful. Relief of airway obstruction should be attempted *only* if signs of *complete* airway obstruction are observed. These signs include ineffective cough (loss of sound), increased respiratory difficulty accompanied by stridor, development of cyanosis, and loss of consciousness. The EMS system should be activated as rapidly as possible by a second rescuer.

The Heimlich maneuver (subdiaphragmatic abdominal thrusts) is recommended for relief of complete upper airway obstruction in a child.[74] These thrusts increase intrathoracic pressure, creating an artificial cough that forces air and may force foreign bodies out of the airway. In the infant a combination of back blows and chest thrusts is recommended for relief of *complete* foreign-body airway obstruction. Although there is a paucity of data regarding relief of foreign-body airway obstruction in infants, existing scientific data do not suggest that back blows and chest thrusts are ineffective for this age group. Since the introduction of the first AHA BLS guidelines recommending back blows and chest thrusts, deaths due to foreign-body airway obstruction in infants and children aged 0 to 4 years have decreased by 60% from more than 450 per year to less than 170 per year.[71,73,75] There have been no scientific reports of complications from or failure of this technique when used in infants. Alternatively, rupture of the stomach, diaphragm, esophagus, and jejunum has been reported following the Heimlich technique.[76,77] Since the infant liver is large and unprotected by the rib cage, the risk of liver injuries may be high if the Heimlich maneuver were recommended for infants. Fatal liver lacerations in several infants have been linked to the application of sudden blunt abdominal trauma during child abuse.[78] For these reasons use of back blows

and chest thrusts is recommended for relief of complete foreign-body airway obstruction in infants. Further data are needed to distinguish opinions and anecdotal experience from fact.

After maneuvers to relieve airway obstruction, the airway is opened using tongue-jaw lift. If the obstructing body is visible, it is removed. If no spontaneous breathing is observed, the airway is opened and rescue breathing is attempted. If the chest does not rise, the head is repositioned, the airway is opened, and rescue breathing is again attempted. If rescue breathing is still unsuccessful (ie, if the chest does not rise), maneuvers to relieve foreign-body obstruction should be repeated.

Manual Removal of Foreign Bodies

Blind finger sweeps should *not* be performed in infants and children since the foreign body may be pushed back into the airway, causing further obstruction. When the airway is opened in the *unconscious,* nonbreathing victim, the tongue-jaw lift is used.

- Grasp both the tongue and the lower jaw between the thumb and finger and lift (tongue-jaw lift). This action draws the tongue away from the back of the throat and may itself partially relieve the obstruction.
- If you see the foreign body, remove it.

The Infant: Back Blows and Chest Thrusts

The following sequence is used to clear a foreign-body obstruction from the airway of an infant. Back blows are delivered while the infant is supported in the prone position (face down) straddling the rescuer's forearm, with the head lower than the trunk. Chest thrusts are delivered while the infant is supine, held on the rescuer's forearm, with the infant's head lower than the body. The rescuer should perform the following steps to relieve airway obstruction in the *conscious* infant:

1. Hold the infant face down, resting on the forearm. Support the infant's head by firmly holding the jaw. Rest your forearm on your thigh to support the infant. The infant's head should be lower than the trunk.
2. Deliver up to five back blows forcefully between the infant's shoulder blades, using the heel of the hand (Fig 11, top).
3. After delivering the back blows, place your free hand on the infant's back, holding the infant's head. The infant is effectively sandwiched between your two hands and arms. One hand supports the head and neck, jaw, and chest while the other supports the back.
4. Turn the infant while the head and neck are carefully supported, and hold the infant in the supine position, draped on the thigh. The infant's head should remain lower than the trunk.

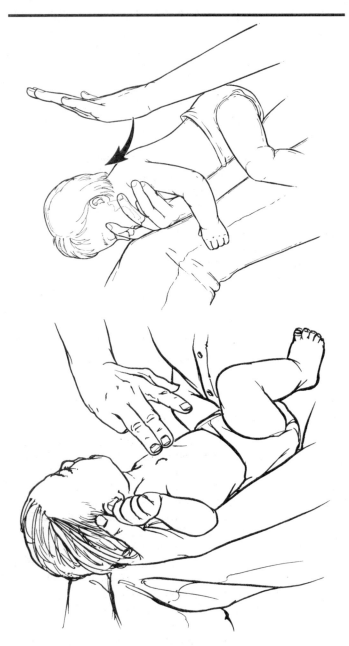

Fig 11. Back blows (top) and chest thrusts (bottom) to relieve foreign-body airway obstruction in the infant.

5. Give up to five quick downward chest thrusts in the same location and manner as chest compressions — two fingers placed on the lower half of the sternum, approximately one finger's breadth below the nipples (Fig 11, bottom).

If the rescuer's hands are small or the infant is large, these maneuvers may be hard to perform. If so, place the infant supine on the lap, with the head lower than the trunk and the head firmly supported. After you have given up to five back blows, turn the infant as a unit to the supine position and give up to five chest thrusts.

Steps 1 through 5 should be repeated until the object is expelled or the infant loses consciousness. If the infant loses consciousness, open the airway using a tongue-jaw lift and remove the foreign object if you see it and attempt rescue breathing and relief of airway obstruction.

If the victim is or becomes unconscious;

1. Open the infant's airway. If the loss of consciousness is witnessed, and foreign-body obstruction is suspected, lift the chin using a tongue-jaw lift and if you see a foreign object, remove it with a finger sweep.
2. Attempt rescue breathing.
3. If the first attempt is unsuccessful, reposition the head and reattempt ventilation.
4. If ventilation is unsuccessful, give five back blows and five chest thrusts.
5. Open the mouth using a tongue-jaw lift and remove the foreign object if you see it.
6. Repeat steps 2 through 4 until ventilation is successful (chest rises).
7. Activate the EMS system after approximately 1 minute, then resume efforts.
8. If the victim resumes effective breathing, place in the recovery position and monitor closely until rescue personnel arrive.

The Child: The Heimlich Maneuver

Abdominal Thrusts With Victim Conscious (Standing or Sitting)

Perform the following steps to relieve complete airway obstruction in the *conscious* victim:

1. Stand behind the victim, arms directly under the victim's axillae encircling the victim's torso.
2. Place the thumb side of one fist against the victim's abdomen in the midline slightly above the navel and well below the tip of the xiphoid process.
3. Grasp the fist with the other hand and exert a series of quick upward thrusts (Fig 12). Do not touch the xiphoid process or the lower margins of the rib cage because force applied to these structures may damage internal organs.
4. Each thrust should be a separate, distinct movement, intended to relieve the obstruction. Continue abdominal thrusts until the foreign body is expelled or the patient loses consciousness.
5. If the victim loses consciousness, open the airway using a tongue-jaw lift and if you see the obstructing object, remove it with a finger sweep.
6. Attempt rescue breathing. If the chest fails to rise, reposition the head and reattempt rescue breathing again. If the airway remains obstructed in the unconscious victim, repeat the Heimlich maneuver (see below).

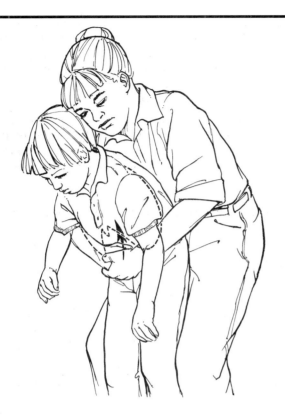

Fig 12. Abdominal thrusts with victim standing or sitting (conscious).

Abdominal Thrusts for the Victim Who Is Unconscious or Who Becomes Unconscious

The rescuer should perform the following steps:

1. Place the victim supine.
2. If the loss of consciousness is witnessed and foreign-body airway obstruction is suspected, open the airway using a tongue-jaw lift and remove the object with a finger sweep if you see it.
3. Attempt rescue breathing. If ventilation is unsuccessful, reposition the head and reattempt ventilation. If ventilation is still unsuccessful, continue with steps 4 through 8 below.
4. Kneel beside the victim or straddle the victim's hips.
5. Place the heel of one hand on the child's abdomen in the midline slightly above the navel and well below the rib cage and xiphoid process. Place the other hand on top of the first.
6. Press both hands into the abdomen with a quick upward thrust (Fig 13). Each thrust is directed upward in the midline and should not be directed to either side of the abdomen. Perform a series of five thrusts. Each thrust should be a separate and distinct movement.
7. Open the airway by grasping both the tongue and lower jaw and lifting the mandible (tongue-jaw lift). If you see the foreign body, remove it using a finger sweep.

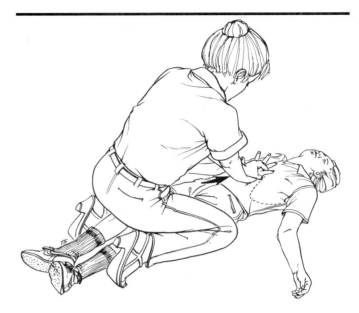

Fig 13. Abdominal thrusts with victim lying (conscious or unconscious).

8. Repeat steps 3 through 6 until ventilation is successful.

BLS in Trauma

Prompt assessment and intervention are essential for successful treatment of childhood trauma (see also chapter 8). Resuscitation should begin as soon as possible after injury, preferably at the scene. Improper resuscitation and failure to adequately open and maintain the airway have been identified as major causes of preventable trauma death.[79]

The pediatric trauma victim requires meticulous support of airway, breathing, and circulation. The child's small airways may become obstructed by soft tissue swelling, blood, vomitus, or dental fragments, so these causes of airway obstruction should be anticipated. Whenever head or neck injury is suspected, the cervical spine must be completely immobilized when the airway is opened. This is best accomplished by a combined jaw-thrust and spinal stabilization maneuver, using only the amount of manual control necessary to prevent cranial-cervical motion[80] (Fig 14). The head tilt–chin lift is contraindicated in trauma victims because it may worsen existing cervical spinal injury. Care must be taken to ensure that the neck is maintained in a neutral position because the prominent occiput of the child predisposes the neck to slight flexion when the child is placed on a flat surface.[81]

If two rescuers are present, the first rescuer opens the airway with a jaw-thrust maneuver while the second rescuer ensures that the cervical spine is absolutely immobilized in a neutral position. Traction on or movement of the neck must be avoided because it may result in conversion of a partial spinal cord injury to a complete injury. Once the airway is controlled, the cervical spine should be immobilized using a semirigid cervical collar and a spine board, linen rolls, and tape, and oxygenation and ventilation should be supported.[82] See chapter 8.

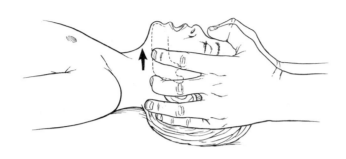

Fig 14. Combined jaw thrust–spine stabilization maneuver for the pediatric trauma victim.

References

1. Walsh CK, Krongrad E. Terminal cardiac electrical activity in pediatric patients. *Am J Cardiol.* 1983;51:557-561.
2. Zaritsky A, Nadkarni V, Getson P, Kuehl K. CPR in children. *Ann Emerg Med.* 1987;16:1107-1111.
3. Friesen RM, Duncan P, Tweed WA, Bristow G. Appraisal of pediatric cardiopulmonary resuscitation. *Can Med Assoc J.* 1982;126:1055-1058.
4. Torphy DE, Minter MG, Thompson BM. Cardiorespiratory arrest and resuscitation of children. *Am J Dis Child.* 1984;138:1099-1102.
5. Gausche M, Seidel JS, Henderson DP, et al. Pediatric deaths and emergency medical services (EMS) in urban and rural areas. *Pediatr Emerg Care.* 1989;5:158-162.
6. Eisenberg M, Bergner L, Hallstrom A. Epidemiology of cardiac arrest and resuscitation in children. *Ann Emerg Med.* 1983;12:672-674.
7. Coffing CR, Quan L, Graves JR, et al. Etiologies and outcomes of the pulseless, nonbreathing pediatric patient presenting with ventricular fibrillation. *Ann Emerg Med.* 1992;21:1046. Abstract.
8. Gillis J, Dickson D, Rieder M, Steward D, Edmonds J. Results of inpatient pediatric resuscitation. *Crit Care Med.* 1986;14:469-471.
9. Lewis JK, Minter MG, Eshelman SJ, Witte MK. Outcome of pediatric resuscitation. *Ann Emerg Med.* 1983;12:297-299.
10. O'Rourke PP. Outcome of children who are apneic and pulseless in the emergency room. *Crit Care Med.* 1986;14:466-468.
11. Schoenfeld PS, Baker MD. Management of cardiopulmonary and trauma resuscitation in the pediatric emergency department. *Pediatrics.* 1993; 91:726-729.
12. Hazinski MF, Chahine AA, Holcomb GW III, Morris JA Jr. Outcome of cardiovascular collapse in pediatric blunt trauma. *Ann Emerg Med.* In press.
13. Quan L, Wentz KR, Gore EJ, Copass MK. Outcome and predictors of outcome in pediatric submersion victims receiving prehospital care in King County, Washington. *Pediatrics.* 1990;86:586-593.
14. Kyriacou DN, Kraus JF, Arcinue E. Effect of immediate resuscitation on childhood outcomes after aquatic submersion injury. *Ann Emerg Med.* 1992; 21:1046. Abstract.
15. Division of Injury Control, Center for Environmental Health and Injury Control, Centers for Disease Control. Childhood injuries in the United States. *Am J Dis Child.* 1990;144:627-646.
16. DiGuiseppi CG, Rivara FP, Koepsell TD, Polissar L. Bicycle helmet use by children: evaluation of a community-wide helmet campaign. *JAMA.* 1989;262:2256-2261.

17. Rice DP, Mackenzie EJ, and Associates. *Cost of Injury in the United States: A Report to Congress.* Atlanta, Ga: Division of Injury, Epidemiology, and Control, Center for Environmental Health and Injury Control, Centers for Disease Control; 1989.
18. Haddon W, Suchman EA, Klein O. *Accident Research: Methods and Approaches.* New York, NY: Harper and Row; 1964.
19. Guyer B, Ellers B. Childhood injuries in the United States: mortality, morbidity, and cost. *Am J Dis Child.* 1990;144:649-652.
20. Cushman R, James W, Waclawik H. Physicians promoting bicycle helmets for children: a randomized trial. *Am J Public Health.* 1991;81:1044-1046.
21. Centers for Disease Control. Fatal injuries to children — United States, 1986. *JAMA.* 1990;264:952-953.
22. The National Committee for Injury Prevention and Control. Traffic injuries. In: *Injury Prevention: Meeting the Challenge. Am J Prev Med.* 1989;5(suppl):115-144.
23. Safety Belt USA: Unpublished reports, Virginia Commonwealth University, Transportation Center. 1990.
24. Robertson LS. Crash involvement of teenaged drivers when driver education is eliminated from high school. *Am J Public Health.* 1980;70:599-603.
25. Margolis LH, Kotch J, Lacey JH. Children in alcohol-related motor vehicle crashes. *Pediatrics.* 1986;77:870-872.
26. Thompson RS, Rivara FP, Thompson DC. A case-control study of the effectiveness of bicycle safety helmets. *N Engl J Med.* 1989;320:1361-1367.
27. DiGuiseppi CG, Rivara FP, Koepsell TD. Attitudes toward bicycle helmet ownership and use by school-age children. *Am J Dis Child.* 1990;144:83-86.
28. The National Committee for Injury Prevention and Control. Residential injuries. In: *Injury Prevention: Meeting the Challenge. Am J Prev Med.* 1989;5(suppl):153-162.
29. *An Evaluation of Residential Smoke Detector Performance Under Actual Field Conditions.* Washington, DC: Federal Emergency Management Agency; 1980.
30. *Facts About Kids and Handguns.* Washington, DC: Center to Prevent Handgun Violence; May 1990.
31. Fingerhut LA, Kleinman JC, Godfrey E, Rosenberg H. Firearm mortality among children, youth and young adults, 1-34 years of age, trends and current status: United States, 1979-1988. *Monthly Vital Stat Rep.* 1991;39:1-16. No. 11.
32. Fingerhut LA, Ingram DD, Feldman JJ. Firearm homicide among black teenage males in metropolitan counties: comparison of death rates in two periods, 1983 through 1985 and 1987 through 1989. *JAMA.* 1992;267:3054-3058.
33. Wintemute GJ. Firearms as a cause of death in the United States, 1920-1982. *J Trauma.* 1987;27:532-536.
34. Weil DS, Hemenway D. Loaded guns in the home: analysis of national random survey of gun owners. *JAMA.* 1992;267:3033-3037.
35. *Caught in the Crossfire: A Report on Gun Violence in Our Nation's Schools.* Washington, DC: Center to Prevent Handgun Violence; September 1990.
36. Callahan CM, Rivara FP. Urban high school youth and handguns: a school-based survey. *JAMA.* 1992;267:3038-3042.
37. Weapon-carrying among high-school students: United States, 1990. *MMWR.* 1991;40:681-684.
38. Wintemute GJ, Teret SP, Kraus JF, Wright MA, Bradfield G. When children shoot children: 88 unintended deaths in California. *JAMA.* 1987;257:3107-3109.
39. *Child's Play: A Study of 266 Unintentional Handgun Shootings of Children.* Washington, DC: Center to Prevent Handgun Violence; 1990.
40. *The Killing Seasons: A Study of When Unintentional Handgun Shootings Among Children Occur.* Washington, DC: Center to Prevent Handgun Violence; 1990.
41. Beaver BL, Moore VL, Peclet M, Haller JA Jr, Smialek J, Hill JL. Characteristics of pediatric firearm fatalities. *J Pediatr Surg.* 1990;25:97-99.
42. Brent DA, Perper JA, Allman CJ, Mortiz GM, Wartella ME, Zelenak JP. The presence and accessibility of firearms in the homes of adolescent suicides: a case-control study. *JAMA.* 1991;266:2989-2995.
43. Christoffel KK. Toward reducing pediatric injuries from firearms: charting a legislative and regulatory course. *Pediatrics.* 1991;88:294-305.

44. American Academy of Pediatrics Committee on Injury and Poison Prevention. Policy statement: firearm injuries affecting the pediatric population. *AAP News.* 1992;8:22-33.

45. Christoffel KK. Pediatric firearm injuries: time to target a growing population. *Pediatr Ann.* 1992;21:430-436.

46. Seidel JS. Emergency medical services and the pediatric patient: are the needs being met? II: training and equipping emergency service providers for pediatric emergencies. *Pediatrics.* 1986;78:808-812.

47. Applebaum D. Advanced prehospital care for pediatric emergencies. *Ann Emerg Med.* 1985;14:656-659.

48. Seidel JS. EMS-C in urban and rural areas: the California experience. In: Haller JA Jr, ed. *Emergency Medical Services for Children: Report of the 97th Ross Conference on Pediatric Research.* Columbus, Ohio: Ross Laboratories; 1989:22-30.

49. Seidel JS, Henderson DP, eds. *Emergency Medical Services for Children: A Report to the Nation.* Washington DC: National Center for Education in Maternal and Child Health; 1991.

50. Durch JS, Lohr KN, eds. *Emergency Medical Services for Children.* Washington, DC: National Academy Press; 1993.

51. Ruben HM, Elam JO, Ruben AM, Greene DG. Investigation of upper airway problems in resuscitation, I: studies of pharyngeal x-rays and performance by laymen. *Anesthesiology.* 1961;22:271-279.

52. Tendrup TE, Kanter RK, Cherry RA. A comparison of infant ventilation methods performed by prehospital personnel. *Ann Emerg Med.* 1989;18:607-611.

53. Melker R, Cavallaro D, Krischer J. One rescuer CPR–a reappraisal of present recommendations for ventilation. *Crit Care Med.* 1981;9:423.

54. Melker RJ. Asynchronous and other alternative methods of ventilation during CPR. *Ann Emerg Med.* 1984;13(pt 2):758-761.

55. Melker RJ, Banner MJ. Ventilation during CPR: two-rescuer standards reappraised. *Ann Emerg Med.* 1985;14:397-402.

56. Cavallaro DL, Melker RJ. Comparison of two techniques for detecting cardiac activity in infants. *Crit Care Med.* 1983;11:189-190.

57. Lee CJ, Bullock LJ. Determining the pulse for infant CPR: time for a change? *Milit Med.* 1991;156:190-199.

58. Nagel EL, Fine EG, Krischer JP, Davis JH. Complications of CPR. *Crit Care Med.* 1981;9:424.

59. Spevak MR, Kleinman PK, Belanger PL, Richmond MD. Does cardiopulmonary resuscitation cause rib fractures in infants? Postmortem radiologic-pathologic study. *Radiology.* 1990;177P:162. Abstract. (National Program, RSNA '90)

60. Feldman KW, Brewer DK. Child abuse, cardiopulmonary resuscitation, and rib fractures. *Pediatrics.* 1984;73:339-342.

61. Zaritsky A. Selected concepts and controversies in pediatric cardiopulmonary resuscitation. *Crit Care Clin.* 1988;4:735-754.

62. Berkowitz ID, Chantarojanasiri T, Koehler RC, et al. Blood flow during cardiopulmonary resuscitation with simultaneous compression and ventilation in infant pigs. *Pediatr Res.* 1989;26:558-564.

63. Krischer JP, Fine EG, Weisfeldt ML, Guerci AD, Nagel E, Chandra N. Comparison of prehospital conventional and simultaneous compression-ventilation cardiopulmonary resuscitation. *Crit Care Med.* 1989;17:1263-1269.

64. Dean JM, Koehler RC, Schleien CL, et al. Age-related changes in chest geometry during cardiopulmonary resuscitation. *J Appl Physiol.* 1987;62:2212-2219.

65. Dean JM, Koehler RC, Schleien CL, Atchison D, et al. Improved blood flow during prolonged cardiopulmonary resuscitation with 30% duty cycle in infant pigs. *Circulation.* 1991;84:896-904.

66. Deshmukh HG, Weil MH, Gudipati CV, Trevino RP, Bisera J, Rackow EC. Mechanism of blood flow generated by precordial compression during CPR, I: studies on closed-chest precordial compression. *Chest.* 1989;95:1092-1099.

67. Finholt DA, Kettrick RG, Wagner HR, Swedlow DB. The heart is under the lower third of the sternum: implications for external cardiac massage. *Am J Dis Child.* 1986;140:646-649.

68. Phillips GW, Zideman DA. Relation of infant heart to sternum: its significance in cardiopulmonary resuscitation. *Lancet.* 1986;1:1024-1025.

69. Orlowski JP. Optimal position for external cardiac massage in infants and children. *Crit Care Med.* 1984;12:224.

70. Thaler MM, Krause VW. Serious trauma in children after external cardiac massage. *N Engl J Med.* 1962;267:500-501.

71. National Safety Council. How people died accidentally in 1983. In: *Accident Facts 1984.* Chicago, Ill: National Safety Council; 1984.

72. Harris CS, Baker SP, Smith GA, Harris RM. Childhood asphyxiation by food: a national analysis and overview. *JAMA.* 1984;251:2231-2235.

73. Reilly JS. Prevention of aspiration in infants and young children: federal regulations. *Ann Otol Rhinol Laryngol.* 1990;99:273-276.

74. Heimlich HJ. A life-saving maneuver to prevent food-choking. *JAMA.* 1975;234:398-401.

75. National Safety Council. How people died in home accidents: 1978. In: *Accident Facts 1979.* Chicago, Ill: National Safety Council; 1979:81-82.

76. Fink JA, Klein RL. Complications of the Heimlich maneuver. *J Pediatr Surg.* 1989;24:486-487.

77. Van der Ham AC, Lange JF. Traumatic rupture of the stomach after Heimlich maneuver. *J Emerg Med.* 1990;8:713-715.

78. Cooper A, Floyd T, Barlow B, et al. Major blunt abdominal trauma due to child abuse. *J Trauma.* 1988;28:1483-1487.

79. Dykes EH, Spence LJ, Young JG, Bohn DJ, Filler RM, Wesson DE. Preventable pediatric trauma deaths in a metropolitan region. *J Pediatr Surg.* 1989;24:107-110.

80. Cooper A, Foltin G, Tunik M. Airway control in the unconscious child victim: description of a new maneuver. *Ped Emerg Care.* In press.

81. Herzenberg JE, Hensinger RN, Dedrick DK, Phillips WA. Emergency transport and positioning of young children who have an injury of the cervical spine: the standard backboard may be hazardous. *J Bone Joint Surg Am.* 1989;71:15-22.

82. Soud T, Pieper P, Hazinski MF. Pediatric trauma. In: Hazinski MF, ed. *Nursing Care of the Critically Ill Child.* 2nd ed. St Louis, Mo: CV Mosby Co; 1992:842-843.

Airway and Ventilation

Chapter 4

Respiratory problems are common in infants and children and are an important cause of in- and out-of-hospital cardiopulmonary arrest in the pediatric age group. Assessment and treatment decisions must be made quickly to prevent progression and deterioration to respiratory failure and cardiopulmonary arrest. If respiratory failure or respiratory arrest is promptly treated, intact survival of the child is likely. However, once respiratory arrest progresses to pulseless *cardiac* arrest, outcome is poor.[1-7] Therefore, early recognition and effective management of respiratory problems are fundamental to pediatric advanced life support.

This chapter reviews the techniques and adjuncts used in airway management and the priorities of assessment and treatment of the infant and child with respiratory insufficiency or failure. Timely and appropriate use of these techniques and adjuncts is critical to the survival of the patient.

Anatomic and Physiologic Considerations

The pediatric airway differs from the adult airway in several important anatomic and physiologic ways.[8] Anatomic differences of the upper airway include the following:

- The airway of the infant or child is much smaller than that of the adult.
- The tongue in the infant, relative to the oropharynx, is larger compared with that of an adult.
- The larynx in infants and toddlers is relatively cephalad in position.
- The epiglottis in infants and toddlers is short, narrow, and angled away from the long axis of the trachea.
- The vocal cords have a lower attachment anteriorly.
- In children younger than 10 years, the narrowest portion of the airway is below the vocal cords at the level of the nondistensible cricoid cartilage, and the larynx is funnel shaped. In teenagers and adults, the narrowest portion of the airway is at the glottic inlet (Fig 1), and the larynx is cylinder shaped.

These anatomic differences have the following important clinical consequences:

- Relatively small amounts of edema or obstruction can significantly reduce pediatric airway diameter and increase resistance to airflow and therefore the work of breathing.
- Posterior displacement of the tongue may cause severe airway obstruction. Controlling the position of the tongue with the laryngoscope blade may be difficult during tracheal intubation.

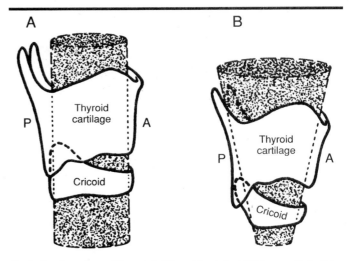

Fig 1. Configuration of the adult (A) and the infant (B) larynx. Note the cylinder shape of the adult larynx. The infant larynx is funnel shaped because of a narrow, undeveloped cricoid cartilage. A indicates anterior; P, posterior. Reproduced with permission from Coté and Todres.[9]

- The high position of the larynx makes the angle between the base of the tongue and glottic opening more acute. As a result, straight laryngoscope blades are more useful than curved blades in creating a direct visual plane from the mouth to the glottis.
- Controlling the epiglottis with a laryngoscope blade may be more difficult.
- A blindly placed endotracheal tube may become caught at the anterior commissure of the vocal cords.
- Endotracheal tube size must be selected based on the size of the cricoid ring rather than the glottic opening. An air leak, observed at a peak inspiratory pressure of 20 to 30 cm H_2O, should be present after intubation if the endotracheal tube size is appropriate.

In the infant and young child, the subglottic airway is smaller and more compliant and the supporting cartilage less developed than in the adult. Therefore, the airway can easily become obstructed by the presence of mucus, blood, or pus; edema; active constriction; external compression (eg, vascular ring or tumor); or pressure differences created during spontaneous respiratory efforts in the presence of upper or lower airway obstruction (Fig 2). Even a minor reduction in diameter of the small pediatric airway results in a clinically significant reduction in cross-sectional area and a concomitant increase in resistance to airflow and work of breathing (Fig 3).

Resistance to airflow is inversely proportional to the fourth power of the airway radius when *laminar flow* is present (ie, during quiet breathing). Thus, even under ideal conditions, *any* reduction in airway size results in an

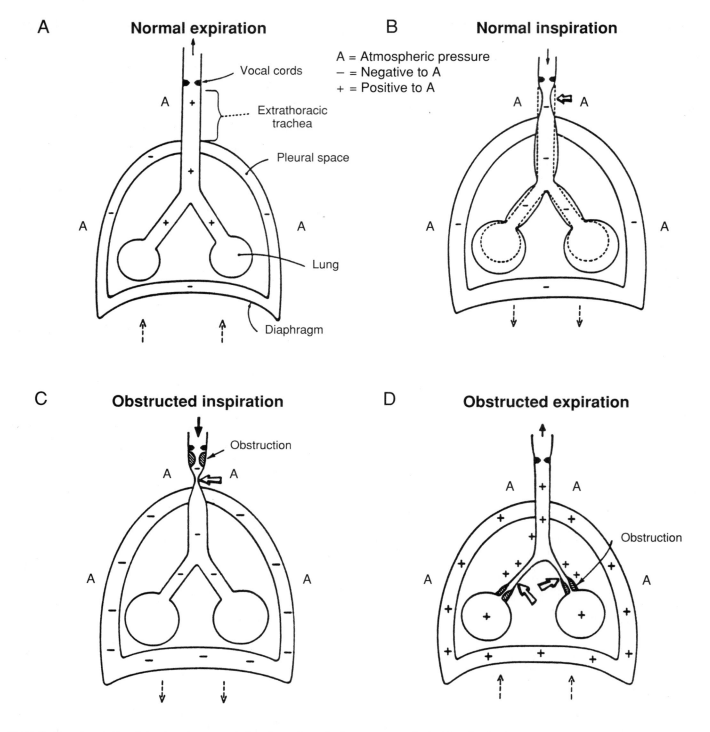

A — **Normal expiration**

Vocal cords

A = Atmospheric pressure
− = Negative to A
+ = Positive to A

Extrathoracic trachea

Pleural space

Lung

Diaphragm

B — **Normal inspiration**

C — **Obstructed inspiration**

Obstruction

D — **Obstructed expiration**

Obstruction

Fig 2. **A**, At end-expiration, intrapleural pressure is less than atmospheric pressure, so it should maintain airway patency. In infants the highly compliant chest does not provide the support required. Thus airway closure occurs with each breath. Intraluminal pressures are slightly positive in relation to atmospheric pressure, so air is forced out of the lungs. Descent of the diaphragm and contraction of the intercostal muscles develop a greater negative intrathoracic pressure relative to intraluminal and atmospheric pressure. **B**, The net result is a longitudinal stretching of the larynx and trachea, dilation of the intrathoracic trachea and bronchi, movement of air into the lungs, and some dynamic collapse of the extrathoracic trachea (arrow). The dynamic collapse is due to the increased compliance of the trachea and the negative intraluminal pressure in relation to atmospheric pressure. **C**, Respiratory dynamics occurring with upper airway obstruction; note the severe dynamic collapse of the extrathoracic trachea below the level of obstruction. This collapse is greatest at the thoracic inlet, where the largest pressure gradient exists between negative intratracheal pressure and atmospheric pressure (arrow). **D**, Respiratory dynamics occurring with lower airway obstruction. Breathing through a partially obstructed lower airway (such as occurs in bronchiolitis or asthma) results in greater positive intrathoracic pressures, with dynamic collapse of the intrathoracic airways (prolonged expiration or wheezing [arrows]). Reproduced with permission from Coté and Todres.[9]

exponential increase in resistance to airflow and work of breathing. However, when airflow is *turbulent,* eg, during crying, resistance to airflow is inversely proportional to the *fifth* power of the radius. For this reason, the infant or child with airway obstruction should be kept as calm and quiet as possible to prevent generation of turbulent air-flow, increased airway resistance (Fig 3), and markedly increased work of breathing.[9]

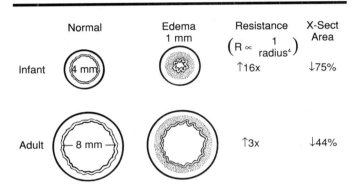

Fig 3. Effects of edema on airway resistance in the infant versus the adult. Normal airways are represented on the left, edematous airways (with 1 mm of circumferential edema) on the right. Resistance to flow is inversely proportional to the *fourth* power of the lumen radius for lami-nar flow and to the *fifth* power for turbulent flow. The net result is a 75% decrease in cross-sectional area and a 16-fold increase in resistance in the infant versus 44% and threefold in the adult during quiet breathing. Turbulent flow in the child (eg, crying) would increase the work of breathing 32-fold. Reproduced with permission from Coté and Todres.[9]

The ribs and sternum normally support the lungs and help them remain expanded. The intercostal muscles and diaphragm alter intrathoracic volume and pressure, causing air to move into the lungs. In infants the ribs and intercostal cartilage are highly compliant and fail to support the lungs adequately.[10,11] As a result, functional residual capacity is reduced when respiratory effort is diminished or absent. If the airway is obstructed, active inspiration often results in paradoxical chest movement with sternal and intercostal retractions rather than chest and lung expansion. In addition, the lack of lung support makes the tidal volume of infants and toddlers almost totally dependent on movement of the diaphragm. When diaphragm movement is impeded by high intrathoracic pressure (eg, pulmonary hyperinflation, such as occurs in asthma) or by gastric distention, respiration is compro-mised because the intercostal muscles cannot lift the chest wall.

The high compliance of the pediatric airway makes it very susceptible to dynamic collapse in the presence of airway obstruction.[12] Upper airway obstruction — eg, epiglottitis, croup, or presence of an extrathoracic foreign body — may cause tracheal collapse during inspi-ration (Fig 2C). An intrathoracic foreign body or a disease such as bronchiolitis or asthma (Fig 2D) often causes lower airway obstruction during exhalation. The applica-tion of positive end-expiratory pressure (PEEP) often improves air exchange by opposing the forces causing dynamic airway collapse (Fig 4).

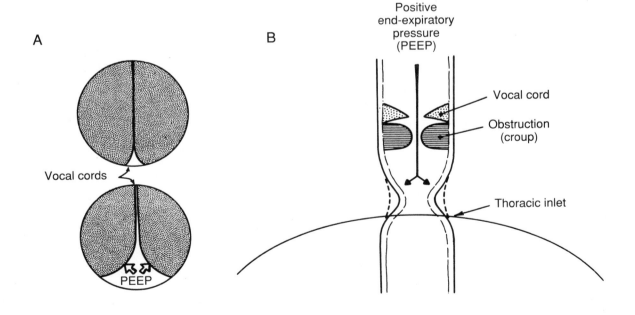

Fig 4. In the presence of upper airway obstruction caused by laryngospasm (A) or mechanical obstruction (B), application of approximately 10 cm H_2O positive end-expiratory pressure (PEEP) during spontaneous breathing often relieves obstruction (arrows) by keeping the vocal cords apart (Fig A) and the airway patent (broken lines, Fig B). If this simple maneuver does not relieve obstruction, positive-pressure ventilation may be necessary. Reproduced with permission from Coté CJ. Pediatric anesthesia. In: Miller RD, ed. *Anesthesia.* 3rd ed. New York, NY: Churchill Livingstone; 1990:911.

The pediatric patient has a high oxygen demand per kilogram of body weight because the child's metabolic rate is high. Oxygen consumption in infants is 6 to 8 mL/kg per minute compared with 3 to 4 mL/kg per minute in adults.[13,14] Therefore, in the presence of apnea or inadequate alveolar ventilation, hypoxemia develops more rapidly in the child than in the adult.

An illness leading to respiratory distress or failure may cause hypoxemia by several mechanisms:

- The disease process decreases lung compliance and/or increases airway resistance, resulting in increased work of breathing and increased oxygen demand.
- The disease process directly interferes with exchange of oxygen or carbon dioxide.
- Mismatch of ventilation and perfusion causes shunting of pulmonary blood through the lung so that hypoxemia and (to a lesser extent) hypercarbia occur.

Ventilatory function may also be compromised by depression of central control of ventilation by hypoxemia, hypothermia, street drugs or drug intoxication, medications, metabolic derangements (eg, hypoglycemia), or central nervous system injury, dysfunction, or seizures. Respiratory rate and effort must be carefully monitored in patients with drug intoxication or head injury because apnea is relatively common in these patients. Fortunately, cervical spine injuries are relatively uncommon in infants and children. However, high spinal injury (C4 and above) may cause apnea by disrupting the innervation of the diaphragm.

Airway Adjuncts for the Spontaneously Breathing Patient in Respiratory Distress

General Principles

The goals of emergency airway management are to *anticipate* and *recognize* respiratory problems and to support or replace those functions that are compromised or lost. In an emergency, determining the cause of respiratory dysfunction may be impossible and even unnecessary before initiating some or all of the steps of emergency airway management.

Oxygen, in the highest possible concentration, should be administered to all seriously ill or injured patients with respiratory insufficiency, shock, or trauma, even if measured arterial oxygen tension is high. In these patients, oxygen delivery to tissues may be limited by inadequate pulmonary gas exchange or inadequate circulatory volume, cardiovascular function, or blood volume distribution. Humidification should be added as soon as practical to prevent obstruction of the small airways by dried secretions. Heated humidification systems are preferable to

cool mist systems, since the latter may produce hypothermia in the small victim.

A number of factors contribute to severe progressive hypoxemia and tissue hypoxia during cardiac arrest. At best, mouth-to-mouth ventilation provides an inspired oxygen concentration of 16% to 17% with a maximal alveolar tension of 80 mm Hg in larger children. Since even optimal chest compressions generate only a fraction of the normal cardiac output, oxygen delivery to tissues is markedly diminished. In addition, CPR is associated with right-to-left pulmonary shunting caused by ventilation-perfusion mismatch.

Alert children experiencing respiratory difficulty should be allowed to remain in a position of comfort since they usually assume a position that promotes optimal airway patency and minimizes respiratory effort. Anxiety increases oxygen consumption and possibly respiratory distress (Fig 2). Alert children in respiratory distress should therefore be allowed to remain with their parents, and airway equipment (including oxygen) should be introduced in a nonthreatening manner. If a child is upset by one method of oxygen support (such as a mask), alternative methods (eg, a face tent or a "blow-by" stream of humidified oxygen held by a parent toward the child's mouth and nose) should be attempted.

If the child is *somnolent* or *unconscious,* the airway may become obstructed by a combination of neck flexion, relaxation of the jaw, posterior displacement of the tongue against the posterior wall of the pharynx, and collapse of the hypopharynx.[15,16] Noninvasive methods of opening the airway (see chapter 3) should precede the use of adjuncts.[17,18] If necessary, the airway should be cleared by removing secretions, mucus, or blood from the oropharynx and nasopharynx with suction.

Assisted ventilation must be provided if spontaneous ventilation is inadequate (as judged by insufficient chest movement and inadequate breath sounds) despite a patent airway. In most respiratory emergencies, infants and children can be successfully ventilated with a bag-valve–mask device, even in the presence of airway obstruction.[19] Gentle positive-pressure breaths administered with a bag-valve–mask device should be carefully timed to augment the child's inspiratory efforts. If the breaths are not coordinated with the child's efforts, ventilation may be ineffective and may result in coughing, vomiting, laryngospasm, and gastric distention with further impedance of effective ventilation.

Noninvasive Respiratory Monitoring

Pulse oximetry is an important noninvasive technique for monitoring the child with respiratory insufficiency because it provides continuous evaluation of arterial oxygen saturation.[20] Pulse oximetry does not indicate the adequacy of ventilation but may provide an early indication of respiratory deterioration and development of hypoxemia and should be used throughout stabilization and transport.[21] Pulse oximeters only enable evaluation of *oxygenation;* they *do not* reflect effectiveness of *ventilation* (carbon dioxide elimination).

The pulse oximeter consists of two light-emitting diodes and a photodetector in a sensor. Oxygenated hemoglobin primarily absorbs infrared light, but reduced (nonoxygenated) hemoglobin primarily absorbs red light. When the light-emitting diodes of the oximeter are placed directly across a pulsatile tissue bed from the photodetector, the absorption of emitted light can be determined by a microprocessor.[22]

Since the light absorption of methemoglobin and carboxyhemoglobin is different from that of normal hemoglobin, the pulse oximeter will not accurately reflect hemoglobin saturation in the presence of methemoglobinemia or carbon monoxide poisoning.[22] If these conditions are present, hemoglobin saturation must be determined by measurement of a blood sample using oximetry.

The pulse oximeter requires pulsatile blood flow to determine oxygen saturation. It will not provide useful data in the child with shock and poor perfusion. If the pulse oximeter does not detect the pulse signal, there may be a mechanical problem or a problem with the interface, or the child may be in a low-perfusion state that requires urgent treatment.

If infant sensors are unavailable, an adult sensor may be placed around the hand or foot of an infant. If intense vasoconstriction is present and a pulsatile signal is not detected in the extremities, an infant pulse oximeter probe may be applied to the ear lobe. If the patient is unconscious, the probe may also be applied to the nares, the cheek at the corner of the mouth, and even to the tongue.[23,24]

Different brands of pulse oximeters vary greatly in their speed of response to the development of hypoxemia.[25,26] The validity of oximeter data must be confirmed by evaluating the patient's appearance and comparing the heart rate recorded by the oximeter with that recorded by the electrocardiogram. If the heart rates do not correlate or the patient's appearance does not correspond to the level of oxygenation, the accuracy of the oximeter must be questioned.

An end-tidal carbon dioxide detector may reflect trends in the patient's $PaCO_2$ and may allow verification of correct endotracheal tube placement in infants larger than 2 kg during stabilization and transport in the prehospital or hospital setting.[27] End-tidal carbon dioxide monitoring may be misleading during resuscitation of pulseless arrest. A detectable level confirms endotracheal placement. However, extremely low end-tidal carbon dioxide tension in this setting probably reflects decreased pulmonary blood flow rather than esophageal tube placement.[28]

Arterial Blood Gas Analysis

Arterial blood gas analysis is the most accurate method of determining arterial oxygen and carbon dioxide tensions and pH. Usually blood gas analysis is extremely helpful in determining the effectiveness of oxygenation and ventilation and in quantifying respiratory or metabolic acidosis and response to therapy. During CPR, however, arterial PO_2 and pH may not accurately reflect tissue oxygenation and pH but indicate effectiveness (or ineffectiveness) of *perfusion*[29,30] (see "Acid-Base Balance," chapter 6).

Oxygen Delivery Systems

If spontaneous ventilation is effective, oxygen may be administered via a number of different delivery systems. The choice of delivery system is determined by the child's clinical status and the desired concentration of oxygen. Oxygen delivery systems can be divided into low-flow and high-flow systems.[31] In a low-flow system, room air is entrained because the gas flow is insufficient to meet all inspiratory flow requirements. In a high-flow system, the flow rate and reservoir capacity provide adequate gas flow to meet the total inspired flow requirements of the patient, so entrainment of room air does not occur. No matter which system is used, the delivered oxygen concentration is determined by the patient's minute ventilation and gas flow delivery rate. Low-flow systems theoretically provide an oxygen concentration of 23% to 90%, although they do not do so reliably. High-flow systems can reliably deliver either low or high inspired oxygen concentrations. These systems should therefore be used in the emergency setting.

Oxygen Mask

Several types of oxygen masks may be used to administer humidified oxygen in a wide range of concentrations. The soft vinyl pediatric mask is often poorly tolerated by infants and toddlers but may be accepted by older children.

The simple oxygen mask is a low-flow device that delivers 35% to 60% oxygen with a flow rate of 6 to 10 L/min. The inspired oxygen concentration can be increased only modestly (up to approximately 60%) because the inspiratory entrainment of room air occurs through exhalation ports in the side of the mask and between the mask and the face. Oxygen concentration delivered to the patient will be reduced if the patient's spontaneous inspiratory flow requirement is high, the mask is loose, or the oxygen flow into the mask is low. A minimum oxygen flow of 6 L/min must be used to maintain an increased inspired oxygen concentration and prevent rebreathing of exhaled carbon dioxide.

A *partial rebreathing mask* consists of a simple face mask with a reservoir bag (Fig 5). It reliably provides an inspired oxygen concentration of 50% to 60% (compared with 30% to 60% for standard masks). During exhalation,

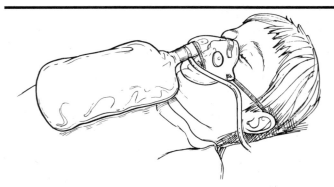

Fig 5. Partial rebreathing mask.

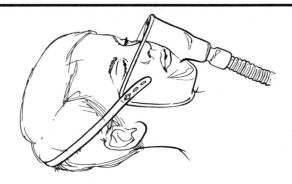

Fig 6. Face tent or shield.

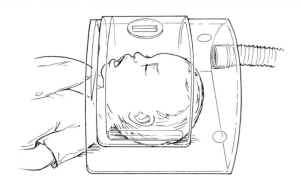

Fig 7. Oxygen hood.

the first third of the exhaled gases flows into the reservoir bag and combines with fresh oxygen. Since the initial portion of the exhaled gas remains in the upper airway and is not involved in respiratory gas exchange during the prior breath, it remains oxygen rich. During inspiration the patient draws gas predominantly from the fresh oxygen inflow and from the reservoir bag, so entrainment of room air through the exhalation ports is minimized. Rebreathing of exhaled carbon dioxide from the mask is prevented if the oxygen flow rate into the bag is consistently maintained above the patient's minute ventilation. If the oxygen flow rate is sufficient and the mask fit secure, the reservoir bag will not empty completely during inspiration. An oxygen flow rate of 10 to 12 L/min generally is required.

A *nonrebreathing mask* consists of a face mask and reservoir bag with the following additions: (1) a valve incorporated into the exhalation port to prevent entrainment of room air during inspiration and (2) a valve placed between the reservoir bag and the mask to prevent flow of exhaled gas into the bag. On inspiration the patient draws 100% oxygen from the reservoir bag and the fresh oxygen inflow. Oxygen flow into the mask is adjusted to prevent collapse of the bag. An inspired oxygen concentration of 95% can be achieved with an oxygen flow of 10 to 12 L/min and the use of a well-sealed face mask.

A Venturi-type mask is designed to reliably and predictably provide controlled low-to-moderate (25% to 60%) inspired oxygen concentrations.

Face Tent

A face tent or face shield (Fig 6) is a high-flow, soft plastic "bucket" that is often better tolerated by children than a face mask. However, even with a high oxygen flow (10 to 15 L/min), stable inspired oxygen concentrations greater than 40% cannot be reliably provided. An advantage of the face tent is that it permits access to the face (eg, for suctioning) without interrupting the oxygen flow to the child.

Oxygen Hood

An oxygen hood is a clear plastic shell that encompasses the patient's head (Fig 7). It is well tolerated by infants; allows easy access to the chest, trunk, and extremities; and permits control of inspired oxygen concentration, gas temperature, and humidity. A gas inflow rate equal to or greater than 10 to 15 L/min maintains approximately the same oxygen concentration within the hood as at the gas source. An inspired oxygen concentration of 80% to 90% may be achieved. As a rule, the hood is not large enough to be used with children older than approximately 1 year.

Oxygen Tent

The oxygen tent is a clear plastic shell that encloses the child's upper body. It can be used to deliver more than 50% oxygen with high flows but cannot reliably provide a stable inspired oxygen concentration. Room air is drawn into the tent whenever the tent is entered, and the child's inspired oxygen concentration therefore falls. The tent limits access to the patient. If humidified oxygen is used, the resulting mist may limit observation of the patient. In practice, a tent does not provide satisfactory supplementation of inspired oxygen if greater than 30% inspired oxygen is required.

Nasal Cannula

A nasal cannula is a simple low-flow oxygen delivery device suitable for infants and children who require only minimal amounts of supplemental oxygen. The cannula consists of two short plastic prongs arising from a hollow face piece. The prongs are inserted into the anterior nares, and oxygen is delivered into the nasopharynx. The inspired oxygen concentration cannot be simply or reliably determined just from nasal oxygen flow rate because it is influenced by other factors, including nasal resistance, oropharyngeal resistance, inspiratory flow rate, and tidal volume. A high oxygen flow rate (>4 L/min) irritates the nasopharynx and may not appreciably improve oxygenation. A nasal cannula does not provide humidified oxygen.

Nasal Catheter

A nasal catheter is a flexible, lubricated oxygen catheter with multiple holes in the distal 2 cm. The catheter is placed in one nostril and advanced posteriorly into the pharynx behind the uvula. This method of oxygen delivery is discouraged because it has no advantage over the nasal cannula, may cause hemorrhage from trauma to enlarged adenoids, and may produce gastric distention or rupture if the catheter is inadvertently placed in the esophagus.

Oropharyngeal Airway

An oropharyngeal airway consists of a flange, a short bite-block segment, and a curved body usually made of plastic and shaped to provide an air channel and suction conduit through the mouth. The curved body of the oropharyngeal airway is designed to fit over the back of the tongue to hold it and the soft hypopharyngeal structures away from the posterior pharyngeal wall. Use of an oropharyngeal airway is indicated for the *unconscious* infant or child if procedures to open the airway (eg, head tilt–chin lift or jaw thrust) fail to provide and maintain a clear, unobstructed airway. An oropharyngeal airway should *not* be used in a *conscious* or semiconscious patient since it may stimulate gagging and vomiting. Airway sizes range from 4 to 10 cm in length (Guedel sizes 000 to 4), which should fit children of all ages. The proper size may be estimated by placing the oropharyngeal airway next to the face (Fig 8A). With the flange at the corner of the mouth, the tip of the airway should reach the angle of the jaw (Fig 8B). If the oropharyngeal airway is too large, it may obstruct the larynx, make a tight mask fit difficult, and traumatize laryngeal structures (Fig 8C). If the oropharyngeal airway is too small or is inserted improperly, it will push the tongue posteriorly into the pharynx, obstructing the airway (Fig 8D).

The oropharyngeal airway should be inserted while a tongue depressor holds the tongue on the floor of the mouth. If a tongue depressor is unavailable, the airway may be inverted for insertion into the mouth, using the curved portion as a tongue depressor. As the airway approaches the back of the oropharynx, it is rotated 180° into proper position. The head and jaw must be positioned properly to maintain a patent airway even after insertion of an oropharyngeal airway.

Nasopharyngeal Airway

A nasopharyngeal airway is a soft rubber or plastic tube that provides a conduit for airflow between the nares and the posterior pharyngeal wall (Fig 9A). A shortened endotracheal tube may also be used as a nasopharyngeal airway. Responsive patients generally tolerate this type of airway better than an oropharyngeal airway. Nasopharyngeal airways are available in sizes 12F to 36F. A 12F nasopharyngeal airway (approximately the size of a 3-mm endotracheal tube) will generally fit the nasopharynx of a full-term infant. The outside airway diameter should not be so large as to cause sustained blanching of the alae nasi. The proper airway length is approximately equal to the distance from the tip of the nose to the tragus of the ear. The airway is lubricated and inserted through a nostril in a posterior direction perpendicular to the plane of the face and passed gently along the floor of the nasopharynx (Fig 9B). The airway should be inserted gently since it can irritate the mucosa or lacerate adenoidal tissue and cause a nosebleed that may aggravate airway obstruction and complicate airway management. The small internal diameter of a nasopharyngeal airway can become obstructed by mucus, blood, vomitus, or the soft tissues of the pharynx, so its patency must be frequently evaluated. Suctioning of the airway may be necessary to ensure patency. A shortened endotracheal tube may provide an airway of sufficient size that it is unlikely to become obstructed (Fig 9A). Care must be taken to firmly reinsert the 15-mm adapter to prevent accidental advancement of the shortened endotracheal tube beyond the nares.

Suction Devices

Suctioning of secretions, blood, vomitus, or meconium from the oropharynx, nasopharynx, or trachea may be necessary to achieve a patent airway. Suction may be created by a vacuum outlet or an electric or battery-powered portable suction device. Portable suction devices are easy to transport but may not provide adequate suction power. A suction force of 80 to 120 mm Hg is generally necessary to suction the airway of an infant or child. A wall-mounted suction unit should provide an airflow of more than 30 L/min at the end of the delivery tube and a vacuum of more than 300 mm Hg when the tube is clamped at full suction.[32]

Flexible plastic suction catheters are useful for aspiration of thin secretions from an endotracheal tube, the trachea, the nasopharynx, or the mouth. Rigid wide-bore suction cannulas (tonsil tips) provide more effective suctioning of the pharynx and are useful for removing thick secretions and particulate matter. Since vagal stimulation, with resultant bradycardia, may occur from stimulation of the posterior pharynx, larynx, or trachea, the heart rate should always be monitored during suctioning.

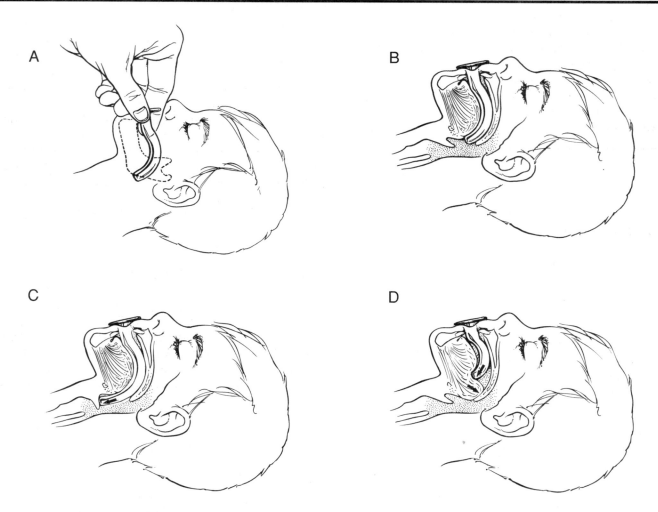

Fig 8. A through D, Proper airway selection. An airway of the proper size should relieve obstruction caused by the tongue without damaging laryngeal structures. The appropriate size can be estimated by holding the airway next to the child's face (8A): the tip of the airway should end just cephalad to the angle of the mandible (broken line), resulting in proper alignment with the glottic opening (8B). If the oral airway inserted is too large, the tip will align posterior to the angle of the mandible (8C) and obstruct the glottic opening by pushing the epiglottis down (8C, arrow). If the oral airway inserted is too small, the tip will align well above the angle of the mandible (8D) and exacerbate airway obstruction by pushing the tongue into the oropharynx (8D, arrows). Adapted with permission from Coté and Todres.[9]

Sterile technique should be used during endotracheal suctioning to reduce the likelihood of airway contamination. A side opening at the proximal end of the suction catheter is used to control negative pressure. The catheter should be gently inserted into the airway just beyond the end of the endotracheal tube *without* application of suction. Suction is then applied by occluding the side opening while withdrawing the catheter with a rotating, twisting motion. To prevent trauma to the carina or main bronchi, the suction catheter should not routinely be inserted more than 1 to 2 cm beyond the end of the endotracheal tube. Suction attempts should not exceed 5 seconds and should be preceded and followed by a short period of ventilation with 100% oxygen to avoid hypoxemia. The heart rate and the child's clinical appearance should be monitored during suctioning. If bradycardia develops or clinical appearance deteriorates, suction-ing should be interrupted and the patient ventilated with a high oxygen concentration until the heart rate and appearance return to normal.

Management of Respiratory Failure or Arrest

If potential respiratory failure is identified, supportive measures must be immediately instituted. The approach to the treatment of respiratory failure is the same as that of basic life support:

- Open the **A**IRWAY
- Support **B**REATHING using an appropriate adjunct that will deliver the highest available oxygen concentration and maintain adequate ventilation
- Assess **C**IRCULATION

Potential respiratory failure is not always readily apparent from a single examination. It is often helpful to interpret physical examination and laboratory data (eg, arterial blood gases) in the context of previous examinations and patient history. When a trend is noted, specific intervention will frequently prevent respiratory failure. *As soon as respiratory failure or inadequate ventilation is identified clinically or by blood gas analysis, rapid initiation of assisted ventilation is the only appropriate therapy.*

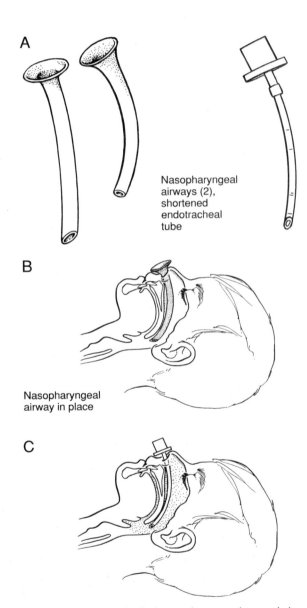

Shortened endotracheal tube used as nasopharygeal airway

Fig 9. A, Nasopharyngeal airway. A shortened endotracheal tube may be substituted (to reduce resistance). B, Placement of a nasopharyngeal airway. Note that the standard 15-mm adapter must be firmly reinserted into the endotracheal tube. C, Cut-off endotracheal tube used as a nasopharyngeal airway.

Ventilation Face Masks

A ventilation face mask allows the rescuer to ventilate and oxygenate a patient and can be used for patients with an oropharyngeal or nasopharyngeal airway in place during spontaneous, assisted, or controlled ventilation.

A ventilation mask consists of a rubber or plastic body, a standardized 15-mm/22-mm connecting port, and a rim or face seal. Most disposable masks used for infants and children have a soft, inflatable cuff with a relatively large undermask volume. In infants and toddlers, the undermask volume should be as small as possible to decrease dead space and minimize rebreathing of exhaled gases. Ideally the mask should be transparent, permitting the rescuer to observe the color of the child's lips and condensation on the mask (indicating exhalation) and to detect regurgitation.

Face masks are available in a variety of sizes. The proper mask size is selected to provide an airtight seal. The mask should extend from the bridge of the nose to the cleft of the chin, enveloping the nose and mouth but avoiding compression of the eyes (Fig 10). If an airtight seal is not maintained, the inspired oxygen concentration is lowered during spontaneous respiration, and assisted or controlled ventilation cannot be effectively provided.

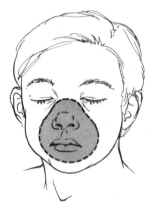

Fig 10. Proper area of the face for face mask application. Note that no pressure is applied to the eyes.

Bag-Valve–Mask Ventilation

Two hands must be used to provide bag-valve–mask ventilation. The mask is held on the face with one hand as a head tilt–chin lift maneuver is performed (Fig 11); the other hand compresses the ventilation bag. In infants and toddlers, the jaw is supported with the base of the middle or ring finger. Pressure in the submental area should be avoided because it can cause airway compression and obstruction. In older children, the fingertips of the third, fourth, and fifth fingers are placed on the ramus of the mandible to hold the jaw forward and extend the head. This creates a one-handed jaw-thrust maneuver. When

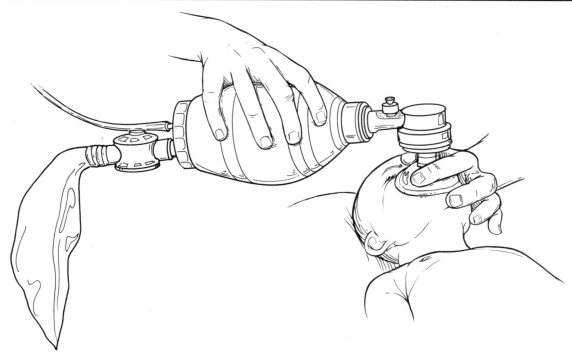

Fig 11. One-handed face mask application technique. Note that the fingers avoid pressure on the soft tissues of the neck, which could cause laryngeal/tracheal compression.

single-operator efforts are not adequate, effective ventilation can often be achieved by two people.[33] One rescuer uses both hands to open the airway and make an air-tight mask-to-face seal while the second rescuer compresses the ventilation bag (Fig 12).

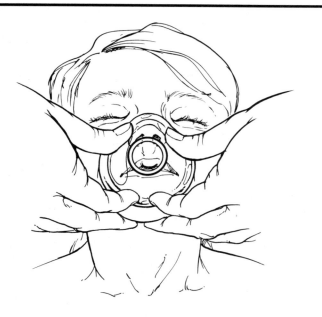

Fig 12. Two-handed face mask application technique. A second person is needed to ventilate the child.

During mask ventilation it may be necessary to gently move the head and neck through a range of positions to determine the optimum position for airway patency and effectiveness of bag-valve–mask ventilation. A neutral sniffing position, without hyperextension of the head, is usually appropriate for infants and toddlers. Extreme hyperextension is avoided in infants since it may produce airway obstruction. Children older than 2 years may require some anterior displacement of the cervical spine to obtain optimal airway patency. This displacement may be achieved by placing a folded towel under the neck and head (Fig 13A through C).

If effective ventilation is not achieved (ie, the chest does not rise), reposition the head, ensure that the mask is fitted snugly against the face, lift the jaw, and consider suctioning the airway. Also ensure that the bag (and gas source) is functioning properly.

If the child demonstrates spontaneous ventilatory effort and partial airway obstruction, application of 5 to 10 cm H_2O continuous positive airway pressure (CPAP) via a face mask may maintain adequate airway patency and oxygenation without the need for assisted ventilation (Fig 4). This requires a tight mask fit and a breathing circuit capable of delivering CPAP.

Inflation of the stomach frequently occurs during assisted or controlled ventilation with a face mask. Gastric distention is especially likely when assisted or controlled ventilation is provided in the presence of partial airway obstruction or low lung compliance or if excessive inspiratory flow rate or ventilation pressure is provided.

Gastric distention should be avoided or promptly treated, since it predisposes the patient to regurgitation and aspiration of stomach contents and may prevent adequate ventilation by limiting downward displacement of the diaphragm.

Gastric inflation and passive regurgitation in the *unconscious* infant or child may be minimized by applying cricoid pressure (Sellick maneuver) during assisted or controlled ventilation (Fig 14).[34-36] This maneuver occludes the proximal esophagus by displacing the cricoid cartilage posteriorly; the esophagus is compressed between the cricoid ring and the cervical spine. The cricoid cartilage is the first tracheal ring, located by

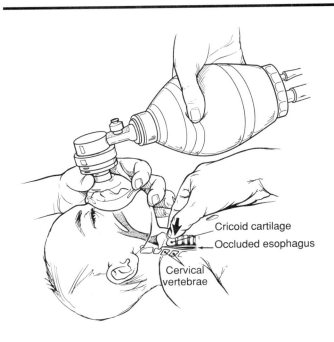

Fig 14. Cricoid pressure (Sellick maneuver).

palpating a prominent horizontal band inferior to the thyroid cartilage and cricothyroid membrane. Cricoid pressure is applied by a second rescuer using one fingertip in infants and the thumb and index finger in children. Excessive pressure must be avoided because it may produce tracheal compression and obstruction in infants.

Self-inflating Bag-Valve Ventilation Devices

A self-inflating bag-valve device with a face mask provides a rapid means of ventilating a patient in an emergency and does not require an oxygen source.[31] The bag recoil allows the self-inflating bag to refill independent of inflow from a gas source. During reinflation the gas intake valve opens, entraining room air or supplemental oxygen if a fresh oxygen inflow reservoir is provided (Fig 15A). During bag compression the gas intake valve closes and a second valve opens to permit gas flow to the patient. During patient exhalation the bag outlet valve (nonrebreathing valve) closes and the patient's exhaled gases are vented to the atmosphere to prevent rebreathing and retention of carbon dioxide. Inability to ventilate or rebreathing of carbon dioxide may occur if secretions or vomitus occlude the nonrebreathing valve and interfere with its function. Self-inflating bags are available in a variety of sizes.

A self-inflating bag-valve device delivers room air (21% oxygen) unless supplemental oxygen is provided. At an oxygen inflow of 10 L/min, pediatric self-inflating bag-valve devices without oxygen reservoirs deliver 30% to 80% oxygen to the patient.[37] To deliver a consistently higher oxygen concentration, a bag-valve device should be equipped with an oxygen reservoir. Reservoir-

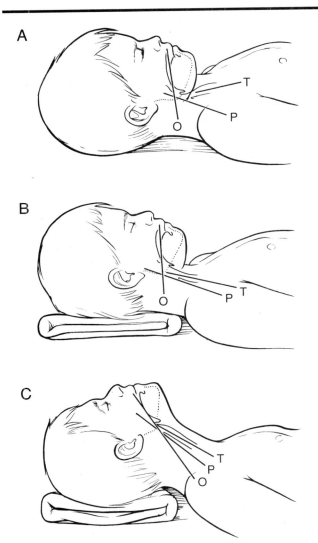

Fig 13. Correct positioning of the child more than 2 years of age for ventilation and tracheal intubation. **A,** With the patient on a flat surface (eg, bed or table), the oral (O), pharyngeal (P), and tracheal (T) axes pass through three divergent planes. **B,** A folded sheet or towel placed under the occiput of the head aligns the pharyngeal and tracheal axes. **C,** Extension of the atlanto-occipital joint results in alignment of the oral, pharyngeal, and tracheal axes. Reproduced with permission from Coté and Todres.[9]

equipped bag-valve devices can provide oxygen concentrations of 60% to 95%. A minimum oxygen inflow of 10 to 15 L/min is required to maintain adequate oxygen volume in the reservoir.[37] Adult self-inflating bag-valve devices, which have larger reinflating bags, require an oxygen inflow of 15 L/min or greater to reliably deliver high oxygen concentrations. High oxygen flow rates may cause some spring-loaded ball or disk outlet valves to chatter or stick. If this occurs, the flow should be reduced to the maximum rate that can be provided without chattering or sticking.

Before initiating ventilation the provider should confirm that oxygen is flowing into the bag by listening over the tail of the bag for the sound of oxygen flow. The sound of oxygen flow should also be verified whenever the patient's condition deteriorates.

Many self-inflating bags are equipped with a pressure-limited pop-off valve set at 35 to 45 cm H_2O to prevent barotrauma. Bags used for resuscitation should have *no pop-off valve* or one that is easily occluded, since pressures required for ventilation during CPR may exceed the pop-off limit, particularly during bag-mask ventilation.[38] When lung compliance is poor or airway resistance is high, an automatic pop-off may result in insufficient delivered tidal volume, as indicated by inadequate chest expansion.[38] Occlusion of the pop-off valve may remedy the problem and can be accomplished by depressing the valve with a finger during ventilation or by twisting the pop-off valve into a closed position. Peak ventilation pressure can best be monitored with a manometer placed in line with the bag-valve device.

The bag-valve device used must be appropriate to patient size and condition so that the operator has a feel for the patient's lung compliance. Sudden decreases in lung compliance may indicate main bronchus intubation (usually right), an obstructed endotracheal tube (caused by secretions, blood, or a kink), or pneumothorax. When assisted ventilation is provided, the administered tidal volume should be approximately 10 to 15 mL/kg. Neonatal-size (250 mL) ventilation bags are usually inadequate to support effective tidal volume and the longer inspiratory times required by full-term neonates and infants.[39] Resuscitation bags used for ventilating full-term neonates and infants should have a minimum volume of 450 mL. Studies using infant manikins have shown that effective infant ventilation can be accomplished with pediatric (and larger) resuscitation bags.[40] When larger bags are used, only the force and tidal volume necessary to produce effective chest expansion should be used.

Self-inflating bag-valve devices with a fish-mouth or leaf-flap–operated outlet (nonrebreathing) valve should not be used to provide supplemental oxygen during *spontaneous* ventilation. Although these valves can open during inspiration, allowing the child to inspire the oxygen-enriched gas mixture contained in the bag, many infants cannot generate the increased inspiratory effort required to open the outlet valve. Bag-valve devices with spring-

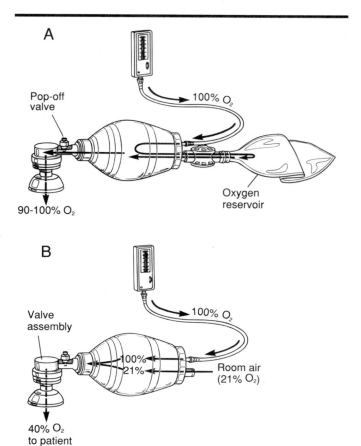

Fig 15. Self-inflating bag-valve device (A) with and (B) without an oxygen reservoir. Oxygen is entering both bags in this illustration.

loaded disk- or ball-operated outlet valves will *not* open during patient inspiration; air/oxygen is delivered only when the bag is compressed.

Positive end-expiratory pressure (PEEP) may be provided during controlled or assisted ventilation by adding a compatible spring-loaded ball or disk or a magnetic-disk PEEP valve to the bag-valve outlet. Bag-valve devices equipped with PEEP valves should *not* be used to provide CPAP in the spontaneously breathing child since high negative inspiratory pressure is required to open the outlet valve.

Anesthesia Ventilation Systems

Anesthesia ventilation systems[41] consist of a reservoir bag, an overflow port, a fresh gas inflow port, and a standard 15-mm/22-mm connector for mask or tracheal tube connection (Fig 16). The overflow port usually includes an adjustable clamp or valve. The reservoir bag volume for infants is 500 mL; for children, 1000 to 2000 mL; and for adults, 3000 to 5000 mL.

More experience is required to effectively control these ventilation devices than to control the self-inflating bag since the fresh gas flow, the outlet control valve, and proper face mask fit must all be carefully adjusted to

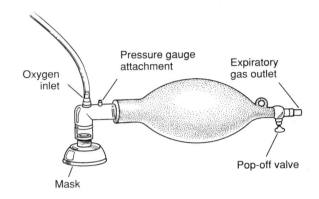

Fig 16. Anesthesia ventilation bag.

achieve ventilation. For these reasons the anesthesia bag should be used only by trained and experienced persons. The composition of inspired gas will be determined by fresh gas flow since a nonrebreathing valve is absent. The pop-off valve must be adjusted to maintain gas volume in the reservoir bag yet permit a high oxygen inflow rate to wash out exhaled gases. If the pop-off valve is partially closed and offers too much resistance to flow, high airway pressure may be generated, with the potential development of barotrauma and its complications. Insufficient washout of exhaled gases may also result in rebreathing and hypercapnia. The oxygen inflow must not be reduced to compensate for a pop-off valve that is too tightly closed. If the valve is opened too far, the reservoir bag will collapse and effective patient ventilation will be impossible until the reservoir refills. Similarly, it is inappropriate to completely close the pop-off valve to compensate for an insufficient oxygen inflow rate. In both instances, rebreathing of exhaled gases may occur, leading to hypercarbia and acidosis. An in-line pressure manometer should be used as a guide to prevent barotrauma. However, effective ventilation is determined by observation of adequate chest movement rather than by reading a pressure manometer.

Fresh gas flow should be adjusted to at least 2 L/min in patients weighing less than 10 kg, 4 L/min in patients weighing 10 to 50 kg, and 6 L/min in patients weighing more than 50 kg. An increase in the fresh gas flow rate decreases the rebreathing of carbon dioxide and is therefore an effective method of preventing hypercarbia.

Anesthesia ventilation systems can be used to provide supplemental oxygen during spontaneous respiration, even in small infants, since there are no flow valves to be opened during inspiration. In this situation the fresh gas flow rate must be at least three times the patient's minute ventilation or removal of exhaled CO_2 may be inefficient. PEEP or CPAP may be provided through this bag by partial closure of the adjustable pop-off valve until the desired level of PEEP is achieved (5 to 10 cm). A mask must also be used.

Endotracheal Airway

Ventilation via an endotracheal tube is the most effective and reliable method of assisted ventilation because

- The airway is isolated, ensuring adequate ventilation and oxygen delivery
- Potential pulmonary aspiration of gastric contents is reduced
- Interposition of ventilations with chest compressions can be accomplished efficiently
- Inspiratory time and peak inspiratory pressures can be controlled
- PEEP can be delivered, if needed, through use of a PEEP valve in the exhalation port

Indications for endotracheal intubation include

- Inadequate central nervous system control of ventilation
- Functional or anatomic airway obstruction
- Loss of protective airway reflexes
- Excessive work of breathing, which may lead to fatigue and respiratory insufficiency
- Need for high peak inspiratory pressure or PEEP to maintain effective alveolar gas exchange
- Need for mechanical ventilatory support
- Potential occurrence of any of the above if patient transport is needed

The Endotracheal Tube

The endotracheal tube should be sterile, disposable, and constructed of translucent polyvinyl chloride with a radiopaque marker. An endotracheal tube of uniform internal diameter is preferable to a tapered tube. The Cole shouldered tracheal tube is not recommended because it may cause laryngeal injury. A standard 15-mm adapter is firmly affixed to the proximal end for attachment to a ventilating device. The distal end of the endotracheal tube may provide an opening in the side wall (Murphy eye) to reduce the risk of right-upper-lobe atelectasis. The Murphy eye also reduces the likelihood of complete endotracheal tube obstruction if the end opening is occluded. The endotracheal tube should have distance markers (in centimeters) for use as reference points during placement and to facilitate detection of unintentional endotracheal tube movement. A vocal cord marker may also be present at the level of the glottic opening to ensure that the tip of the tube is in a midtracheal position (Fig 17).

A cuffed endotracheal tube should have a low-pressure, high-volume cuff and is generally indicated for children aged 8 to 10 years or older. In children younger than 8 to 10 years, the normal anatomic narrowing at the level of the cricoid cartilage provides a functional "cuff." If a cuff is present, inflation is appropriate if an audible air leak is present when ventilation to a pressure of 20 to 30 cm H_2O is provided. An appropriately selected uncuffed endotracheal tube should also allow an air leak at the cricoid ring at a peak inflation pressure of 20 to 30 cm H_2O.

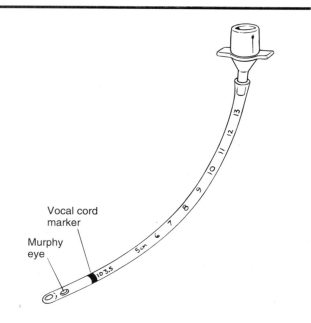

Vocal cord marker

Murphy eye

Fig 17. Endotracheal tube with distance markers.

The absence of an air leak may indicate that the cuff is inflated excessively, that the endotracheal tube is too large, or that laryngospasm is occurring around the endotracheal tube. These conditions may lead to excessive pressure on surrounding tissues. However, if successful intubation has been difficult, even a "tight" endotracheal tube should be left in place until the patient has been stabilized.

A 3-mm or 3.5-mm internal diameter (i.d.) endotracheal tube is adequate for term newborns and small infants, a 4-mm i.d. endotracheal tube during the first year of life, and a 5-mm i.d. endotracheal tube in the second year of life. A simple visual estimate of appropriate endotracheal tube size can be made by choosing a tube with an outside diameter approximating the diameter of the child's little finger. Several other methods and formulas have been developed for estimating the correct endotracheal tube size. In one such formula (used for children older than 2 years) the endotracheal tube size (i.d. in millimeters) may be approximated as follows:

$$\text{Endotracheal Tube (mm i.d.)} = \frac{\text{Age (y)}}{4} + 4$$

An alternative method of endotracheal tube size selection is based on the relationship between the child's length and endotracheal tube size. Length-based determination of endotracheal tube size is more accurate than age-based determination.[42,43] Resuscitation tapes based on length may help identify the correct endotracheal tube size. These strategies only estimate proper tube size. Endotracheal tubes 0.5 mm smaller and larger than the estimated appropriate size should be readily available.

Recommended endotracheal tube sizes are provided in the Table.

The proper distance (depth) of insertion in centimeters (alveolar ridge to midtrachea) *for children older than 2 years* can be approximated by adding one half the patient's age to 12:

$$\frac{\text{Age (y)}}{2} + 12$$

Use of this formula will generally result in placement of the tip of the endotracheal tube above the carina. Alternatively, the distance of insertion (in centimeters) can be estimated by multiplying the internal diameter of the tube by 3. For example:

i.d. = 3.5 mm
Depth of insertion = 3.5 x 3 = 10.5 cm

The Laryngoscope

The laryngoscope consists of a handle with a battery and a blade with a light source. The blade is used to expose the glottis by moving the tongue laterally, placing the blade tip in the vallecula, and lifting the base of the tongue onto the floor of the mouth. If the glottic opening is not exposed by this maneuver, the blade is advanced so that it lifts the epiglottis directly. Adult and pediatric laryngoscope handles fit all blades interchangeably and differ only in diameter and length. The laryngoscope blade may be curved or straight (Fig 18). Several sizes are available. A straight blade is preferred for infants and toddlers since it provides better visualization of the relatively cephalad and anterior glottis, but a curved blade is often preferred for older children since its broader base and flange facilitate displacement of the tongue and improve visualization of the glottis.

Laryngoscopy permits a visual axis through the mouth and pharynx to the larynx, through which an endotracheal tube, a suction catheter, or Magill forceps can be passed for tracheal intubation, suctioning, or extraction of foreign material, respectively.

Preparation for Intubation

Before tracheal intubation is attempted, ventilation is provided with a bag-valve–mask device using 100% oxygen. Monitoring of the heart rate and (if possible) oxygen saturation by pulse oximetry should be performed during the procedure since ventilation will be interrupted. Intubation attempts should be brief, since those lasting longer than 30 seconds may produce profound hypoxemia, especially in infants, whose small lung volumes and increased oxygen requirements rapidly consume oxygen reserves.

The laryngoscope and suction equipment should be checked *before* laryngoscopy to ensure that they are in working order. A variety of blades should be available for

Guidelines for Laryngoscope, Endotracheal Tube, and Suction Catheter Sizes

Patient Age	Laryngoscope	Endotracheal Tube Size I.D. (mm)	Distance (cm) Midtrachea to Teeth/Gums	Suction Catheter (F)
Premature infant	Miller 0*	2.5,3.0 uncuffed	8	5-6
Term infant	Miller 0-1* Wis-Hipple 1 Robertshaw 0	3.0,3.5 uncuffed	9-10	6-8
6 months		3.5, 4.0 uncuffed	10	8
1 year	Wis-Hipple 1½ Robertshaw 1	4.0, 4.5 uncuffed	11	8
2 years	Miller 2 Flagg 2	4.5, 5.0 uncuffed	12	8
4 years		5.0, 5.5 uncuffed	14	10
6 years		5.5 uncuffed	15	10
8 years	Miller 2 Macintosh 2	6.0 cuffed or uncuffed	16	10
10 years		6.5 cuffed or uncuffed	17	12
12 years	Macintosh 3	7.0 cuffed	18	12
Adolescent	Macintosh 3 Miller 3	7.0, 8.0 cuffed	20	12

*Oxyscope modifications are available for Miller 0 and 1 blades. They may reduce the likelihood of hypoxemia during laryngoscopy in infants.

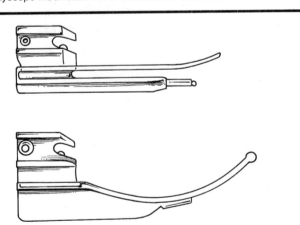

Fig 18. Laryngoscope blades, straight and curved.

selection of the proper blade size. The blade is attached to the handle by inserting its U-shaped indentation onto the small bar at the end of the handle. After the indentation is aligned with the bar, the blade is pressed forward, clipped onto the bar, and elevated until it snaps into position perpendicular to the handle (Fig 19). If the light on the flange of the blade is dim, flickers, or does not illuminate, the blade may be improperly seated on the handle, or the bulb or batteries (contained in the handle) may be faulty. Fiberoptic technology is also available for laryngoscopic illumination.

A malleable yet rigid stylet may be inserted into the endotracheal tube before intubation to shape the tube to the desired configuration. To avoid airway trauma during intubation, the tip of the stylet *must not* extend beyond the distal end of the endotracheal tube. The stylet should be lightly lubricated with a water-soluble lubricant to facilitate its withdrawal once the endotracheal tube is positioned.

Heart rate should be continuously monitored during intubation since mechanical stimulation of the airway or hypoxemia may induce bradyarrhythmias in the infant and young child. If bradycardia occurs (heart rate less than 60 beats per minute in the infant or child, or a heart rate consistently below the patient's baseline), the procedure should be interrupted and the patient ventilated with 100% oxygen by face mask and bag-valve device. The incidence of reflex bradyarrhythmias during intubation may be reduced by pretreatment with intravenous atropine (0.02 mg/kg). However, prevention of bradycardia by this means may impede the detection of hypoxemia (bradycardia is also a sign of hypoxemia). The administration of atropine is recommended during intubation of the spontaneously breathing infant or child. However, in an emergency (eg, an apneic patient) intubation should proceed without atropine if its administration would delay intubation.

A pulse oximeter can monitor oxygen saturation noninvasively and should be used whenever possible during intubation. Individual oximeters vary widely in the rapidity of response to the development of hypoxemia.[26,31,44] Pulse oximetry should always be used to confirm clinical assessment.

Continuous evaluation of oxygen saturation monitoring is especially important if the heart rate response to hypoxemia has been blunted by atropine. An intubation attempt must be interrupted if the patient develops significant hypoxemia, cyanosis, pallor, or a decreased heart rate. The patient should be immediately ventilated with 100% oxygen before another attempt.

Intubation Technique

To directly visualize the glottis, the axes of the mouth, pharynx, and trachea must be aligned (Fig 13). If cervical spine injury is suspected, the neutral position must be maintained using manual cervical stabilization. In children older than 2 years without suspected cervical spine trauma, anterior displacement of the neck or cervical spine (so-called head extension) and simultaneous extension of the neck (ie, lifting the chin into the "sniffing position") can be facilitated by placing the child's head on a small pillow. Infants and toddlers younger than 2 years should be placed on a flat surface for intubation with the chin lifted into the sniffing position.[45] These young patients do not require anterior neck displacement, because such displacement occurs naturally when the relatively prominent occiput is placed on a flat surface with the child supine. Proper alignment of the mouth, pharynx, and trachea may also be achieved by placing a small pillow or blanket under the torso of the infant or toddler (up to 2 years of age).

Orotracheal intubation is preferred during resuscitation because it can be performed more rapidly than nasotracheal intubation. The laryngoscope handle is held in the left hand, and the blade is inserted into the mouth in the midline following the natural contour of the pharynx to the base of the tongue (Figs 19 and 20). Once the tip of the blade is at the base of the tongue (in the vallecula, ie, the space between the epiglottis and the base of the tongue) and the epiglottis is visualized, control of the tongue is achieved by moving the proximal end of the blade to the right side of the mouth and sweeping the tongue toward the middle. Alternatively, the blade may be inserted in the right side of the mouth to the base of the tongue. Once the epiglottis is visualized, the proximal end of the blade and the handle are swept to the midline. This movement toward the midline provides a channel in the right third of the mouth through which the endotracheal tube will be passed while direct visualization of the laryngeal structures is maintained.

The risk of laryngeal trauma is increased if the blade is first inserted into the esophagus and then slowly withdrawn to visualize the glottis. This practice should be avoided.

Either a curved or straight blade may be used for intubation of children. The tip of a curved blade is inserted into the vallecula to displace the tongue anteriorly (Fig 20). Ideally with a straight blade the tip of the blade is used to lift the epiglottis and visualize the glottic opening (Fig 20). The tip should rest beyond the vallecula. After

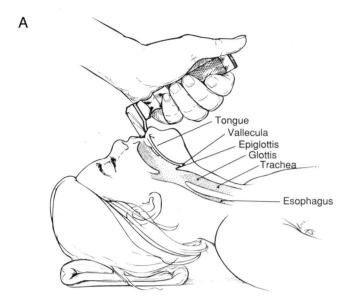

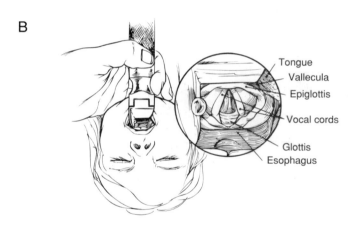

Fig 19. A, Introduction of the laryngoscope with anatomic landmarks; B, operator's view of the anatomy. Gloves should be worn.

the blade is properly positioned, traction is exerted upward in the direction of the long axis of the handle to displace the base of the tongue and the epiglottis anteriorly, exposing the glottis. The handle and blade *must not* be used in a prying or levering motion, nor should the upper gums or teeth be used as a fulcrum, since this may damage the teeth and reduce the ability to visualize the larynx.

To avoid visual obstruction of the glottic opening by the endotracheal tube, the endotracheal tube is inserted from the right corner of the mouth, not down the barrel of the laryngoscope blade. In this way the rescuer should be able to see the endotracheal tube as it passes through the glottic opening. It may be helpful if an assistant displaces the corner of the mouth on the right to enable the visualization of the passage of the tube. In addition,

A

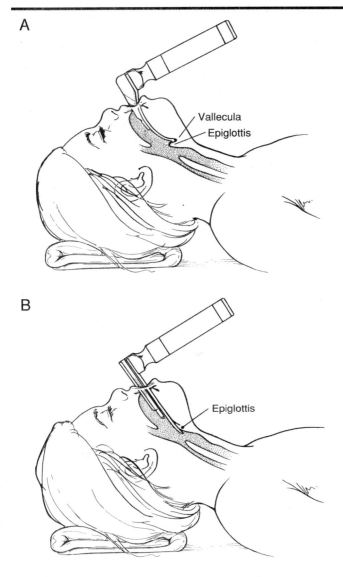

Vallecula
Epiglottis

B

Epiglottis

Fig 20. Position of laryngoscope blade when using (A) a curved blade versus (B) a straight blade. Note that a straight blade may often be used in the same manner as a curved blade, ie, its tip placed in the vallecula.

application of cricoid pressure by an assistant may facilitate visualization of the glottic opening. The black glottic marker of the tube is placed at the level of the vocal cords; this places the tip of the endotracheal tube in midtracheal position. Cuffed endotracheal tubes are inserted until the cuff is positioned just below the vocal cords.

Immediately after intubation, the position of the endotracheal tube tip must be clinically assessed by

- Observation for symmetrical chest movements
- Auscultation for equal breath sounds over each lateral chest wall high in the axillae
- Documentation of absent breath sounds over the stomach
- Notation of the end-tidal carbon dioxide level (if available)

In low cardiac output states, endotracheal CO_2 levels may be minimal, especially in infants.[27] If these clinical criteria are not met or if epigastric distention occurs during positive-pressure ventilation via the tube, esophageal intubation is suspected. The endotracheal tube should be removed and ventilation maintained with a bag-valve–mask device. If chest movement or breath sounds are asymmetrical, bronchial intubation is suspected. The endotracheal tube should be slowly withdrawn until equal breath sounds are heard bilaterally and chest expansion is symmetrical. Proper position of the endotracheal tube should be confirmed by chest x-ray as soon as possible.

If the endotracheal tube is properly placed but lung expansion is inadequate, or if inadequate oxygenation or ventilation is documented by pulse oximetry, end-tidal CO_2 monitoring, or arterial blood gas analysis, one of the following problems should be considered:

- The endotracheal tube is too small, producing a large air leak. Replacement of the tube with a larger one may be necessary. In the child older than 8 to 10 years, the endotracheal tube cuff should be inflated until the air leak just disappears (at 20 to 30 cm H_2O).
- The pop-off valve on the resuscitation bag is not depressed or occluded, and ventilation is escaping into the atmosphere. This problem is most likely to occur when the child's lung compliance is poor (eg, near-drowning, pulmonary edema[38]) or when airway resistance is high (eg, bronchiolitis, asthma). An increase in inflation and cuff pressures may be required to produce effective ventilation in these patients.
- A leak is present at any of several connections in the bag-valve device. Leaks may be detected by separating the bag-valve device from the patient and occluding the endotracheal connection while the bag is compressed.
- The operator is providing inadequate tidal volume. This is easily confirmed: a larger volume breath is provided while the rescuer observes movement of the chest wall and auscultates breath sounds.
- Lack of lung expansion or lung collapse is occurring for other reasons (eg, pneumothorax, obstructed endotracheal tube, etc).

After intubation, the endotracheal tube should be secured to the patient's face with adhesive liquid (eg, tincture of benzoin) and taped securely to prevent unintentional extubation. Before the endotracheal tube is taped in place, correct position should again be confirmed by auscultation. The distance marker at the lips should be noted in the chart to allow detection of unintentional endotracheal tube displacement. (See the Table for distance from midtrachea to teeth.)

Esophageal Obturator Airway

Esophageal obturator airways (EOAs) are not recommended for the pediatric patient because of the variability in esophageal lengths and face mask sizes required for this age group.

Oxygen-Powered Breathing Devices

Oxygen-powered breathing devices are not recommended for pediatric use because the tidal volume is difficult to control and high airway pressures may produce gastric distention or a tension pneumothorax.

Tension Pneumothorax

Tension pneumothorax may complicate trauma or positive-pressure ventilation. It should be suspected in the victim of blunt trauma or in any intubated patient who deteriorates suddenly during positive-pressure ventilation (including overzealous ventilation by bag and mask). As pressure builds within the chest, the extraordinary mobility of the pediatric mediastinum results in extreme mediastinal shift, with resultant compromise in venous return, cardiac output, and air entry. Clinical signs of tension pneumothorax include severe respiratory distress, hyperresonance to percussion and diminished breath sounds on the affected side, and deviation of the trachea and mediastinal structures away from the affected side.

Treatment consists of immediate needle decompression. This should be done without confirmatory chest x-ray since delay can be fatal. An 18- to 20-gauge over-the-needle catheter is inserted through the second intercostal space, over the top of the third rib, in the midclavicular line. A gush of air will be heard after successful needle decompression. A chest tube should be placed as soon as it is feasible.

Cricothyrotomy

Cricothyrotomy is rarely required but may enable oxygen administration to children with complete upper airway obstruction caused by a foreign body, severe orofacial injuries, infection, or laryngeal fracture. Standard methods of opening the airway, including repositioning of the head and jaw, use of an oropharyngeal or nasopharyngeal airway, and tracheal intubation, will permit adequate oxygenation and ventilation in most circumstances. Successful cricothyrotomy has been reported in laboratory animals but only anecdotally in children; further data are needed on the use of this technique for the pediatric age group.[46-49]

Theoretically, cricothyrotomy should facilitate effective delivery of oxygen to most patients with upper airway obstruction since the most common site of pediatric airway obstruction is at or above the glottis. If a foreign body is located below the level of the cricoid cartilage (inferior to the cricothyroid membrane), cricothyrotomy probably will be ineffective. However, since a rescuer cannot predict the exact site of obstruction, cricothyrotomy should not be withheld if other methods have failed to establish a patent airway.

Cricothyrotomy may be performed either surgically (incision) or with a needle (puncture). In the pediatric patient, particularly the infant and toddler, risk of injury to vital structures such as the carotid arteries or jugular veins is significant during surgical cricothyrotomy. Therefore, this procedure should be performed only by persons with surgical training. The technique of needle cricothyrotomy is presented here for highly skilled medical providers who encounter complete upper airway obstruction that is unresponsive to standard treatment techniques.

A roll of sheets or towels is placed under the child's shoulders to position the larynx as far anterior as possible. The cricothyroid membrane is located. It extends from the cricoid to the thyroid cartilage (Fig 21) and can be palpated with a fingernail. Locate an anterior and midline transverse indentation between the two cartilages (Fig 22A and B). The relatively avascular cricothyroid membrane can be punctured and the underlying trachea entered percutaneously. Initially a small-bore (20-gauge) needle attached to a syringe is inserted and aspirated to verify proper position (air should appear in the syringe). A large-bore cannula (at least 14-gauge) is then inserted through the cricothyroid membrane (Fig 22C and D). The cannula is directed toward the midline caudally and posteriorly at a 45° angle. Aspiration of air signifies entry into the trachea (Fig 22E and F). The cannula is advanced into the trachea, the needle is removed, and air is again aspirated to confirm intraluminal position. The cannula is then connected to a ventilating device. Intravenous cannulas may be attached to most 3-mm i.d. endotracheal tube adapters (15 mm), thus providing a connection for ventilating devices (22 mm) (Fig 22G and H). The size of 15-mm/3-mm adapters will vary from manufacturer to manufacturer, so the provider should assemble equipment needed for a cricothyrotomy before it is needed.

An alternative method of cricothyrotomy involves a modified Seldinger technique. A needle is inserted through the cricothyroid membrane, and a wire is passed through the needle. A dilator is advanced over the wire to enable ultimate insertion of a 3-mm i.d. tube. Experience with the use of percutaneous dilational cricothyrotomy has been primarily limited to adult patients.[50]

Oxygen administration may be possible through the cricothyrotomy but ventilation is limited. If the patient with total airway obstruction is breathing spontaneously, simple delivery of 100% oxygen via the cricothyrotomy catheter may be all that is required to sustain life. Suboptimal ventilation may be tolerated since short periods of hypercarbia, in the absence of hypoxemia, may be well tolerated by seriously ill infants and children.[51] Fresh gas flow rates should be low (average of approximately 100 mL/kg per minute; total, 1 to 5 L/min) to minimize potential for barotrauma. Exhalation of gas will generally occur through the upper airway and out the oropharynx. If upper airway obstruction is complete, it may be necessary to pause between insufflations to allow passive exhalation.

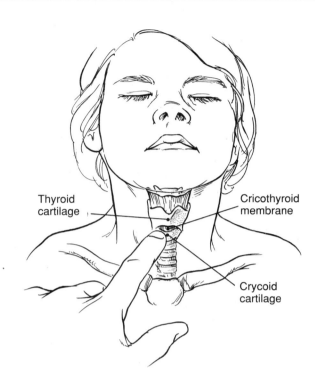

Fig 21. Cricothyroid membrane anatomy. Note that the cricothyroid membrane is between the thyroid and cricoid cartilages.

Percutaneous needle cricothyrotomy with large-bore (14- or 16-gauge) intravenous catheters will result in high resistance to air flow because of the small diameter of the catheters. This high resistance frequently prohibits effective ventilation (ie, maintenance of normal $PaCO_2$) by a bag-valve device coupled to the intravenous catheter with a 3-mm i.d. endotracheal tube connector. However, oxygenation with some degree of moderate hypercarbia may be possible.[48] The pop-off valve of the bag-valve ventilating device must be disabled to provide the high peak inflation pressures needed. A transtracheal cannula of adequate size and an appropriate ventilating device are necessary to achieve effective ventilation and oxygenation with cricothyrotomy. If effective ventilation *and* oxygenation are required via a cricothyrotomy, a transtracheal cannula of 3.0 mm i.d. or larger and a bag-valve device can be used in children and small adults.[49] Effective ventilation (ie, maintenance of a normal $PaCO_2$) via a 14- or 16-gauge intravenous catheter can also be accomplished using specialized high-flow jet oxygen ventilation devices, which are not widely available.[52-54]

Published experience with percutaneous catheter cricothyrotomy in infants and small children in emergency airway management is minimal, and optimal sizes of intravenous catheters for this purpose have not been determined. Significant and life-threatening barotrauma (eg, pneumothorax, pneumomediastinum, subcutaneous emphysema) may result from attempts at jet ventilation if the tip of the catheter is not in the lumen of the trachea.[54-57]

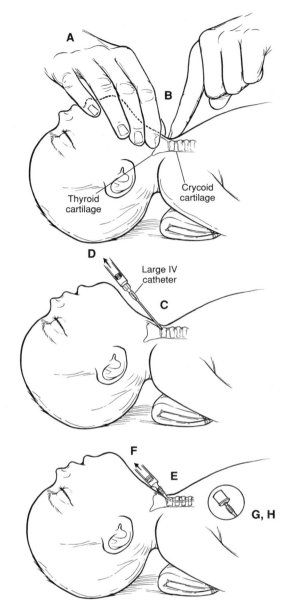

Fig 22. Percutaneous cricothyrotomy. Extend the head in the midline with a rolled towel or folded sheet beneath the shoulders. Stand to the left of the patient and stabilize the trachea with the right hand (A). The cricothyroid membrane is located with the index fingertip of the left hand between the thyroid and cricoid cartilages (B). This space is very narrow (1 mm) in an infant, and only a fingernail can discern it. The trachea is then stabilized between the middle finger and thumb of the left hand while the fingernail of the index finger marks the cricothyroid membrane. A small-bore (20- or 22-gauge) needle attached to a syringe is introduced. If air is aspirated, the small-bore needle is replaced by a large intravenous catheter (12- to 14-gauge) that is inserted through the cricothyroid membrane (C), and air is aspirated (D). The catheter is advanced into the trachea through the membrane, and the needle is removed. Intraluminal position is confirmed when aspiration of air is accomplished via a 3-mL syringe (E, F). Most 3-mm adapters from a pediatric endotracheal tube can be attached to the intravenous catheter (G). Ventilation is accomplished by connecting to a breathing circuit with a standard 22-mm connector (H). Alternatively, the barrel of the 3-mL syringe may remain attached to the intravenous catheter, and an 8-mm endotracheal tube adapter is inserted into the syringe barrel and attached to a ventilating system with a standard 22-mm adapter. Reproduced with permission from Coté et al.[48]

Airway Emergencies in the Patient With an Artificial Airway

Assessment

As previously discussed, airway management is crucial in prevention of cardiac arrest and successful resuscitation of the patient with respiratory failure. The airway must be opened and ventilation must be assisted or controlled. *Frequent reassessment* of the effectiveness of ventilation and oxygenation is essential and includes

- Observation for symmetrical chest wall expansion
- Auscultation for equal breath sounds bilaterally
- Observation for improved patient color and perfusion
- Objective evaluation of arterial oxygenation via pulse oximetry and carbon dioxide elimination via end-tidal CO_2 monitoring
- Objective evaluation of arterial blood oxygen and carbon dioxide tensions

Managing Airway Emergencies

Patients with artificial airways are at risk for a variety of problems that may result in life-threatening loss of artificial airway function, including loss of oxygen supply, occlusion or kinking of the airway, and displacement of the airway. Precautions must be taken to reduce the probability of such events, and patients must be monitored carefully to enable early detection and prompt corrective action should these events occur. The head of the intubated child must remain in a neutral position, since neck flexion may result in endobronchial intubation and neck extension may result in extubation.[58,59] Tracheostomy tubes must be securely tied in place and endotracheal tubes securely taped.

When respiratory distress develops in the patient with an artificial airway, the first priority is rapid assessment of the patient's status. Adequacy of air exchange and oxygenation is evaluated by observation of chest expansion, use of noninvasive monitoring devices (eg, pulse oximeter, expired carbon dioxide monitor), and auscultation of both sides of the chest and both axillae. Breath sounds should be equal and adequate bilaterally. The heart rate should be appropriate for age and clinical condition. This information will determine the urgency of the required response.

The second priority is to determine the likely cause of the problem. Endotracheal tube position is evaluated by visual inspection and auscultation. If a ventilator is being used, it should be temporarily disconnected and the patient *ventilated manually* with a resuscitation bag, using 100% oxygen. Auscultation during manual ventilation and the "feel" for increased resistance while squeezing the resuscitation bag aid in the assessment of airway patency and position. If breath sounds are poor and there is no movement of the chest with manual inflation, the artificial airway has been displaced from the trachea or is obstructed (in which case there will be high resistance to manual inflation). If the artificial airway is obstructed, an attempt should be made to suction it with a relatively large catheter, ensuring that the suction catheter passes beyond the distal end of the tube. After suctioning, manual ventilation is resumed and assessment of breath sounds, airway resistance, and adequacy of chest movement is repeated. If the endotracheal tube appears to be properly positioned and adequate ventilation is obtained by manual inflation, the problem may be located in the ventilator. The patient should be manually ventilated until the problem is identified and corrected.

If the endotracheal tube is occluded and patency cannot be restored by suctioning, the endotracheal tube *must* be removed and replaced. The patient is ventilated by bag and mask until preparations for reintubation are complete. If the endotracheal tube is displaced from the trachea, the tube is removed and the patient manually ventilated with bag and mask until reintubation can be accomplished. Reintubation should be a semielective procedure except in rare situations in which ventilation cannot be achieved by bag and mask.

The management of obstructed tracheostomy tubes is similar to that used for obstructed endotracheal tubes. If the tube is completely occluded and ventilation cannot be accomplished, the tube should be removed and replaced with a new device immediately. If this is not possible, the patient must be ventilated by bag and mask or intubated orally.

Tracheostomy tubes may be plastic or metal (Fig 23). The metal tubes have thin walls and do not have a built-in 15-mm endotracheal tube connector. All metal tubes have an inner cannula that can be easily removed for cleaning or if the tube becomes obstructed. Plastic tubes used in pediatric patients usually do not have inner cannulas. If one of these tubes becomes occluded, it must be removed and replaced with a clean tracheostomy tube. Plastic tracheostomy tubes are usually equipped with a 15-mm connector for easy connection to a standard oxygen delivery system.

The short length of the tracheostomy tube (compared with an endotracheal tube) facilitates suctioning. Suctioning of a tracheostomy tube should take no longer than 3 to 4 seconds. Irrigation of the tube with a small amount of sterile saline may be helpful if secretions are thick.

Tracheostomy tubes are held in position by ties (usually made of twill tape) extending from either side of the tracheostomy tube and fastened around the neck. The ties should be fastened so that only a little finger can pass between the ties and the child's neck. This ensures that the ties are not too tight or too loose, which could lead to unintentional extubation. The ties must be removed or cut before the tube can be removed from the trachea. Once the ties are cut, the tracheostomy tube may be removed from the trachea by simply grasping the tube and guiding it out. A pair of scissors (and a clean

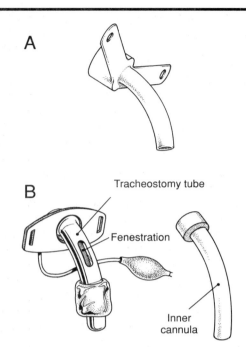

A

B

Tracheostomy tube

Fenestration

Inner
cannula

Fig 23. Tracheostomy tubes: (A) plastic and (B) metal with inner cannula.

tracheostomy tube, prepared with ties) should be kept at the bedside of all patients with tracheostomy tubes. To facilitate access to the tracheostomy tube, the patient should be positioned with the head and neck extended with a rolled sheet or towel beneath the shoulders.

Before a clean tracheostomy tube is inserted, the stoma and trachea should be suctioned with a catheter. This suctioning is particularly important in emergencies, since thick secretions may have accumulated in the trachea around the tube and may be advanced down the trachea by the new tube. The stoma may be held open, if necessary, by gentle downward and lateral traction from two fingers placed below on either side of the tracheostomy. If the patient is not breathing spontaneously, bag-mask ventilation via the upper airway must be provided until preparations for recannulation are complete. Placement of a finger over the stoma may be necessary to prevent air escape and patient hypoventilation. If total upper airway obstruction is present and the tracheostomy stoma is the only functioning airway, mouth-to-stoma ventilation may be necessary.

The new tracheostomy tube is placed in the stoma and gently guided into position in the trachea. The tube usually passes easily if the stoma is well healed. Because metal tubes may be unintentionally pushed into a para-tracheal location, an obturator should be inserted into the metal tracheostomy tube before the tube is inserted into the trachea. During passage of the tracheostomy tube into the trachea, air movement should be heard through the tube (unless an obturator is used). Once the trache-

ostomy tube is in position, its patency should be rapidly assessed, the patient ventilated manually, and the ties secured to maintain the tracheostomy tube in the trachea. Again, the ties should be snug against the neck so that only a little finger can be slipped under the tie but not so tight as to obstruct jugular venous return.

Several techniques may minimize the occasional difficulty encountered during tracheostomy tube replacement. A well-lubricated suction catheter may be passed through the new tracheostomy tube and the end of the catheter inserted through the stoma into the trachea. The tracheostomy tube is then passed into the trachea using the suction catheter as a guide. Gentle but firm pressure may be used to insert the tube through a tight stoma if a catheter is present as a guide. A mixture of sterile water and water-soluble lubricant applied to the stoma and the tracheostomy tube may facilitate tube passage through the stoma.

Alternative methods for recannulation include the use of a smaller tracheostomy tube (which is later replaced with an appropriate size tube) or insertion of an endo-tracheal tube. The advantages of using an endotracheal tube in an emergency include the wide range of sizes available and the beveled tip, which facilitates entry through a tight stoma. In addition, condensation from expired air in the tube provides visual reassurance of the continuity of the lumen of the tube with that of the trachea.

If recannulation cannot be accomplished, the patient should be intubated orally with an endotracheal tube. The tracheostomy tube can then be reinserted under controlled conditions. Alternatively, a flexible bronchoscope of appropriate size may be used as a guide by passing it first through a tracheostomy tube and then through the stoma.

Recannulation of a tracheostomy stoma during the first week after its placement may be difficult. In this circumstance, incorrect placement of the tracheostomy tube into the paratracheal tissues (rather than the trachea) is common and can result in a tension pneumothorax. Most surgeons place temporary traction sutures at the lateral margins of the tracheal incision. Gentle lateral traction on these sutures will help open the stoma and facilitate recannulation. Vigorous traction should not be used since it may damage the trachea or break the sutures. A suction catheter should be used to guide the new tube into place, since a catheter is much less likely to create a false tract. If one or two attempts to replace the tube fail, the patient should be intubated orally and the tracheostomy tube replaced by the surgeon or someone skilled in airway management.

References

1. Lewis JK, Minter MG, Eshelman SJ, Witte MK. Outcome of pediatric resuscitation. *Ann Emerg Med.* 1983;12:297-299.
2. Eisenberg M, Bergner L, Hallstrom A. Epidemiology of cardiac arrest and resuscitation in children. *Ann Emerg Med.* 1983;12:672-674.

3. Ludwig S, Kettrick RG, Parker M. Pediatric cardiopulmonary resuscitation: a review of 130 cases. *Clin Pediatr (Phila)*. 1984;23:71-75.

4. Wark H, Overton JH. A paediatric 'cardiac arrest' survey. *Br J Anaesth*. 1984;56:1271-1274.

5. Torphy DE, Minter MG, Thompson BM. Cardiorespiratory arrest and resuscitation of children. *Am J Dis Child*. 1984;138:1099-1102.

6. O'Rourke PP. Outcome of children who are apneic and pulseless in the emergency room. *Crit Care Med*. 1986;14:466-468.

7. Zaritsky A. Selected concepts and controversies in pediatric cardiopulmonary resuscitation. *Crit Care Clin*. 1988;4:735-754.

8. Eckenhoff JE. Some anatomic considerations of the infant larynx influencing endotracheal anesthesia. *Anesthesiology*. 1951;12:401-410.

9. Coté CJ, Todres ID. The pediatric airway. In Coté CJ, Ryan JF, Todres ID, Groudsouzian NG, eds. *A Practice of Anesthesia for Infants and Children*. 2nd ed. Philadelphia, Pa: WB Saunders; 1993.

10. Mansell A, Bryan C, Levison H. Airway closure in children. *J Appl Physiol*. 1972;33:711-714.

11. Anthonisen NR, Danson J, Robertson PC, Ross WR. Airway closure as a function of age. *Respir Physiol*. 1969;8:58-65.

12. Wittenborg MH, Gyepes MT, Crocker D. Tracheal dynamics in infants with respiratory distress, stridor, and collapsing trachea. *Radiology*. 1967;88:653-662.

13. Cross KW, Tizard JP, Trythall DA. The gaseous metabolism of the newborn infant. *Acta Paediatr*. 1957;46:265-285.

14. Epstein RA, Hyman AI. Ventilatory requirements of critically ill neonates. *Anesthesiology*. 1980;53:379-384.

15. Hudgel DW, Hendricks C. Palate and hypopharynx: sites of inspiratory narrowing of the upper airway during sleep. *Am Rev Respir Dis*. 1988;138:1542-1547.

16. Abernethy LJ, Allan PL, Drummond GB. Ultrasound assessment of the position of the tongue during induction of anaesthesia. *Br J Anaesth*. 1990;65:744-748.

17. Morikawa S, Safar P, DeCarlo J. Influence of the head-jaw position upon upper airway patency. *Anesthesiology*. 1961;22:265-270.

18. Galloway DW. Upper airway obstruction by the soft palate: influence of position of head, jaw, and neck. *Br J Anaesth*. 1990;64:383-384.

19. Davis HW, Gartner JC, Galvis AG, Michaels RH, Mestad PH. Acute upper airway obstruction: croup and epiglottitis. *Pediatr Clin North Am*. 1981;28:859-880.

20. Coté CJ, Rolf N, Liu LM, et al. A single-blind study of combined pulse oximetry and capnography in children. *Anesthesiology*. 1991;74:980-987.

21. McGuire TJ, Pointer JE. Evaluation of a pulse oximeter in the prehospital setting. *Ann Emerg Med*. 1988;17:1058-1062.

22. Tremper KK, Barker SJ. Pulse oximetry. *Anesthesiology*. 1989;70:98-108.

23. Jobes DR, Nicolson SC. Monitoring of arterial hemoglobin oxygen saturation using a tongue sensor. *Anesth Analg*. 1988;67:186-188.

24. Coté CJ, Daniels AL, Connolly M, Szyfelbein SK, Wickens CD. Tongue oximetry in children with extensive thermal injury: comparison with peripheral oximetry. *Can J Anaesth*. 1992;39(pt 1):454-457.

25. Reynolds LM, Nicolson SC, Steven JM, Escobar A, McGonigle ME, Jobes DR. Influence of sensor site location on pulse oximetry kinetics in children. *Anesth Analg*. 1993;76:751-754.

26. Severinghaus JW, Naifeh KH, Koh SO. Errors in 14 pulse oximeters during profound hypoxia. *J Clin Monit*. 1989;5:72-81.

27. Bhende MS, Thompson AE, Cook DR, Saville AL. Validity of a disposable end-tidal CO_2 detector in verifying endotracheal tube placement in infants and children. *Ann Emerg Med*. 1992;21:142-145.

28. Bhende MS, Thompson AE, Orr RA. Utility of an end-tidal CO_2 detector during stabilization and transport of critically ill children. *Pediatrics*. 1992;89:1042-1044.

29. Weil MH, Grundler W, Yamaguchi M, Michaels S, Rackow EC. Arterial blood gases fail to reflect acid-base status during cardiopulmonary resuscitation: a preliminary report. *Crit Care Med*. 1985;13:884-885.

30. Steedman DJ, Robertson CE. Acid-base changes in arterial and central venous blood during cardiopulmonary resuscitation. *Arch Emerg Med*. 1992;9:169-176.

31. McPherson SP. *Respiratory Therapy Equipment*. 3rd ed. St Louis, Mo: CV Mosby Co; 1985:74-112, 178-204.

32. Zander J, Hazinski MF. Pulmonary disorders: airway obstruction. In: Hazinski MF, ed. *Nursing Care of the Critically Ill Child*. 2nd ed. St Louis, Mo: Mosby Year Book; 1992.

33. Jesudian MC, Harrison RR, Keenan RL, Maull KI. Bag-valve-mask ventilation: two rescuers are better than one: preliminary report. *Crit Care Med*. 1985;13:122-123.

34. Sellick BA. Cricoid pressure to control regurgitation of stomach contents during induction of anesthesia. *Lancet*. 1961;2:404-406.

35. Salem MR, Wong AY, Mani M, Sellick BA. Efficacy of cricoid pressure in preventing gastric inflation during bag-mask ventilation in paediatric patients. *Anesthesiology*. 1974;40:96-98.

36. Moynihan RJ, Brock-Utne JG, Archer JH, Feld LH, Kreitzman TR. The effect of cricoid pressure on preventing gastric insufflation in infants and children. *Anesthesiology*. 1993;78:652-656.

37. Finer NN, Barrington KJ, Al-Fadley F, Peters KL. Limitations of self-inflating resuscitators. *Pediatrics*. 1986;77:417-420.

38. Hirschman AM, Kravath RE. Venting vs ventilating: a danger of manual resuscitation bags. *Chest*. 1982;82:369-370.

39. Milner AD, Vyas H, Hopkin IE. Efficacy of facemask resuscitation at birth. *Br Med J Clin Res Ed*. 1984;289:1563-1565.

40. Tendrup TE, Kanter RK, Cherry RA. A comparison of infant ventilation methods performed by prehospital personnel. *Ann Emerg Med*. 1989;18:607-611.

41. Dorsch JA, Dorsch SE. *Understanding Anesthesia Equipment: Construction, Care, and Complications*. 2nd ed. Baltimore, Md: Williams & Wilkins Co; 1984:182-196.

42. Luten RC, Wears RL, Broselow J, et al. Length-based endotracheal tube and emergency equipment selection in pediatrics. *Ann Emerg Med*. 1992;21:900-904.

43. Garland JS, Kishaba RG, Nelson DB, Losek JD, Sobocinski KA. A rapid and accurate method of estimating body weight. *Am J Emerg Med*. 1986;4:390-393.

44. Severinghaus JW, Naifeh KH. Accuracy of response of six pulse oximeters to profound hypoxia. *Anesthesiology*. 1987;67:551-558.

45. Westhorpe RN. The position of the larynx in children and its relationship to the ease of intubation. *Anaesth Intensive Care*. 1987;15:384-388.

46. Klain M, Keszler H, Brader E. High frequency jet ventilation in CPR. *Crit Care Med*. 1981;9:421-422.

47. Klain M, Keszler H, Stool S. Transtracheal high frequency jet ventilation prevents aspiration. *Crit Care Med*. 1983;11:170-172.

48. Coté CJ, Eavey RD, Todres ID, Jones DE. Crycothyroid membrane puncture: oxygenation and ventilation in a dog model using an intravenous catheter. *Crit Care Med*. 1988;16:615-619.

49. Neff CC, Pfister RC, Van Sonnenberg E. Percutaneous transtracheal ventilation: experimental and practical aspects. *J Trauma*. 1983;23:84-90.

50. Florete OG. Airway management. In: Civetta JM, Taylor RW, Kirby RR, et al, eds. *Critical Care*. Philadelphia, Pa: JB Lippincott Co; 1992:1430-1431.

51. Goldstein B, Shannon DC, Todres ID. Supercarbia in children: clinical course and outcome. *Crit Care Med*. 1990;18:166-168.

52. Ravussin P, Bayer-Berger M, Monnier P, Savary M, Freeman J. Percutaneous transtracheal ventilation for laser endoscopic procedures in infants and small children with laryngeal obstruction: report of two cases. *Can J Anaesth*. 1987;34:83-86.

53. Stothert JC Jr, Stout MJ, Lewis LM, Keltner RM Jr. High pressure percutaneous transtracheal ventilation: the use of large gauge intravenous-type catheters in the totally obstructed airway. *Am J Emerg Med*. 1990;8:184-189.

54. Benumof JL, Scheller MS. The importance of transtracheal jet ventilation in the management of the difficult airway. *Anesthesiology*. 1989;71:769-778.

55. Vivori E. Anaesthesia for laryngoscopy. *Br J Anaesth*. 1980;52:638. Letter.

56. Steward DJ, Fearon B. Anaesthesia for laryngoscopy. *Br J Anaesth*. 1981;53:320. Letter.

57. Steward DJ. Percutaneous transtracheal ventilation for laser endoscopic procedures in infants and small children. *Can J Anaesth*. 1987;34:429-430. Letter.

58. Todres ID, deBros F, Kramer SS, Moylan FM, Shannon DC. Endotracheal tube displacement in the newborn infant. *J Pediatr*. 1976;89:126-127.

59. Donn SM, Kuhns LR. Mechanism of endotracheal tube movement with change of head position in the neonate. *Pediatr Radiol*. 1980;9:37-40.

Vascular Access

Chapter 5

Establishment of reliable vascular access is a crucial step in pediatric ALS. If vascular access is accomplished within the first minutes of resuscitation, infusion of medications and fluids is possible, and successful resuscitation may be more likely.[1] Although the endotracheal tube may be used for emergency administration of some medications, intravenous or intraosseous access is preferred for drug delivery and is mandatory for the infusion of fluids, especially when cardiopulmonary compromise results from noncardiac causes, such as trauma or sepsis.[2,3]

Intracardiac administration of drugs is *not* recommended during closed-chest CPR. Intracardiac injections pose risks of coronary artery laceration, cardiac tamponade, and pneumothorax and do not result in more rapid circulation of drugs than the intravenous route.[4] Intracardiac drug administration also requires interruption of external chest compression and ventilation.

Arterial cannulation provides a direct means of continuously measuring blood pressure and sampling blood to evaluate arterial oxygenation and acid-base balance, thus helping to guide postresuscitation therapy. This chapter reviews percutaneous techniques for intravenous, intraosseous, and intra-arterial cannulation and surgical cannulation of the saphenous vein in seriously ill or injured infants and children.

Venous Access

General Principles

Vascular access is vital for drug and fluid administration, but venous access may be difficult to achieve in the pediatric patient.[1] During CPR the preferred venous access site is the largest, most accessible vein that does not require the interruption of resuscitation. If peripheral veins can be readily seen or palpated below the skin surface, peripheral venous access is attempted before other forms of vascular access. Peripheral venipuncture provides a satisfactory route for administration of fluid or drugs if it can be achieved within a few minutes.

Peripheral venipuncture can be performed in veins of the arm, hand, leg, and foot,[5] although cannulation of small vessels may be difficult when veins collapse during shock or cardiopulmonary arrest. In such circumstances attempts at peripheral venous access should be limited to large peripheral veins. The veins selected should be those that are relatively constant with respect to anatomic location, such as the femoral vein, the median cubital vein at the elbow, or the long saphenous vein at the ankle. Cannulation of scalp veins is less desirable than that of other sites during resuscitation, because catheters placed in these extremely small vessels often infiltrate

when fluids or medications are administered rapidly and forcefully, and attempts at cannulation of these vessels may interfere with control of the airway and ventilation. However, scalp veins may be cannulated during postresuscitation stabilization.

The intraosseous route enables infusion of drugs, fluid, and blood products. This route is a reliable alternative to venipuncture in infants and children who are in shock or cardiopulmonary arrest[6] if peripheral venous access cannot be achieved within a few minutes. The intraosseous route provides access to a noncollapsible venous plexus in the medulla of the bone and can usually be established within seconds. The proximal tibia is the preferred site for intraosseous needle insertion in infants and small children. The main contraindication to intraosseous infusion is the presence of a fracture in the pelvis or extremity proximal to or in the bone chosen for intraosseous needle insertion.

If a central venous catheter is in place at the time of arrest, it should be used for drug administration. If central venous access is not in place but can be rapidly and safely achieved by experienced providers, it may be attempted. The femoral, internal jugular, axillary, or subclavian or external jugular veins may be used.[7] The femoral vein is often selected in emergencies because its predictable anatomic location and large size make it the safest and easiest central vein to cannulate and it can be accessed without interfering with resuscitation. If the tip of the femoral venous catheter is inserted to a point above the diaphragm, rapid delivery of resuscitative drugs to the heart occurs during CPR. However, a catheter of this length will create significant resistance to fluid infusion and should not be used in the resuscitation of children who require rapid volume administration. Short (5 to 10 cm) central venous catheters inserted in the femoral vein may be extremely useful under these conditions.

Boluses of fluid during resuscitation are typically administered with hand-held syringes. Once an hourly fluid rate is calculated, infusion pumps should be used to regulate the infusions and prevent inadvertent administration of excessive volumes of fluids. If infusion pumps are unavailable, volume-limiting devices such as minidrip chambers should be used, with the infusion rate carefully controlled by gravity and screw clamp, to prevent infusion of more than 20 mL/kg as a single bolus (approximately 25% of the child's estimated circulating blood volume over less than 20 minutes).

Priorities of Access

The resuscitation team should use a protocol for the establishment of venous access in children (Fig 1). Such a protocol limits the time devoted to futile attempts to achieve peripheral and central venous catheterization.[8]

During CPR in children 6 years old or younger, intraosseous access should be established if reliable venous access cannot be achieved within three attempts or 90 seconds, whichever comes first.[8] Although successful intraosseous cannulation has been reported in children older than 6 years,[9,10] such cannulation becomes progressively more difficult because the tibial bone marrow becomes smaller and more difficult to cannulate as patient age increases. If intraosseous access is attempted in older patients, using a threaded cannula will facilitate passage of the needle through the cortex, and alternative sites (including the iliac crest) may need to be considered. Although it may be possible to achieve intraosseous access in victims older than 6 years, other forms of vascular access can likely be accomplished more quickly and with less difficulty. In children older than 6 years, percutaneous central venous access or saphenous vein cutdown should be established if reliable venous access cannot be obtained within the first 90 seconds of resuscitation. Attempts at peripheral and central venous access in the head, neck, and chest should be limited during CPR to avoid interruption of ventilation and chest compressions.

During the 1980s a small number of resuscitation studies in adult animal models suggested that central venous drug administration produced more rapid onset of action and higher peak drug levels than peripheral venous administration.[11-13] However, these differences have not been demonstrated in pediatric animal arrest models.[14] In pediatric animal and human resuscitation studies, peripheral venous, central venous, and intraosseous drug administration result in comparable onset of drug action and peak drug levels, particularly if the drug is followed by a bolus of several milliliters of normal saline.[14-16] These pediatric studies have led to de-emphasis of central venous cannulation and emphasis on the need to follow each drug administered by any vascular route with a bolus of at least 5 mL of normal saline.[17] This bolus will move the drugs into the central circulation and speed their delivery to the heart.

Although a single study performed in an adult canine arrest model suggests more rapid circulation of drugs administered via the superior vena cava versus the inferior vena cava,[18] there is no evidence in human or pediatric models of CPR to suggest a clinical difference between superior vena cava or inferior vena cava drug administration. The preferred site of vascular access remains the largest vein that can be rapidly accessed without interfering with CPR. Healthcare providers should attempt vascular access using the technique and site with which they are most familiar and skilled.

Intravenous or intraosseous drug administration is preferable to endotracheal drug administration. However, if it is expected that vascular access will not be achieved within 3 to 5 minutes, epinephrine should be administered by the endotracheal route. Other low-volume, lipid-soluble

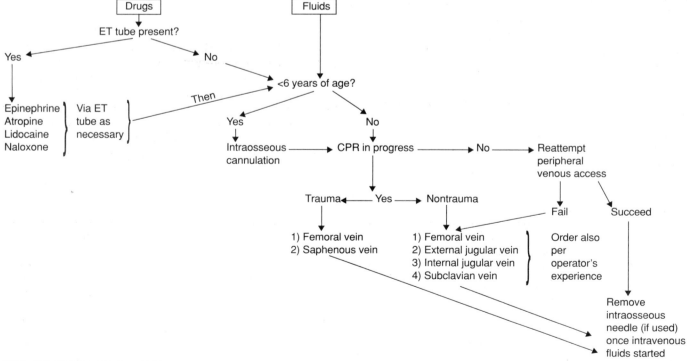

Fig 1. Priorities for vascular access.

resuscitative drugs, including atropine, lidocaine, and naloxone, can also be administered by this route (see chapter 6).[19]

Ideally all catheters should be inserted using sterile technique. However, ideal technique is often not possible during emergencies. Therefore, once the patient is stable, replacement of catheters under sterile conditions should be considered.

Cannulation of Peripheral Veins

Peripheral venous cannulation is associated with few complications. However, these catheters can be difficult to insert in patients with cardiopulmonary compromise, especially infants and toddlers. In general, the size of cannula selected is the largest that can be reliably inserted in a large vein. It may be necessary to attempt blind insertion of a cannula into a vein that cannot be seen or palpated, based on typical anatomic location of the vein. For example, the median cubital vein at the elbow and the long saphenous vein at the ankle are relatively constant in location. Drugs administered via a peripheral vein during CPR should always be followed by a flush to move the drugs into the central circulation.

Complications

Complications of peripheral venous access procedures include hematoma formation, cellulitis, thrombosis, phlebitis, pulmonary thromboembolism, air embolism, catheter-fragment embolism, infiltration, and skin slough.[7] Severe complications, however, are relatively infrequent. Infusion of certain fluids or medications (such as calcium, dopamine, or epinephrine) may contribute to the development of vasculitis. When possible, these substances should be diluted and administered through the largest vein available.

Devices

Four types of venous cannulas are used in infants and children:

- Over-the-needle catheters
- Catheter-over-wire or catheter-through-introducing sheath
- Butterfly needles
- Through-the-needle catheters

Over-the-needle catheters are most commonly used for peripheral venous access and are presented here. Through-the-needle catheters, catheters-over-wires, and catheters-through-sheaths are included in the section "Cannulation of Central Veins."

Butterfly Needles. Butterfly needles are useful in obtaining blood specimens for laboratory analysis but tend to infiltrate easily. Over-the-needle catheters are preferred for primary venous access in patients with trauma, shock, or cardiopulmonary arrest.

Over-the-Needle Catheters. Over-the-needle catheters can be inserted into any vein, ie, the antecubital fossa, in the dorsum of the hands or feet, and the external jugular and saphenous veins. Ideally the catheter has a clear hub, so blood flashback can be observed when the vein is successfully entered. Over-the-needle catheters are available in a variety of sizes (Table). The size of the catheter used during resuscitation should be the largest catheter that can be quickly inserted to establish reliable, unobstructed flow. Small catheters may be used until a larger vein is cannulated with a larger catheter.

During insertion, the bevel of the needle is aimed downward[5] (Fig 2) to facilitate entrance into constricted peripheral veins that may be encountered in patients with trauma, shock, and cardiopulmonary arrest. Over-the-needle catheters may also be temporarily placed into a central vein to allow initial drug and fluid administration until a longer catheter is inserted (see also "Cannulation of Central Veins").

Sites

Upper Extremity. The cephalic, basilic, and median cubital veins in the forearm provide a route for rapid delivery of drugs and fluid to the central circulation but may be difficult to locate in well-nourished infants (Fig 3). Of these veins, the median antecubital vein is probably easiest to cannulate. In the dorsum of the hand, the most commonly used veins include tributaries of the cephalic and basilic veins as well as the dorsal venous arch.

Equipment for Venous Cannulation

Age (y)	Weight (kg)	Butterfly Needles (gauge)	Over-the-Needle Catheters (gauge)	Venous Catheters				Catheter Introducers			
				French Size	Length (cm)	Wire Diameter [mm (in)]	Needle (gauge)	French Size	Length (cm)	Wire Diameter [mm (in)]	Needle (gauge)
<1	<10	21, 23, 25	20, 22, 24	3.0	8	0.46 (.018)	21	4.0	6	0.53 (.021)	20
								4.5	6	0.53 (.021)	20
1-12	10-40	16, 18, 20	16, 18, 20	4.0	12	0.53 (.021)	20	5.0	13	0.64 (.025)	19
								5.5	13	0.64 (.025)	19
								6.5	13	0.64 (.025)	19
>12	>40	16, 18, 20	14, 16, 18	5.0	20	0.89 (.035)	18	7.0	13	0.89 (.035)	18
				6.3	20		18	8.0	13	0.89 (.035)	18

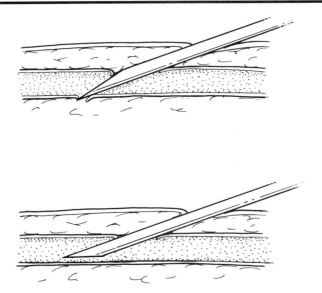

Fig 2. Top, When the venipuncture is performed with the needle point *bevel up*, the needle point pierces the deep wall of the vessel before blood return is apparent. Bottom, With the needle point inserted *bevel down*, the point of the needle enters the mid-lumen of the tiny vein.

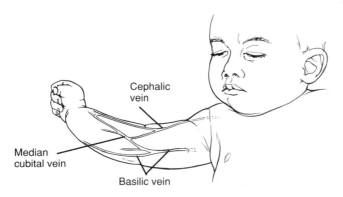

Fig 3. Veins of the upper extremity.

Lower Extremity. The saphenous veins, the median marginal veins, and the veins of the dorsal arch of the lower extremities may be accessed for cannulation (Fig 4). Of these veins, the great saphenous vein at the ankle is probably easiest to cannulate.

Scalp Veins. The small superficial veins of the scalp are rarely useful during resuscitative efforts but may be used to administer fluids and medications during post-resuscitation stabilization.

Technique for Upper or Lower Extremity Peripheral Venous Cannulation Using an Over-the-Needle Catheter

Note: Whenever possible, hand washing and sterile technique should be performed. During resuscitation, however, vascular access must be achieved as quickly as possible, so some of the following steps (indicated by *)

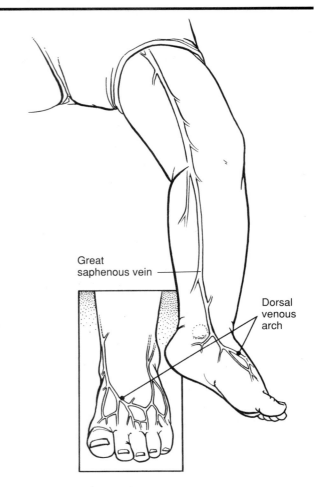

Fig 4. Veins of the lower extremity.

may have to be omitted. Universal precautions should always be taken.

1. Immobilize the extremity to be used and locate and stretch the vein. If the antecubital fossa vein is cannulated, a soft roll of gauze may be placed behind the elbow to hyperextend it. If the dorsal hand veins are cannulated, hold the hand firmly with the wrist flexed. If the dorsal foot veins are cannulated, hold the foot firmly with the ankle extended.
2. Apply a tourniquet proximal to the vein.
*3. Wash hands.
4. Put on gloves.
5. Cleanse the skin over the vein with an antiseptic solution.
*6. Flush the needle/catheter to be used with sterile saline and disconnect the syringe, leaving fluid in the lumen of the needle.
*7. Puncture the skin slightly distal or lateral to the side of the proposed venipuncture site using an 18- or 20-gauge needle to facilitate entry of the catheter through the skin. Pull the skin to the side before puncture, then release. Do not enter the vein with this needle.

8. Insert the needle/catheter through the puncture site with the bevel of the needle facing downward. Slowly advance it into the vein until blood flows back freely.

9. Advance the catheter/needle a few millimeters further to ensure that the catheter is in the vein. Advance the remainder of the catheter over the needle and into the vein. Remove the needle and confirm free backflow of blood through the catheter toward the bevel.

10. Remove the tourniquet.

11. Tape the catheter firmly in place, evacuate any air in the connecting tubing, attach an infusion set, and apply a sterile dressing to the insertion site.[20]

Technique for Scalp Vein Cannulation Using a Butterfly or Over-the-Needle Catheter

Note: Whenever possible, hand washing and sterile technique should be performed. During resuscitation, however, vascular access must be achieved as quickly as possible, so some of the following steps (indicated by *) may be omitted. Universal precautions should always be taken.

1. Restrain the patient.
2. Shave the selected site and surrounding skin.
3. Place a rubber band tourniquet around the head.
*4. Wash hands.
5. Put on gloves.
6. Cleanse the skin with an antiseptic solution.
*7. Flush the needle/catheter and tubing with sterile saline and disconnect the syringe, leaving fluid in the system.
8. Palpate the desired vein and stretch the skin over the vein, identifying the direction of blood flow. Identify the temporal artery and avoid it.
9. Introduce the needle through the skin with the bevel pointed downward directly over the vein or adjacent to the vein and slowly advance the needle into the vein until blood flows back freely into the tubing or connection hub.
10. Advance the needle a few millimeters further to ensure that the catheter is in the vein. If an over-the-needle catheter is used, thread the remainder of the catheter into the vein, remove the needle, and confirm the free backflow of blood from the catheter.
11. Remove the tourniquet.
12. Reconnect the syringe and test the position of the needle by injecting a small amount of sterile saline.
13. Tape the needle or catheter firmly in place, evacuate any air in the connecting tubing, attach an infusion set, and apply a sterile occlusive dressing to the insertion site.[20]

A similar technique may be used to insert a butterfly needle or over-the-needle catheter into a peripheral vein.

Intraosseous Cannulation (Cannulation of Intramedullary Sinuses)

Intravenous access is difficult to achieve in an emergency, and delay in obtaining this access can compromise the effectiveness of resuscitation.[1,21] Intraosseous access, initially described in the 1940s,[9,10] provides a safe and reliable method for rapidly achieving a route for administration of drugs, fluids, and blood products into a noncollapsible marrow venous plexus during resuscitation of children, particularly those 6 years old or younger. Intraosseous access can be reliably achieved in 30 to 60 seconds in most cases, even by healthcare providers with minimal experience.[15,22-26]

In general, any intravenous drug or fluid required during the resuscitation of children can be safely administered by the intraosseous route. Reports of successful administration of catecholamines, calcium, antibiotics, digitalis, heparin, lidocaine, atropine, sodium bicarbonate, phenytoin, neuromuscular blocking agents, crystalloids, colloids, and blood can be found in the literature.[27-38] Continuous infusions of catecholamines can also be accomplished by the intraosseous route.[27] Onset of action and drug levels following intraosseous infusion during CPR are comparable to those achieved following intravenous administration, and levels similar to those achieved after central venous administration have been documented in pediatric arrest models.[16] Fluid required for rapid volume resuscitation and administration of viscous drugs and solutions should be administered under pressure to overcome resistance of emissary veins that lead from the intramedullary cavity to the general circulation via microscopic channels in the bony cortex.[39,40]

Complications

Animal studies have shown that local effects of intraosseous infusion on the bone marrow and long-term effect on bone growth are minimal.[41,42] Microscopic pulmonary fat and bone marrow emboli have been reported but do not appear to be clinically significant.[43] Complications following intraosseous infusion have been reported in fewer than 1% of patients,[44-46] but they are often more serious than those associated with peripheral vein infusion. Reported complications include tibial fracture, compartment syndrome, skin necrosis, and osteomyelitis.[44-47] Although uncommon, these complications may be severe. Therefore, intraosseous infusion should be reserved for the treatment of critically ill infants and children and used as a temporary measure until other venous access sites become available.[24,25]

Devices

Two types of intraosseous needles[26,48] are available for use in infants and children: specially designed intraosseous infusion needles and Jamshidi-type bone marrow aspiration needles. Short, wide-gauge spinal needles with internal stylets are not recommended for intraosseous use because they are thin-walled and bend easily. They can be used in an emergency if no alternative is available. Standard hypodermic needles should *not* be used for intraosseous infusion, because they often become clogged with bone and bone marrow.

Drugs administered via the intraosseous route must be followed by a sterile saline flush of at least 5 mL to ensure that the drug is delivered to the central circulation. Fluids must be administered under pressure using an infusion pump or pressure bag or with manual injection using a syringe.

Site

The flat, anteromedial surface of the tibia, approximately 1 to 3 cm below the tibial tuberosity, is the preferred site for infants and children less than 6 years of age, since the marrow cavity in that location is very large and the potential for injury to adjacent tissues is minimal.

Technique of Intraosseous (Intramedullary) Cannulation

Note: Whenever possible, hand washing and sterile technique should be performed. During resuscitation, however, vascular access must be achieved as quickly as possible, so some of the following steps (indicated by *) may have to be omitted. Universal precautions should always be taken.

1. Locate the site of cannulation. The tibial tuberosity is identified by palpation, and the site of intraosseous cannulation is approximately 1 to 3 cm below this tuberosity on the medial surface of the tibia, approximately one finger's width below and just medial to the tibial tuberosity. At this site the tibia is just under the skin surface.
*2. Wash hands.
3. Put on gloves.
4. Cleanse the skin over the insertion site with an antiseptic solution.
5. Check the needle and ensure that the bevels of the outer needle and internal stylet are properly aligned.
6. Grasp the thigh and knee above and lateral to the insertion site with the palm of the nondominant hand. Wrap the fingers and thumb around the knee to stabilize the proximal tibia. Do not allow any portion of your hand to rest behind the insertion site. The leg should be supported on a firm surface.
7. Palpate the landmarks and again identify the flat surface of the tibia just below and medial to the tibial tuberosity.
8. Insert the needle through the skin over the flat anteromedial surface of the tibia already identified.
9. Advance the needle through the bony cortex of the proximal tibia, directing the needle perpendicular

(90°) to the long axis of the bone or slightly caudad (toward the toes) to avoid the epiphysial plate, using a gentle but firm twisting or drilling motion (Fig 5).

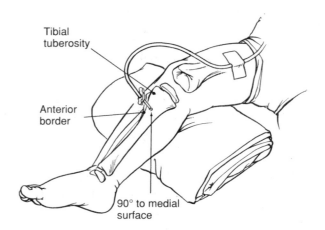

Fig 5. Intraosseous cannulation technique.

10. Stop advancing the needle when a sudden decrease in resistance to forward motion of the needle is felt. This decrease in resistance usually indicates entrance into the bone marrow cavity. It is possible to aspirate bone marrow at this point. Any aspiration of bone marrow must be followed by irrigation to prevent obstruction of the needle with marrow.
11. Unscrew the cap and remove the stylet from the needle.
12. Stabilize the intraosseous needle and slowly inject 10 mL of normal saline through the needle. Check for any signs of increased resistance to injection, increased circumference of the soft tissues of the calf, or increased firmness of the tissue.
13. If the test injection is successful, disconnect the syringe, evacuate any air remaining in the connection tubing, and join an infusion set to the needle. Secure the needle and tubing with tape and support it with a bulky dressing.
14. If the test injection is unsuccessful (ie, infiltration of the normal saline into the leg tissue is observed), remove the needle and attempt the procedure on the other leg.

Insertion is successful and the needle is clearly in the marrow cavity if the following conditions are present[27]:

• A sudden decrease in resistance to insertion occurs as the needle passes through the bony cortex into the marrow
• The needle can remain upright without support
• Marrow can be aspirated into a syringe joined to the needle, although this is not consistently achieved
• Fluid flows freely through the needle without evidence of subcutaneous infiltration.

If the needle becomes obstructed with bone or bone marrow, it can be replaced with a second needle passed through the same cannulation site, provided no evidence of infiltration is observed. If evidence of infiltration is observed or if the test injection fails, a second attempt at intraosseous cannulation should be performed on the contralateral tibia.

Cannulation of Central Veins

Central venous cannulation enables delivery of the infusate directly into the central circulation and delivery of medications at or near their site of action. Although central venous drug administration produces more rapid onset of drug action and higher peak drug levels than peripheral venous drug administration in adult resuscitation models,[11-13] this advantage does not appear to be present in pediatric animal models or clinical studies.[3,14] Central venous cannulation allows monitoring of central venous pressure during postresuscitation stabilization. In addition, there is little risk of infiltration of drugs that are administered by this route.

Complications

Complications of central venous cannulation include local and systemic infection, venous or arterial bleeding, arterial cannulation, thrombosis, phlebitis, pulmonary thromboembolism, hydrothorax, hemothorax, cardiac tamponade, arrhythmias, air embolism, and catheter-fragment embolism.[5,49,50] The incidence of these complications is determined by the site, the experience of the clinician, and the clinical condition of the patient. Hemorrhage has been reported in nonarrest studies after injury to the adjacent carotid artery during catheterization of the internal jugular vein.[51] Pneumothorax, hemothorax, and chylothorax are more likely complications after subclavian vein or internal jugular vein cannulation on the left side, because the cupula of the lung is higher on the left side than on the right.

Complications of central venous catheterization are more common in the pediatric age group than in adult patients. As a result, this form of intravenous access should be used only when the potential benefits outweigh the risks (eg, peripheral venous access cannot be achieved, or central venous pressure monitoring is required). The procedure should be performed or directly supervised by an experienced clinician who is knowledgeable about the unique features of central venous anatomy in infants and children.[51-53]

Devices and Techniques

Through-the-Needle Catheters. Access to the central circulation can be achieved through the femoral, external jugular, internal jugular, axillary, and subclavian veins. Although through-the-needle catheters can be used, the Seldinger technique (see below) is often preferable. If a through-the-needle catheter is used, a 19-gauge catheter

(17-gauge needle) or a 16-gauge catheter (14-gauge needle) provides a wide bore for rapid administration of drugs or fluids in children. Although a 22-gauge catheter (19-gauge needle) is easier to place in infants than a larger catheter, its small diameter precludes its use for rapid volume administration.

Great care must always be exercised during placement of a through-the-needle catheter because the catheter tip can be sheared off by the sharp needle.[49,50] If any resistance is encountered during catheter advancement, the catheter should *not* be withdrawn through the needle. Instead, the entire assembly should be withdrawn as a unit to prevent catheter shearing and potential fragment embolism.

Modified Seldinger Technique for Insertion of Catheters and Introducing Sheaths. Pressure-monitoring catheters are catheters of relatively low compliance that allow measurement of central venous or intracardiac pressures. A catheter-introducing sheath consists of a dilator within a large-bore sheath. Once the catheter-introducer is placed into a central vein, the dilator is removed and the sheath may be used for fluid infusion or to guide the insertion of a central venous catheter.

The Seldinger (guidewire) technique[54] is especially useful for establishing vascular access in children. This technique allows the introduction of catheters (Table 1) into the central venous circulation after initial venous entry using a small-gauge, thin-walled needle or an over-the-needle catheter. Once free flow of blood is achieved using the small needle or catheter, a guidewire is threaded through the needle or catheter into the vessel, and the small-gauge needle or catheter is withdrawn over the guidewire while the guidewire is held in place (Fig 6). A large catheter or a catheter-introducing sheath is then passed over the guidewire into the vessel, and the guidewire is withdrawn. If the catheter-introducing sheath is used, both the sheath and the dilator are passed over the guidewire. The guidewire and dilator are then removed simultaneously, leaving the sheath in the large vein.

Sites

Femoral Vein. The inferior vena cava is cannulated via the femoral vein. The femoral vein is used most frequently during emergency central venous cannulation because it is relatively easy to access. This site is associated with a lower rate of complications than other sites[55] and is distant from major sites of activity during resuscitation. The Seldinger technique provides the most reliable access into the central venous system via the femoral vein during an acute emergency.

Superior Vena Cava. The superior vena cava may be cannulated via the external jugular, internal jugular, axillary, or subclavian vein. Internal jugular and subclavian vein cannulation should be performed only by persons specifically trained and skilled in the technique, because the complication rate is significant when cannulation is attempted by inexperienced persons.

Cannulation of the external jugular vein is relatively safe because the vein is superficial and easily visible. The major disadvantages of this site are (1) potential compromise of the airway by extension and rotation of the neck to expose the vein and (2) a low success rate in achievement of central placement of the catheter because of the acute angle of entry of the external jugular vein into the subclavian vein.[56,57]

The anatomy of the internal jugular vein and its relation to the carotid artery, the sternocleidomastoid muscle, and the clavicle are shown in Fig 7. Despite the risk of bleeding, cannulation of the internal jugular vein can be successful, even in newborns. The right internal jugular vein is preferred to the left because there is less chance of causing a pneumothorax or damage to the thoracic duct and a greater chance that the catheter will pass directly from the innominate vein into the superior vena cava instead of the right subclavian vein. Three approaches are possible for internal jugular venous cannulation: the posterior, the anterior, and the central (middle) routes.[57] No one approach is clearly superior to the others.[58-62] The high central route appears to be the most widely used for

entry into the internal jugular vein, but the choice should be made based on the experience of the operator.

Subclavian vein cannulation in infants and children can be performed by the infraclavicular route[63-65] but in the past has been associated with a high complication rate when performed during emergencies.[66] Thus, subclavian vein cannulation is not recommended for small children unless alternate routes are unavailable. The risk of complications is lower in older children (1 year or older), but the subclavian vein still is not the ideal site of vascular access during resuscitation.

Techniques

Femoral Vein (Fig 8A and B)

Note: Whenever possible, hand washing and sterile technique should be performed. During resuscitation, however, vascular access must be achieved as quickly as possible, so some of the following steps (indicated by *) may have to be omitted. Universal precautions should always be taken.

1. Restrain the leg with slight external rotation
2. Identify the femoral artery by palpation or, if pulses are absent, by finding the midpoint between the

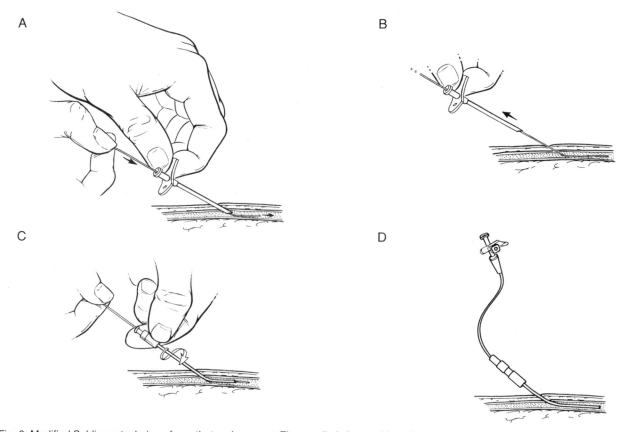

Fig. 6. Modified Seldinger technique for catheter placement. The needle is inserted into the target vessel, and the flexible end of the guidewire is passed freely into the vessel (A). The needle is then removed, leaving the guidewire in place (B). The catheter is advanced with a twisting motion into the vessel (C). Finally, the wire is removed and the catheter connected to an appropriate flow or monitoring device (D). Reproduced from Schwartz AJ, Coté CJ, Jobes DR, Ellison N. Scientific Exhibit. Central venous catheterization in pediatrics. Gloves should be worn.

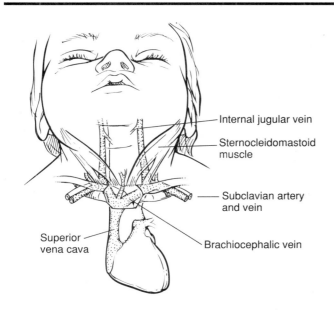

Fig 7. The internal jugular vein and its relationship to the surrounding anatomy.

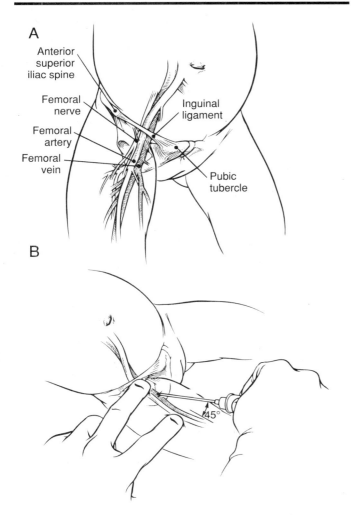

Fig 8. Femoral vein (A) anatomy and (B) cannulation technique.

anterior superior iliac spine and the symphysis pubis. (When chest compression is performed, pulsations in the femoral area may originate from either the femoral vein or the femoral artery,[67] and needle puncture should be attempted at the point of pulsation.)

*3. Scrub hands.

4. Put on gloves.

5. Cleanse the skin with an antiseptic solution.

6. Cover the area with a sterile drape.

*7. Anesthetize the skin with 1% lidocaine if the child is responsive to pain.

8. Flush the needle, syringe system, and catheter with sterile saline.

9. Introduce a thin-walled needle or over-the-needle catheter one finger's breadth below the inguinal ligament, just medial to the femoral artery. Apply gentle negative pressure to an attached 3-mL syringe and slowly advance the needle, directing the needle toward the umbilicus at a 45° angle. Once a free flow of blood is obtained, as indicated by a backflash of blood into the syringe, disconnect the syringe and place a finger over the needle hub to prevent entrainment and potential embolism of air. If no backflash of blood is obtained, continue gentle aspiration and slowly withdraw the needle and syringe, as this may unkink a vein that has become kinked upon entry.

10. Once the needle is in the vein, advance a guidewire through the needle during a positive-pressure breath or spontaneous exhalation, remove the needle over the guidewire (leaving the guidewire in place), then pass a catheter or catheter-introducing sheath over the wire. Advance the catheter into the inferior vena cava to the right atrium (the distance must be previously determined from surface landmarks). The guidewire may then be removed.

11. Secure the catheter or introducer in place with suture material or tape, evacuate any air remaining in the connecting tubing, attach an infusion set, and apply a sterile, occlusive dressing to the catheter insertion site.[20]

12. Obtain a chest radiograph to verify that the catheter tip is correctly positioned at the inferior vena cava–right atrial junction.

External Jugular Vein (Fig 9). The external jugular vein, while an excellent portal to the central venous circulation, is itself a peripheral vein. It generally is used only when cannulation of other peripheral veins at more accessible sites (ie, an upper or lower extremity) is unsuccessful. The external jugular vein should *not* be used as a primary site for peripheral venous cannulation during resuscitation of patients with respiratory failure or airway compromise, because cannula insertion requires extension and rotation of the neck. This manipulation will interfere with resuscitative efforts.

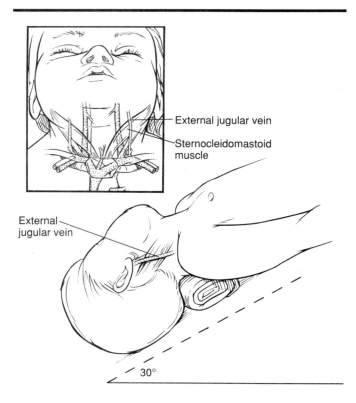

Fig 9. External jugular vein cannulation.

Note: Whenever possible, hand washing and sterile technique should be performed. During resuscitation, however, vascular access must be achieved as quickly as possible, so some of the following steps (indicated by *) may have to be omitted. Universal precautions should always be taken.

1. Restrain the child in a 30° head-down (Trendelenburg) position with the head turned away from the side to be punctured. Auscultate and document bilateral breath sounds before the procedure is initiated. The right side is preferred for access.
2. Identify the external jugular vein.
*3. Scrub hands.
4. Put on gloves.
5. Prepare the skin with an antiseptic solution.
6. Cover the area with a sterile drape.
*7. Anesthetize the skin with 1% lidocaine if the child is responsive to pain.
8. Flush the needle, catheter, and syringe system with sterile saline.
9. Using sterile technique, puncture the skin slightly distal to or to one side of the visible external jugular vein with a 16- or 18-gauge needle to facilitate entry of the catheter through the skin. Do not enter the vein with the needle.
10. Temporarily occlude the vein just above the clavicle by applying gentle pressure with the tip of the long finger of the nondominant hand to mimic the effect of a tourniquet.
11. Stretch the skin over the vein just below the angle of the mandible using the thumb of the nondominant hand to immobilize the vein, after allowing it to distend fully.
12. If peripheral cannulation is desired, insert a short-length over-the-needle catheter into the vein and proceed as described for peripheral venous cannulation. If central venous access is desired, insert a long-length through-the-needle catheter or catheter-over-guidewire and proceed as described for cannulation of the internal jugular vein.
13. Secure the catheter firmly in place with suture material or tape, evacuate any air remaining in the connecting tubing, attach an infusion set, and apply a sterile, occlusive dressing to the insertion site.[20] Auscultate and document breath sounds.
14. If central venous catheterization is attempted, obtain a chest radiograph to verify that the catheter tip is correctly positioned above the junction of the superior vena cava and right atrium and to rule out pneumothorax or hemothorax.

Internal Jugular Vein (Fig 10). The following technique is common to the anterior, central, and posterior routes of internal jugular vein cannulation. The right side of the neck is preferred for several reasons: the dome of the right lung and pleura is lower than the left, so the risk of pneumothorax is reduced, the path to the right atrium is more direct, and the risk of injury to the thoracic duct is minimal.

Note: Whenever possible, hand washing and sterile technique should be performed. During resuscitation, however, vascular access must be achieved as quickly as possible, so some of the following steps (indicated by *) may have to be omitted. Universal precautions should always be taken.

1. If no cervical spine injury is present, hyperextend the patient's neck by placing a towel roll transversely beneath the shoulders.
2. Restrain the child in a 30° head-down (Trendelenburg) position with the head turned slightly away from the side of cannulation.[68] The right side is preferred. Auscultate and document bilateral breath sounds before the procedure is initiated.
3. Identify the anatomic landmarks of the sternocleidomastoid muscle and the clavicle.
*4. Scrub hands.
5. Put on gloves.
6. Cleanse the skin with an antiseptic solution.
7. Cover the area with a sterile drape.
*8. Anesthetize the skin with 1% lidocaine if the child is responsive to pain.
9. Flush the needle, syringe, and catheter system with sterile saline.

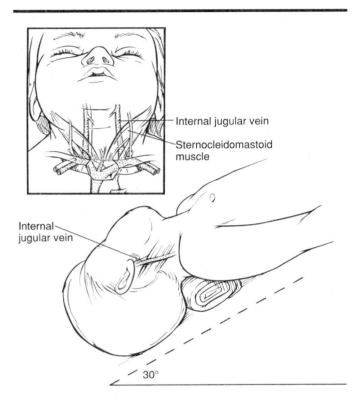

Fig 10. Internal jugular vein cannulation.

10. Using sterile technique, introduce a thin-walled needle into the neck near the intended site of cannulation. Applying gentle negative pressure to an attached 3-mL syringe, slowly advance the needle, directing it into the vein using the anterior, central, or posterior approach. (See below for specific technique.) Once a free flow of blood is obtained (indicated by a backflash into the syringe), disconnect the syringe and place a finger over the needle hub to prevent the entrainment and potential embolism of air.

11. During a positive-pressure breath or spontaneous exhalation, advance the guidewire into the right atrium, insert a guidewire through the needle, remove the needle over the guidewire, and pass a catheter or catheter-introducing sheath over the wire. Advance the catheter to the superior vena cava–right atrial junction (the distance must be previously determined from surface landmarks). The guidewire or introducer may then be removed and an infusion set attached after evacuation of any remaining air from the connecting tubing.

12. Aspirate blood from each port of the central line. Alternatively, lower the intravenous fluid reservoir below head level and allow blood to flow back freely into the intravenous tubing before initiating fluid infusion through the catheter. If blood return does not occur, the catheter may be lodged against the wall of a vessel or against the wall of the right atrium. The catheter should then be slightly withdrawn, and

aspiration repeated (this withdrawal/aspiration may be performed twice). If blood return is still not observed, it must be assumed that the catheter is not in the vessel. The catheter should be removed and another attempt made.

13. Once aspiration of blood and free flow of infusate are documented, secure the catheter in place with suture material and apply a sterile, occlusive dressing.[20] Auscultate and document bilateral breath sounds.

14. Obtain a chest radiograph to verify that the catheter tip is correctly positioned at the junction of the superior vena cava and right atrium and to rule out pneumothorax and hemothorax.

Three common approaches for internal jugular vein cannulation are provided below. The provider should become familiar with one technique rather than randomly attempting all three.

1. *Anterior route.* Palpate the carotid artery medially at the anterior border of the sternocleidomastoid muscle with the index and third fingers. Introduce the needle at the midpoint of this anterior border at a 30° angle with the coronal plane. Direct the needle caudad in the sagittal plane toward the ipsilateral nipple (Fig 11A).

2. *Central route.* Identify a triangle formed by the two portions (sternoclavicular heads) of the sternocleidomastoid muscle with the clavicle at its base. Introduce the needle at the apex of this triangle at a 30° angle to the coronal plane. Direct the needle caudad toward the ipsilateral nipple. If the vein is not entered, withdraw the needle and redirect the needle more toward the ipsilateral shoulder (Fig 11B).

3. *Posterior route.* Introduce the needle deep into the sternal head of the sternocleidomastoid muscle at the junction of the middle and lower thirds of the posterior margin (eg, just above the point where the external jugular vein crosses this muscle). Direct the needle toward the suprasternal notch (Fig 11C).

Subclavian Vein (Fig 12A and B)

Note: Whenever possible, hand washing and sterile technique should be performed. During resuscitation, however, vascular access must be achieved as quickly as possible, so some of the following steps (indicated by *) may have to be omitted. Universal precautions should always be taken.

1. If no cervical spine injury is present, hyperextend the patient's neck and open the costoclavicular angles by placing a towel roll directly beneath and parallel to the thoracic spine.

2. Restrain the child in a 30° head-down (Trendelenburg) position with the head turned away from the side to be punctured. Auscultate and document bilateral breath sounds before the procedure is initiated. The right side is preferred.

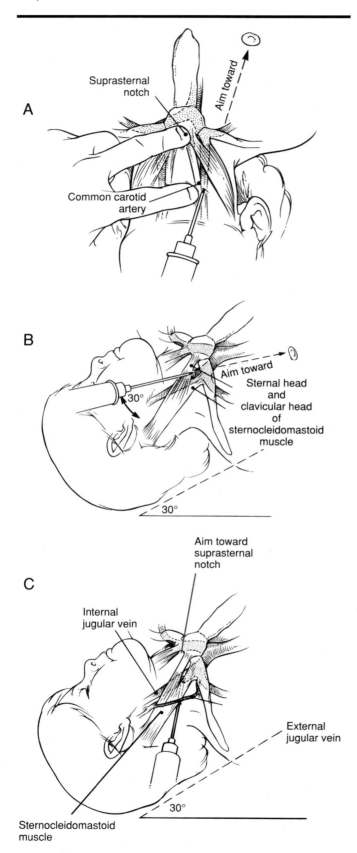

Fig 11. Internal jugular vein technique. A, Anterior route; B, central route; C, posterior route.

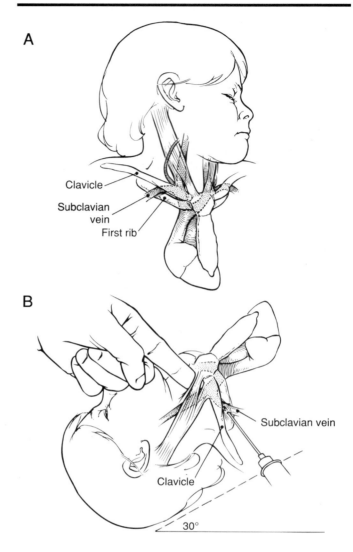

Fig 12. Subclavian vein. A, Anatomy; B, technique.

3. Identify the junction of the middle and medial thirds of the clavicle.
*4. Scrub hands.
5. Put on gloves.
6. Cleanse the skin with an antiseptic solution.
7. Cover the area with a sterile drape.
*8. Anesthetize the skin with 1% lidocaine if the child is responsive to pain.
9. Flush the needle, catheter, and syringe with sterile saline.
10. Using sterile technique, introduce a thin-walled needle just under the clavicle at the junction of the middle and medial thirds of the clavicle. Slowly advance the needle while applying gentle negative pressure with an attached syringe, directing the needle toward a fingertip placed in the suprasternal notch. The syringe and needle should be parallel to the frontal plane, directed medially and slightly cephalad, beneath the clavicle toward the posterior

aspect of the sternal end of the clavicle, ie, the lower end of the fingertip in the sternal notch. Once a free flow of blood is obtained, as indicated by a backflash into the syringe, it may be necessary to rotate the bevel to a caudad position to facilitate placement of the catheter or guidewire into the superior vena cava. Disconnect the syringe and place a finger over the needle hub to prevent the entrainment and potential embolism of air.

11. During a positive-pressure breath or spontaneous exhalation, insert a guidewire through the needle, remove the needle over the guidewire, advance the guidewire into the right atrium.

12. Pass a dilator over the wire and remove the dilator.

13. Pass a catheter or a catheter-introducing sheath over the wire. Advance the catheter to the superior vena cava–right atrial junction (the insertion distance must be previously determined from surface landmarks). The guidewire or introducer may then be removed and an infusion set attached after any remaining air is evacuated from the connecting tubing.

14. Demonstrate free blood return from all ports of the catheter and, subsequently, free flow of infusate. If blood does not immediately flow back freely, the catheter may be lodged against a vessel wall or the wall of the right atrium. The catheter should then be withdrawn slightly and aspiration repeated (this withdrawal/aspiration may be performed twice). If blood return is still not observed, it must be assumed that the catheter is not in the vessel and the catheter should be removed.

15. Once free blood return and free flow of infusate are documented, secure the catheter or catheter-introducing sheath in place with suture material and apply a sterile, occlusive dressing.[20] Auscultate and document bilateral breath sounds.

16. Obtain a chest radiograph to verify that the catheter tip is correctly positioned at the superior vena cava–right atrial junction and to rule out pneumothorax and hemothorax.

Saphenous Vein Cutdown

If peripheral venous, central venous, and intraosseous cannulation cannot be performed, a venous cutdown is an alternative means of vascular access. However, percutaneous central venous cannulation is usually more successful and is associated with a lower rate of complications than saphenous vein cutdown.[69] In addition, a saphenous vein cutdown may take longer than 10 minutes to perform (even in experienced hands), may last no longer than percutaneous cannulation, and is associated with a higher infection rate than other methods of venous access.[69,70]

Site

The long saphenous vein that courses anterior to the medial malleolus at the ankle is the preferred site for cutdown (Fig 13).

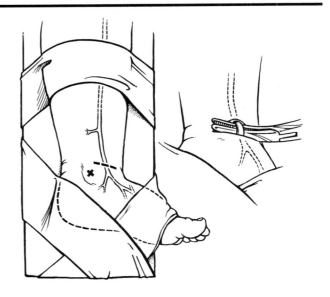

Fig 13. Saphenous vein cutdown.

Technique

Note: Whenever possible, hand washing and sterile technique should be performed. During resuscitation, however, vascular access must be achieved as quickly as possible, so some of the following steps (indicated by *) may have to be omitted. Universal precautions should always be taken.

1. Identify a proposed incision site perpendicular to the long axis of the tibia, one finger's breadth (approximately 2 cm) superior and anterior to the medial malleolus in children and one half finger's breadth (approximately 1 cm) anterior and superior in infants.

2. Apply a tourniquet proximal to the proposed incision site.

*3. Scrub hands.

4. Put on gloves.

5. Cleanse the skin with an antiseptic solution.

6. Cover the area with a sterile drape.

7. Using sterile technique, infiltrate the skin with 1% lidocaine (if the child responds to pain) and make an incision through the skin perpendicular to the long axis of the tibia. Carefully dissect the subcutaneous tissue with the tips of a small curved hemostat to expose the superficial fascia.

8. Pierce the superficial fascia with the tips of the hemostat and spread it gently, parallel to the long axis of the tibia. Pass the hemostat (with the tips up) to the bone, spread the tips, and raise the hemostat

from the incision site. The saphenous vein should be picked up by the hemostat. Alternatively, the adjacent tissues may be dissected with the tips of the hemostat to identify the saphenous vein before it is elevated.

9. Once the vein has been isolated, place a ligature or tie around the distal end of the vein and anchor the vein in place. Place a second ligature or tie around the proximal end of the vein, but leave it untied.

10. Make an anterior venotomy through the vein with a No. 11 scalpel blade inserted perpendicular to the long axis of the vessel into the upper (most superficial) third of the vessel. Thread a catheter into the proximal limb of the vein through the venotomy site. Tie the proximal ligature around the vein and the catheter within to hold the catheter in place. Tie the distal ligature around the catheter. Alternatively, catheterize the exposed vein under direct visualization, using an over-the-needle catheter.

11. Remove the tourniquet, evacuate any air remaining in the connecting tubing, attach an infusion set, suture the incision site, and apply a sterile, occlusive dressing.[20]

Arterial Access

After spontaneous circulation has been restored, insertion of an arterial catheter enables continuous monitoring of blood pressure and blood sampling.[71] Arterial catheters may be extremely useful for patient monitoring, but their use is associated with complications including localized or generalized infection, air or particulate embolization, and thrombosis of the artery with associated tissue necrosis or ischemia and growth failure in the affected limb.[72,73] In children the most common complications of *radial* artery catheterization include minor skin lesions, localized necrosis, and radial artery occlusion.[74] Factors associated with the highest risk of radial artery occlusion include patient age of less than 5 years, cutdown insertion, and duration of cannulation of more than 4 days.[74] Recent studies have documented a lower incidence of complications[75] and greater longevity (patency) of radial artery catheters[76] when a continuous infusion with heparinized saline (5 U/mL at 1-2 mL/h) is provided.[75,76] Unfortunately, temporary total occlusion of the radial artery has been reported in as many as 63% of infants following percutaneous radial artery catheterization.[77] Although this complication typically resolves spontaneously, it underscores the need to closely monitor distal extremity perfusion following arterial cannulation. If significant compromise of perfusion is observed, the arterial catheter should be removed and placed in another site if necessary.

Site

Arterial catheters can be placed percutaneously in the radial, brachial, axillary, femoral, dorsalis pedis, and posterior tibial arteries.[78] Temporal artery cannulation should

not be attempted, because it may be associated with severe cerebral thromboembolic complications, thought to be caused by migration of thrombus to the internal carotid circulation.[79-81] The radial artery and femoral artery are preferred sites of cannulation.

Technique

The technique for cannulation of the radial artery is described here[82-84] (see Fig 14). A similar technique is used for cannulation of other arteries.

The main source of blood flow for the fingers is the superficial palmar arch. In most (88%) people this arch is supplied predominantly with flow from the ulnar artery.[85] Approximately 12% of normal adult patients demonstrate *radial artery–dominant* palmar arch flow, and 1.6% of normal adults demonstrate *radial-dependent* flow with no other collateral circulation.[85] This latter group (1.6%) of the population would be at high risk for development of hand ischemia after radial artery catheterization, particularly if complicated by radial artery occlusion.

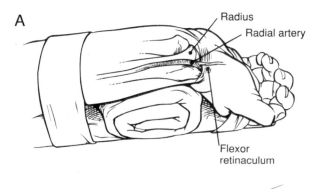

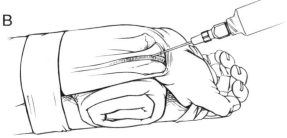

Fig 14. Radial artery (A) anatomy and (B) cannulation.

Collateral circulation to the hand may be evaluated before radial artery cannulation using a modified Allen test[86] or Doppler flow evaluation[85] (see box). However, the predictive value of a positive Allen test in detecting poor collateral flow may be extremely low, because hyperextension of the fingers frequently produces a false-positive Allen test.[85,87] In addition, false-negative Allen tests have been reported in a substantial number of patients shown to have radial-dependent palmar flow and inadequate (ulnar) collateral circulation by Doppler flow evaluation.[87,88] Doppler studies may be more reliable than the modified Allen test,[85] although the accuracy of Doppler flow evaluation has not been determined. Regardless of the method of evaluation of collateral flow before cannulation, it is imperative that hand circulation be closely monitored following radial artery catheterization. If any evidence of hand ischemia is observed, the catheter should be removed. Consultation with a vascular surgeon may be necessary if evidence of ischemia persists.

Cannulation of the radial artery is accomplished as follows.

Note: Universal precautions should always be taken.

1. Dorsiflex the hand at the wrist 45° to 60° and secure both the hand and the lower forearm to a board. Maintain dorsiflexion with a roll of gauze placed behind the wrist. Tape the hand down, leaving all fingers exposed so that perfusion of the hand can be assessed. Temporarily tape the thumb aside to prevent movement during attempts at arterial cannulation.
2. Locate the radial pulse just proximal to the head of the radius.
3. Scrub hands and put on gloves.
4. Cover the area with a sterile drape.
5. Cleanse the skin with an antiseptic solution.
6. Anesthetize the skin with 1% lidocaine if the child is responsive to pain.
7. Puncture the skin at the site of maximal pulsation with a 20-gauge needle. Advance a 20- to 24-gauge, heparin-flushed catheter at a 30° angle and advance it until blood appears in the hub. Two techniques of arterial cannulation are frequently used:

   • Pass the catheter and needle through the artery to transfix it. Withdraw the needle, and then withdraw the catheter very slowly until there is a free flow of blood. Advance the catheter slowly through the lumen of the artery.
   • Puncture only the anterior wall of the artery. Advance the catheter slowly until blood appears in the needle. Lower the needle carefully to a 10° angle. Ascertain that blood flow is continuing, and advance the catheter slowly over the needle into the lumen of the artery.

8. Remove the needle and attach the catheter to a T-connector to permit continuous infusion of heparinized saline (1 to 5 U/mL).[76]
9. Apply a sterile, occlusive dressing and adhesive tape to the puncture site.[20]
10. Remove the gauze roll and secure the wrist in a neutral position to the board. It may be advisable to label the arterial line to prevent administration of drugs through the catheter.

The catheter should be removed immediately if any evidence of tissue ischemia develops. Urgent consultation with a microvascular surgeon should be obtained if evidence of ischemia continues. Recent results of radial artery repair in infants have been encouraging.[90]

Modified Allen Test

1. Compress/clench the child's hand several times.
2. Elevate the hand above the heart and compress/clench the hand tightly.
3. Occlude both the ulnar and radial arteries and lower the hand to the level of the heart.
4. Open the hand but *do not* hyperextend the fingers. Release pressure over the ulnar artery. If color returns to the hand within 6 seconds while the radial artery remains occluded, the Allen test is *negative,* and circulation through the ulnar artery and palmar arch is thought to be adequate. If the hand fails to reperfuse within 6 seconds, the Allen test is *positive,* and flow through the ulnar artery and palmar arch may be inadequate if the radial artery becomes obstructed.

Doppler Flow Evaluation[85]

1. Place a Doppler probe between the heads of the third and fourth metacarpals on the palm of the hand, perpendicular to the palm.
2. Advance the probe proximally until the pulsatile signal is maximal.
3. Occlude the radial artery while monitoring the Doppler signal. If the pulsatile signal is unchanged or increases in intensity, ulnar and palmar arch circulation are probably adequate. If the pulsatile sound diminishes in intensity, flow through the ulnar artery and palmar arch or collateral circulation may be inadequate if the radial artery becomes obstructed.

Location of Radial Artery

A Doppler flow probe may be used to locate the radial artery and confirm catheter placement.[89] A fiberoptic light source may be placed under the wrist (or foot) of small infants to locate arterial flow.

References

1. Rosetti VA, Thompson BM, Aprahamian C, Darin JC, Mateer JR. Difficulty and delay in intravascular access in pediatric arrests. *Ann Emerg Med.* 1984;13:406. Abstract.
2. Carcillo JA, Davis AL, Zaritsky A. Role of early fluid resuscitation in pediatric septic shock. *JAMA.* 1991;266:1242-1245.
3. Stylianos S, Jacir NN, Hoffman MA, et al. Optimal intravenous site for volume replacement. *J Trauma.* 1992;32:947. Abstract.
4. Redding JS, Asuncion JS, Pearson JW. Effective routes of drug administration during cardiac arrest. *Anesth Analg.* 1967;46:253-258.
5. Filston HC, Johnson DG. Percutaneous venous cannulation in neonates and infants: a method for catheter insertion without 'cut-down.' *Pediatrics.* 1971;48:896-901.
6. Fiser D. Intraosseous infusion. *N Engl J Med.* 1990;322:1579-1581.
7. Gauderer MW. Vascular access techniques and devices in the pediatric patient. *Surg Clin North Am.* 1992;72:1267-1284.
8. Kanter RK, Zimmerman JJ, Strauss RH, Stoeckel KA. Pediatric emergency intravenous access: evaluation of a protocol. *Am J Dis Child.* 1986;140:132-134.
9. Heinild S, Søndergaard T, Tudvad F. Bone marrow infusions in childhood: experiences from 1000 infusions. *J Pediatr.* 1947;30:400-412.
10. Meola F. Bone marrow infusions as a routine procedure in children. *J Pediatr.* 1944;25:13-16.
11. Hedges JR, Barsan WB, Doan LA, et al. Central versus peripheral intravenous routes in cardiopulmonary resuscitation. *Am J Emerg Med.* 1984;2:385-390.

12. Kuhn GJ, White BC, Swetnam RE, et al. Peripheral vs central circulation times during CPR: a pilot study. *Ann Emerg Med.* 1981;10:417-419.

13. Emerman CL, Pinchak AC, Hancock D, Hagen JF. Effect of injection site on circulation times during cardiac arrest. *Crit Care Med.* 1988;16:1138-1141.

14. Fleisher G, Caputo G, Baskin M. Comparison of external jugular and peripheral venous administration of sodium bicarbonate in puppies. *Crit Care Med.* 1989;17:251-254.

15. Glaeser PW, Losek JD, Nelson DB, et al. Pediatric intraosseous infusions: impact on vascular access time. *Am J Emerg Med.* 1988;6:330-332.

16. Andropoulos DB, Soifer SJ, Schreiber MD. Plasma epinephrine concentrations after intraosseous and central venous injection during cardiopulmonary resuscitation in the lamb. *J Pediatr.* 1990;116:312-315.

17. Dolister M, Gaddis GM, Gaddis ML. A comparison of the effects of central versus peripheral drug administration plus different sized postinfusion flushes on drug delivery to the aortic root in canine cardiac arrest models. *Ann Emerg Med.* 1993;22:930. Abstract.

18. Dalsey WC, Barsan WG, Joyce SM, Hedges JR, Lukes SJ, Doan LA. Comparison of superior vena caval and inferior vena caval access using a radioisotope technique during normal perfusion and cardiopulmonary resuscitation. *Ann Emerg Med.* 1984;13:881-884.

19. Johnston C. Endotracheal drug delivery. *Pediatr Emerg Care.* 1992;8:94-97.

20. Maki DG, Ringer M. Evaluation of dressing regimens for prevention of infection with peripheral intravenous catheters: gauze, a transparent polyurethane dressing, and an iodophor-transparent dressing. *JAMA.* 1987;258:2396-2403.

21. Rosetti VA, Thompson BM, Miller J, Mateer JR, Aprahamian C. Intraosseous infusion: an alternative route of pediatric intravascular access. *Ann Emerg Med.* 1985;14:885-888.

22. Smith RJ, Keseg DP, Manley LK, Standeford T. Intraosseous infusions by prehospital personnel in critically ill pediatric patients. *Ann Emerg Med.* 1988;17:491-495.

23. Miner WF, Corneli HM, Bolte RG, Lehnhof D, Clawson JJ. Prehospital use of intraosseous infusion by paramedics. *Pediatr Emerg Care.* 1989;5:5-7.

24. Seigler RS, Tecklenburg FW, Shealy R. Prehospital intraosseous infusion by emergency medical services personnel: a prospective study. *Pediatrics.* 1989;84:173-177.

25. Fuchs S, LaCovey D, Paris P. A prehospital model of intraosseous infusion. *Ann Emerg Med.* 1991;20:371-374.

26. Wagner MB, McCabe JB. A comparison of four techniques to establish intraosseous infusion. *Pediatr Emerg Care.* 1988;4:87-91.

27. Berg RA. Emergency infusion of catecholamines into bone marrow. *Am J Dis Child.* 1984;138:810-811.

28. McNamara RM, Spivey WH, Sussman C. Pediatric resuscitation without an intravenous line. *Am J Emerg Med.* 1986;4:31-33.

29. Glaeser PW, Losek JD. Emergency intraosseous infusions in children. *Am J Emerg Med.* 1986;4:34-36.

30. Walsh-Kelly CM, Berens RJ, Glaeser PW, Losek JD. Intraosseous infusion of phenytoin. *Am J Emerg Med.* 1986;4:523-524.

31. Iserson KV, Criss E. Intraosseous infusions: a usable technique. *Am J Emerg Med.* 1986;4:540-542.

32. McNamara RM, Spivey WH, Unger HD, Malone DR. Emergency applications of intraosseous infusion. *J Emerg Med.* 1987;5:97-101.

33. Harte FA, Chalmers PC, Walsh RF, Danker PR, Sheikh FM. Intraosseous fluid administration: a parenteral alternative in pediatric resuscitation. *Anesth Analg.* 1987;66:687-689.

34. Katan BS, Olshaker JS, Dickerson SE. Intraosseous infusion of muscle relaxants. *Am J Emerg Med.* 1988;6:353-354.

35. Sacchetti AD, Linkenheimer R, Lieberman M, Haviland P, Kryszczak LB. Intraosseous drug administration: successful resuscitation from asystole. *Pediatr Emerg Care.* 1989;5:97-98.

36. Tobias JD, Nichols DG. Intraosseous succinylcholine for orotracheal intubation. *Pediatr Emerg Care.* 1990;6:108-109.

37. Goldstein B, Doody D, Briggs S. Emergency intraosseous infusion in severely burned children. *Pediatr Emerg Care.* 1990;6:195-197.

38. Macgregor DF, Macnab AJ. Intraosseous fluids in emergencies. *Pediatrics.* 1990;85:386-387.

39. Hodge D III, Delgado-Paredes C, Fleisher G. Intraosseous infusion flow rates in hypovolemic "pediatric" dogs. *Ann Emerg Med.* 1987;16:305-307.

40. Cameron JL, Fontanarosa PB, Passalaqua AM. A comparative study of peripheral to central circulation delivery times between intraosseous and intravenous injection using a radionuclide technique in normovolemic and hypovolemic canines. *J Emerg Med.* 1989;7:123-127.

41. Pollack CV Jr, Pender ES, Woodall BN, Tubbs RC, Iyer RV, Miller HW. Long-term local effects of intraosseous infusion on tibial bone marrow in the weanling pig model. *Am J Emerg Med.* 1992;10:27-31.

42. Woodall BN, Pender ES, Pollack CV Jr, Miller H, Tubbs RC, Andrew ME. Intraosseous infusion of resuscitative fluids and drugs: long-term effect on linear bone growth in pigs. *South Med J.* 1992;85:820-824.

43. Orlowski JP, Julius CJ, Petras RE, Porembka DT, Gallagher JM. The safety of intraosseous infusions: risks of fat and bone marrow emboli to the lungs. *Ann Emerg Med.* 1989;18:1062-1067.

44. LaFleche FR, Slepin MJ, Vargas J, Milzman DP. Iatrogenic bilateral tibial fractures after intraosseous infusion attempts in a 3-month-old infant. *Ann Emerg Med.* 1989;18:1099-1101.

45. Moscati R, Moore GP. Compartment syndrome with resultant amputation following intraosseous infusion. *Am J Emerg Med.* 1990;8:470-471.

46. Galpin RD, Kronick JB, Willis RB, Frewen TC. Bilateral lower extremity compartment syndromes secondary to intraosseous fluid resuscitation. *J Pediatr Orthop.* 1991;11:773-776.

47. Christensen DW, Vernon DD, Banner W Jr, Dean JM. Skin necrosis complicating intraosseous infusion. *Pediatr Emerg Care.* 1991;7:289-290.

48. Glaeser PW, Losek JD. Intraosseous needles: new and improved. *Pediatr Emerg Care.* 1988;4:135-136.

49. Wellmann KF, Reinhard A, Salazar EP. Polyethylene catheter embolism: review of the literature and report of a case with associated fatal tricuspid and systemic candidiasis. *Circulation.* 1968;37:380-392.

50. Grabenwoeger F, Bardach G, Dock W, Pinterits F. Percutaneous extraction of centrally embolized foreign bodies: a report of 16 cases. *Br J Radiol.* 1988;61:1014-1018.

51. Nicolson SC, Sweeney MF, Moore RA, Jobes DR. Comparison of internal and external jugular cannulation of the central circulation in the pediatric patient. *Crit Care Med.* 1985;13:747-749.

52. Cobb LM, Vinocur CD, Wagner CW, Weintraub WH. The central venous anatomy in infants. *Surg Gynecol Obstet.* 1987;165:230-234.

53. Stenzel JP, Green TP, Fuhrman BP, Carlson PE, Marchessault RP. Percutaneous central venous catheterization in a pediatric intensive care unit: a survival analysis of complications. *Crit Care Med.* 1989;17:984-988.

54. Seldinger SI. Catheter replacement of the needle in percutaneous arteriography: a new technique. *Acta Radiol.* 1953;39:368-376.

55. Stenzel JP, Green TP, Fuhrman BP, Carlson PE, Marchessault RP. Percutaneous femoral venous catheterizations: a prospective study of complications. *J Pediatr.* 1989;114:411-415.

56. Taylor EA, Mowbray MJ, McLellan I. Central venous access in children via the external jugular vein. *Anaesthesia.* 1992;47:265-266.

57. Defalque RJ. Percutaneous catheterization of the internal jugular vein. *Anesth Analg.* 1974;53:116-121.

58. Rao TL, Wong AY, Salem MR. A new approach to percutaneous catheterization of the internal jugular vein. *Anesthesiology.* 1977;46:362-364.

59. Coté CJ, Jobes DR, Schwartz AJ, Ellison N. Two approaches to cannulation of a child's internal jugular vein. *Anesthesiology.* 1979;50:371-373.

60. Prince SR, Sullivan RL, Hackel A. Percutaneous catheterization of the internal jugular vein in infants and children. *Anesthesiology.* 1976;44:170-174.

61. Hall DM, Geefhuysen J. Percutaneous catheterization of the internal jugular vein in infants and children. *J Pediatr Surg.* 1977;12:719-722.

62. Krausz MM, Berlatzky Y, Ayalon A, Freund H, Schiller M. Percutaneous cannulation of the internal jugular vein in infants and children. *Surg Gynecol Obstet.* 1979;148:591-594.

63. Filston HC, Grant JP. A safer system for percutaneous subclavian venous catheterization in newborn infants. *J Pediatr Surg.* 1979;14:564-570.

64. Eichelberger MR, Rous PG, Hoelzer DJ, Garcia VF, Koop CE. Percutaneous subclavian venous catheters in neonates and children. *J Pediatr Surg.* 1981;16:547-553.

65. Venkataraman ST, Orr RA, Thompson AE. Percutaneous infraclavicular subclavian vein catheterization in critically ill infants and children. *J Pediatr.* 1988;113:480-485.

66. Groff DB, Ahmed N. Subclavian vein catheterization in the infant. *J Pediatr Surg.* 1974;9:171-174.

67. Niemann JT, Rosborough JP, Ung S, Criley JM. Hemodynamic effects of continuous abdominal binding during cardiac arrest and resuscitation. *Am J Cardiol.* 1984;53:269-274.

68. Sulek CA, Weiss L, Gravenstein N, Blackshear RH, Smith S. Influence of head position on relationship between internal jugular vein and carotid artery. *Crit Care Med.* 1993:S218. Abstract.

69. Newman BM, Jewett TC Jr, Karp MP, Cooney DR. Percutaneous central venous catheterization in children: first line choice for venous access. *J Pediatr Surg.* 1986;21:685-688.

70. Iserson KV, Criss EA. Pediatric venous cutdowns: utility in emergency situations. *Pediatr Emerg Care.* 1986;2:231-234.

71. Saladino R, Bachman D, Fleisher G. Arterial access in the pediatric emergency department. *Ann Emerg Med.* 1990;19:382-385.

72. Hack WW, Vos A, Okken A. Incidence of forearm and hand ischaemia related to radial artery cannulation in newborn infants. *Intensive Care Med.* 1990;16:50-53.

73. Guy RL, Holland JP, Shaw DG, Fixsen JA. Limb shortening secondary to complications of vascular cannulae in the neonatal period. *Skeletal Radiol.* 1990;19:423-425.

74. Miyasaka K, Edmonds JF, Conn AW. Complications of radial artery lines in the paediatric patient. *Can Anaesth Soc J.* 1976;23:9-14.

75. Selldén H, Nilsson K, Larsson LE, Ekström-Jodal B. Radial arterial catheters in children and neonates: a prospective study. *Crit Care Med.* 1987;15:1106-1109.

76. Butt W, Shann F, McDonnell G, Hudson I. Effect of heparin concentration and infusion rate on the patency of arterial catheters. *Crit Care Med.* 1987;15:230-232.

77. Hack WW, Vos A, van der Lei J, Okken A. Incidence and duration of total occlusion of the radial artery in newborn infants after catheter removal. *Eur J Pediatr.* 1990;149:275-277.

78. Greenwald BM, Notterman DA, DeBruin WJ, McCready M. Percutaneous axillary artery catheterization in critically ill infants and children. *J Pediatr.* 1990;117:442-444.

79. Simmons MA, Levine RL, Lubchenco LO, Guggenheim MA. Warning: serious sequelae of temporal artery catheterization. *J Pediatr.* 1978;92:284.

80. Prian GW. Complications and sequelae of temporal artery catheterization in the high-risk newborn. *J Pediatr Surg.* 1977;12:829-835.

81. Bull MJ, Schreiner RL, Garg BP, Hutton NM, Lemons JA, Gresham EL. Neurologic complications following temporal artery catheterization. *J Pediatr.* 1980;96:1071-1073.

82. Todres ID, Rogers MC, Shannon DC, Moylan FM, Ryan JF. Percutaneous catheterization of the radial artery in the critically ill neonate. *J Pediatr.* 1975;87:273-275.

83. Cole FS, Todres ID, Shannon DC. Technique for percutaneous cannulation of the radial artery in the newborn infant. *J Pediatr.* 1978;92:105-107.

84. Randel SN, Tsang BH, Wung JT, Driscoll JM Jr, James LS. Experience with percutaneous indwelling peripheral arterial catheterization in neonates. *Am J Dis Child.* 1987;141:848-851.

85. Mozersky DJ, Buckley CJ, Hagood CO Jr, Capps WF Jr, Dannemiller FJ Jr. Ultrasound evaluation of the palmar circulation: a useful adjunct to radial artery cannulation. *Am J Surg.* 1973; 126:810-812.

86. Allen EV. Thrombongiitis obliterans; methods of diagnosis of chronic occlusive arterial lesions distal to the wrist with illustrative cases. *Am J Med Sci.* 1929;178:237-239.

87. Kamienski RW, Barnes RW. Critique of the Allen test for continuity of the palmar arch assessed by Doppler ultrasound. *Surg Gynecol Obstet.* 1976;142:861-864.

88. Little JM, Zylstra PL, West J, May J. Circulatory patterns in the normal hand. *Br J Surg.* 1973;60:652-655.

89. Morray JP, Brandford HG, Barnes LF, Oh SM, Furman EB. Doppler-assisted radial artery cannulation in infants and children. *Anesth Analg.* 1984;63:346-348.

90. LaQuaglia MP, Upton J, May JW Jr. Microvascular reconstruction of major arteries in neonates and small children. *J Pediatr Surg.* 1991;26:1136-1140.

Fluid Therapy and Medications

Chapter 6

This chapter reviews the pharmacology of drugs essential for resuscitation and stabilization of infants and children and includes a discussion of fluid therapy and acid-base balance. Therapeutic considerations, indications, doses, routes of administration, precautions, and clinically recommended available forms of medications used in the resuscitation and advanced life support of infants and children are also presented.

The objectives of fluid administration during resuscitation are

- To restore effective circulating volume in hypovolemic shock states
- To restore oxygen-carrying capacity in hemorrhagic shock states
- To correct metabolic imbalances

The objectives of evaluation of acid-base balance are

- To determine the relative contributions of respiratory and circulatory failure to acidosis
- To identify appropriate treatment for documented respiratory or metabolic acidosis

The objectives of medication administration during resuscitation are

- To increase perfusion pressure during chest compression
- To stimulate spontaneous or more forceful myocardial contractility
- To accelerate the heart rate
- To correct metabolic acidosis
- To suppress ventricular ectopy (see chapter 7)

Volume Expansion

Hypovolemia (see chapter 2) is the most common cause of shock in children worldwide. It frequently results from inadequate fluid intake in the presence of diarrhea, diabetic ketoacidosis, or vomiting or from sudden large volume losses associated with burns or trauma. Although septic, anaphylactic, neurogenic, and so-called distributive forms of shock are not usually classified as hypovolemic shock, all are characterized in large part by relative hypovolemia that results from vasodilation, increased capillary permeability, and plasma loss into the interstitium. All forms of shock except cardiogenic shock require volume administration during initial therapy. Therefore, vascular access must be rapidly established with a large-bore, short-length intravascular catheter. Subsequently at least two large-bore vascular catheters must be secured to provide optimal routes for fluid resuscitation (see chapter 5).

The ideal fluid for volume expansion in children with hypovolemic shock is debatable. Isotonic crystalloid solutions, such as lactated Ringer's and normal saline, are inexpensive and readily available and do not produce allergic reactions. These crystalloid solutions effectively expand the interstitial water space and correct sodium deficits, but they only transiently expand the intravascular (circulating) volume, since only approximately one fourth of administered isotonic crystalloid solution remains in the intravascular compartment for more than a few minutes.[1] A large quantity of crystalloid solution (potentially four or five times the deficit) must therefore be infused to restore intravascular volume. Rapid infusion of this quantity is well tolerated by healthy young patients but may cause pulmonary edema in the critically ill child with underlying cardiac or pulmonary disease.

Colloid solutions remain in the intravascular compartment hours longer than crystalloid solutions.[1] As a result, blood and colloid solutions, such as 5% albumin, fresh frozen plasma, and synthetic colloid solutions (eg, hetastarch, dextran 40, dextran 60) are much more efficient volume expanders than crystalloid solutions. However, the colloid solutions may cause sensitivity reactions and other complications (see below). At least one type of colloid solution should be readily available for resuscitation of children with signs of shock.

Blood products should be administered only when specifically indicated for replacement of blood loss or correction of coagulopathies. Blood and blood products may be useful in the treatment of nontraumatic hypovolemic shock but are not the first choice for volume expansion, because the risk of blood-borne infection cannot be eliminated.[2]

Blood *is* the ideal fluid replacement for volume losses sustained by pediatric trauma victims who demonstrate evidence of hypovolemic shock despite two boluses of crystalloid solution (ie, 40 mL/kg total). Under these circumstances blood should be administered as soon as it is available. Occasionally O-negative blood may be administered upon physician order before crossmatch. Blood component therapy may also be valuable in the correction of coagulopathies, although such treatment may be palliative until the cause of the coagulopathy is identified and treated.

Rapid infusion of blood or blood products, particularly in large volumes, may produce several complications.[2] Hypothermia caused by rapid administration of cold blood products can complicate the management of the trauma or submersion victim who already demonstrates hypothermia from exposure to the environment. Hypothermia adversely affects cardiovascular function and compromises several metabolic functions, including the metabolism of citrate, which is present in stored blood. Inadequate citrate clearance, in turn, causes ionized hypocalcemia. The combined effects of hypothermia and ionized hypocalcemia can result in significant myocardial dysfunction. To minimize these problems, blood and blood products should be warmed before rapid IV administration.

Hypovolemic shock results from depletion of intravascular and extravascular volume. If hypovolemia is severe or sustained, vascular tone may decrease and capillary permeability may increase, resulting in greater depletion of intravascular volume. As a result, volume administration must exceed estimated volume losses to replace the transcapillary fluid loss and fill the expanded vascular compartment.

Volume therapy is indicated when a child demonstrates signs of shock (eg, mottled or pale color, cool skin, diminished peripheral pulses, delayed capillary refill despite normal ambient temperature, mental status change, oliguria). Shock may be present despite a "normal" blood pressure. Prompt and effective treatment of early signs of compensated shock may prevent the development of hypotension (decompensated shock) and associated high morbidity and mortality.

Successful fluid therapy requires frequent patient assessment and infusion of a sufficient volume of fluid to restore effective systemic perfusion. When signs of hypovolemic shock are detected, a fluid bolus is administered and the child's response is assessed. Additional fluid, usually administered in bolus form, should be provided (if needed) until systemic perfusion improves and signs of shock are corrected. Each bolus of fluid should be followed by assessment of systemic perfusion to determine the effectiveness of therapy and the need for additional therapy. Volume replacement is often insufficient during the initial resuscitation of children with shock.[3] Volume administration must be continued until signs of shock are no longer observed.

Bolus fluid resuscitation therapy consists of 20 mL/kg of isotonic crystalloid solution administered as rapidly as possible (in less than 20 minutes) immediately after intravascular or intraosseous access is obtained. Ringer's lactate solution or normal saline is appropriate for initial crystalloid infusion. Large volumes of dextrose-containing solutions should *not* be infused during resuscitation because hyperglycemia may induce osmotic diuresis, produce or aggravate hypokalemia, and worsen ischemic brain injury.[4-8] The mini-drip IV systems used for pediatric fluid therapy may not allow rapid bolus fluid administration. However, placement of a three-way stopcock "in-line" in the intravenous tubing system can facilitate rapid fluid delivery. A 35- to 50-mL syringe can be used to push fluids via this stopcock. The child should be reassessed immediately after a bolus infusion. If signs of shock persist, a second 20-mL/kg bolus should be administered. Additional volume boluses, either colloid or crystalloid, should be infused as indicated by repeated assessments

of the patient. A child with hypovolemic shock often requires 40 to 60 mL/kg during the first hour of resuscitation, and as much as 200 mL/kg may occasionally be required during the first few hours of therapy. When septic shock is present, 60 to 80 mL/kg is often required during the first hour of therapy.[3] When children are seriously injured, hemorrhage may produce ongoing volume loss, requiring urgent surgical intervention. The need for surgical intervention should always be considered in these patients.

The efficacy of intravenous volume administration as part of resuscitation after *cardiac arrest* is controversial. In normovolemic adult animal models, volume administration has been shown to decrease myocardial perfusion by elevating right atrial pressure and decreasing coronary perfusion pressure.[9,10] However, these studies may not apply to pediatric patients with hypovolemic cardiac arrest. During resuscitation, bolus administration of normal saline as indicated by clinical examination is preferable to continuous infusion of a large volume of saline. Administration of a crystalloid bolus (20 mL/kg) should be considered during the resuscitation of the child with prehospital cardiac arrest of unknown or suspicious cause if that child fails to respond to provision of adequate oxygenation, ventilation, chest compressions, and epinephrine. Occasionally, unsuspected child abuse and internal hemorrhage are responsible for hypovolemic shock, which may respond to volume administration plus standard resuscitation therapy. Excessive volume administration should be avoided because it may compromise vital organ blood flow.[9]

Acid-Base Balance

Buffer Systems

Acid-base balance is normally maintained by several buffer systems. A *buffer* is a chemical substance present in a solution such as plasma that decreases the change in pH that would otherwise occur after addition of an acid or a base. Physiologic buffers are usually composed of a weak acid and its alkali salt (eg, H_2CO_3 and HCO_3^-; $H_2PO_4^-$ and HPO_4^{-2}). Note that an acid is a proton (hydrogen ion) donor and a base is a proton (hydrogen ion) acceptor.

The bicarbonate buffer system is the most important system for modulation of rapid changes in pH. Other important buffer systems include proteins, phosphate, and hemoglobin. The bicarbonate–carbonic acid buffer is unique because its acid form (H_2CO_3) is volatile. When the bicarbonate anion reacts with an acid, the CO_2 produced can be excreted by ventilation. This enables complete neutralization of a metabolic acid to its (neutral) salt. Note, however, that ventilation *must* be adequate to permit the lungs to eliminate the CO_2 formed.[11]

The negative logarithm of the H^+ concentration in the blood is expressed as pH. Therefore, a pH of 7 indicates an H^+ concentration of 10^{-7} moles per liter, or 0.0000001 mol/L. Since the pH is inversely related to the logarithm of the H^+ concentration, changes in pH of similar magnitude are not associated with parallel changes in H^+. Decreases in pH are associated with numerically larger changes in H^+ concentration than are increases in pH.

The quantity of bicarbonate required to correct abnormalities in pH must be larger than the magnitude of change occurring in the H^+ concentration. The apparent discrepancy between the dose of bicarbonate infused and the calculated buffer needed to decrease H^+ concentration reflects the efficiency of the other buffer systems, such as intracellular proteins, hemoglobin, and phosphate, in buffering changes in H^+ concentration.

Acidosis and Alkalosis

The normal arterial pH is 7.40, with a range of 7.35 to 7.45. A pH below 7.35 indicates acidemia, and a pH above 7.45 indicates alkalemia. Alterations of acid-base balance may be respiratory or metabolic in origin. These changes in pH are reflected by changes in the concentration of carbon dioxide and sodium bicarbonate. The relation of pH to these alterations is approximated by the following equation:

$$pH \approx \frac{Base}{Acid} \approx \frac{HCO_3^-}{H_2CO_3} \approx \frac{20}{1}$$

Carbonic acid (H_2CO_3), the denominator in the ratio above, is directly related to $PaCO_2$. An increase in $PaCO_2$ produces an increase in H_2CO_3, a diminished base-acid ratio, and therefore a lower pH.

Respiratory-induced alterations of pH result from changes in $PaCO_2$, which reflects the ventilatory status of the patient. Normal values of $PaCO_2$ are 35 to 45 mm Hg. As alveolar ventilation increases, $PaCO_2$ decreases, lowering H_2CO_3 and increasing the ratio of base to acid, so the pH rises. This is defined as respiratory alkalosis.

A $PaCO_2$ above 45 mm Hg indicates the presence of alveolar hypoventilation and respiratory acidosis. Alveolar hypoventilation may be present despite tachypnea, because rapid breathing may be inefficient and associated with low tidal volume. Such tachypnea increases dead-space ventilation and reduces alveolar ventilation and is especially likely to develop in critically ill infants and small children.

Compensation by the respiratory or metabolic system complicates the interpretation of respiratory or metabolic changes in acid-base balance. The patient with shock and lactic acidosis and bicarbonate depletion may exhibit respiratory compensation by hyperventilating to decrease the partial pressure of carbon dioxide ($PaCO_2$). Decreased $PaCO_2$ lowers H_2CO_3, thus maintaining the ratio of base to acid near 20:1 and minimizing changes in pH. This condition is consistent with a primary metabolic acidosis and a compensatory respiratory alkalosis. It is important to note that physiologic compensatory mechanisms never "overcorrect" the pH. For example, renal compensation for chronic respiratory acidosis will correct the pH to *near* normal but will not create an alkalotic pH.

Blood Gas Interpretation

The therapeutic approach to evaluation of acid-base balance is simplified by the application of three rules.

Rule I estimates the impact of changes in $PaCO_2$ on the measured pH.

- **Rule I:** An *acute* change in $PaCO_2$ of 1 mm Hg is associated with an increase or a decrease in pH of 0.008 units.

Thus, when the $PaCO_2$ increases by 10 mm Hg, the pH decreases by 0.08 units.

In application, if the $PaCO_2$ is 40 mm Hg, the pH will be 7.40 (normal) in the absence of metabolic acidosis or alkalosis. However, if the $PaCO_2$ increases to 50 mm Hg acutely, the pH decreases to 7.32, indicating the presence of alveolar hypoventilation and respiratory acidosis. Should the $PaCO_2$ fall acutely to 30 mm Hg, the pH will rise to 7.48, indicating alveolar hyperventilation or respiratory alkalosis.

To assess the respiratory component of acid-base balance from arterial blood gas analysis, the following steps may be used:

1. Calculate the amount by which the reported $PaCO_2$ either falls below or exceeds 40 mm Hg. Subtract the patient's $PaCO_2$ from 40 mm Hg.
2. Predict the pH based on the measured $PaCO_2$ according to Rule I.
3. Compare the measured pH with the predicted pH (step 2).
   - If the predicted pH is equal to the measured pH, all changes in the pH are respiratory in origin.
   - If the measured pH is *greater* than the predicted pH, an associated *metabolic alkalosis* is present.
   - If the measured pH is *less* than that predicted from the $PaCO_2$, an associated *metabolic acidosis* is present.

Treatment of respiratory acidosis is essential in the care of critically ill or injured children. Establishment of a secure airway and hyperventilation with 100% oxygen will decrease the $PaCO_2$ and improve systemic arterial oxygenation to help correct the tissue acidosis. Respiratory acidosis is not treated by administration of sodium bicarbonate. Any effective buffering action by sodium bicarbonate requires adequate ventilation so that the carbon dioxide formed from the $HCO_3^- + H^+$ reaction can be eliminated.[11]

Rule II provides a reasonably accurate method of estimating the magnitude of the metabolic component of any existing acidosis or alkalosis.

- **Rule II:** A pH change of 0.01 units is the result of a base change of 0.67 mEq/L.

Thus, if pH increases by 0.15 units, there is an increase in base of 10 mEq/L. Conversely, if pH falls 0.15 units, there is a decrease in base of 10 mEq/L.

Stated differently, for every 0.01 unit change in pH that is not caused by a change in $PaCO_2$, there is a 0.67 mEq/L change in the base concentration. Thus, a 0.09-unit decrease in pH not caused by a change in $PaCO_2$ results from a decrease of 6 mEq/L (9 x 0.67 mEq/L) in base (bicarbonate, or HCO_3^-).

Base excess and *base deficit* are terms used to describe the amount of base in relation to the amount of fixed acid present in the blood sample. The base excess or base deficit is a *calculated* rather than a *measured* value, indicating the theoretical amount of acid or base that must be added to the blood to restore a normal pH. Since the effects of carbonic acid are not reflected in the calculation, changes in the base deficit or excess are metabolic rather than respiratory in origin. The value is expressed in milliequivalents per liter, with a normal range of –2 to +2 mEq/L.

- A *positive* number reflects a base *excess,* ie, an excess of base. If the base excess is greater than +2 mEq/L, metabolic alkalosis is present, and the magnitude of the base excess (in mEq/L) reflects the milliequivalents of base that must be removed (or neutralized by acid) per liter of blood to restore a normal pH.
- A *negative* number reflects a base *deficit,* a deficit of base. If the base deficit is more negative than –2 mEq/L, metabolic acidosis is present, and the magnitude of the base deficit (in mEq/L) reflects the milliequivalents of base per liter of blood that must be added to restore a normal pH.

Base excess or base deficit is calculated by multiplying the difference between actual pH and the pH predicted from the $PaCO_2$ by 67. The *predicted* pH is always subtracted from the *actual* pH before multiplying the difference by 67. If the actual pH is lower than the predicted pH, the pH difference will be a negative number, indicating a base deficit and the presence of metabolic acidosis.

Example 1: Consider the patient with a $PaCO_2$ of 50 mm Hg and a pH of 7.26.

- According to Rule I, the 10 mm Hg rise in $PaCO_2$ above 40 mm Hg indicates respiratory acidosis. If the hypercarbia is uncomplicated by the presence of metabolic acidosis or alkalosis, the actual pH can be predicted from the $PaCO_2$. The 10 mm Hg rise in $PaCO_2$ is expected to decrease a normal pH of 7.40 by 0.08 units (10 × 0.008), for a predicted pH of 7.32.
- However, the actual pH is 7.26.
- The difference between the predicted and the actual pH is then determined (using Rule II) to quantify the base excess or deficit.

— The predicted pH of 7.32 is subtracted from the actual pH of 7.26, resulting in a negative number, –0.06 units, indicating a base deficit and the presence of a metabolic acidosis.
— The magnitude of the base deficit is calculated by multiplying –0.06 × 67 (every 0.01 unit change in pH results from a base change of 0.67 mEq/L).
— Since the pH has changed –0.06 units or –6 × 0.01 units, the base deficit will result from the product of –0.06 × 100 × 0.67, or –0.06 × 67).
— The base deficit is –4.02 mEq/L, rounded to –4 mEq/L, indicating the presence of metabolic acidosis.

- Therefore, the patient demonstrates combined *respiratory* and *metabolic* acidosis.

The substantial base deficit typically observed during cardiac arrest is caused by loss of bicarbonate ions through the buffering of fixed acids. Bicarbonate is located primarily in the *extracellular* fluid compartment, which constitutes approximately 30% of body weight (ie, 0.3 × body weight).[12] This distribution of bicarbonate (0.3 × kg weight) may be used to calculate bicarbonate therapy using Rule III.

- **Rule III:** The total body bicarbonate deficit equals the base deficit (mEq/L) × the patient's weight (in kg) × 0.3.

Example 2: Consider a 25-kg patient with a $PaCO_2$ of 40 mm Hg and a pH of 7.18.

- The $PaCO_2$ is normal. The predicted pH is 7.4.
- The unexplained pH difference of –0.22 units (7.18 minus 7.40) must be attributed to a metabolic acidosis with a calculated base deficit of –14.7 mEq/L (–0.22 × 67).
- Respiratory compensation may be created using mechanical ventilation, and the metabolic acidosis may be partially treated with bicarbonate according to Rule III. Since the base deficit is –14.7 mEq/mL and extracellular fluid equals 30% of body weight, the bicarbonate dose in milliequivalents is calculated as follows:

Base deficit	×	Weight (kg)	×	Distribution of bicarbonate	=	Dose of bicarbonate (mEq)
14.7	×	25	×	0.3	=	100 mEq

Complete correction of the calculated base deficit is not indicated, so generally one fourth to one half of the calculated dose of bicarbonate is administered. One fourth of the calculated dose is approximately equal to a bicarbonate dose of 1 mEq/kg — the dose most frequently used for the treatment of moderate metabolic acidosis. Mechanical ventilation and mild hyperventilation should be used to correct the acidosis. Additional bicarbonate administration may be considered if significant metabolic acidosis persists.

General Guidelines for Administration of Medications

The venous system is the preferred route for drug administration in emergencies but may be difficult to access.[13,14] When venous access is not available, the endotracheal route can be used to deliver epinephrine, atropine, naloxone, and lidocaine.[15] Optimal doses of drugs given by the endotracheal route in pediatric patients have not been established. Some studies suggest that an endotracheal dose must be larger than a conventional IV dose to produce hemodynamic effects similar to those achieved with IV drug administration,[16-19] although clinical data in humans with cardiac arrest is limited.[20] In the absence of definitive *pediatric* data, the current recommended IV dose should be considered the *minimum* dose recommended for endotracheal administration; doses higher than those administered intravenously are often required. To be absorbed, endotracheal medications must be delivered beyond the endotracheal tube into the tracheobronchial tree.[18,21] This delivery is best achieved by diluting the medication to a volume of 3 to 5 mL of normal saline and instilling it into the endotracheal tube.[18,22] Alternatively, the drug may be instilled through a catheter that has been passed beyond the distal tip of the endotracheal tube. The medication must be followed by a flush of 3 to 5 mL of normal saline. Endotracheal drug administration must be followed by several positive-pressure ventilations using a hand resuscitation bag.

During external chest compressions, central venous administration of medications may theoretically provide a more rapid onset and a higher peak concentration than peripheral venous injection.[23,24] In a single study of adult animals, drug injection into the central supradiaphragmatic venous system achieved better drug delivery into the circulation than IV injection below the diaphragm.[25] However, these differences have not been demonstrated in pediatric resuscitation models[26] and may not be important during pediatric CPR. In a pediatric animal model, drug infusion into a peripheral vein provided drug distribution comparable to that achieved by central venous administration.[26] Since it is not clear whether the site of injection is important during resuscitation of the infant or small child, either peripheral or central venous drug administration is acceptable. If the peripheral route is used, drugs should be followed by a saline flush of at least 5 mL to move the drug from the peripheral to the central circulation.

Medications, including catecholamines, are well absorbed from the bone marrow[27-29] (see chapter 5). Therefore, intraosseous infusion can be considered equivalent to IV injection and is preferable to the endotracheal route for drug administration during resuscitation of children, particularly those 6 years of age and younger.

Direct intracardiac injections should *not* be performed because they are associated with significant complications, including coronary artery laceration, cardiac tamponade, and intractable arrhythmias. In addition, intracardiac injections require interruption of cardiac compressions.

Catecholamines (epinephrine, dopamine, dobutamine, isoproterenol) may be diluted in a number of IV solutions for continuous infusion, including 5% dextrose and water, normal saline, or Ringer's lactate solution. When drug infusion is initiated, the IV tubing should be flushed with the catecholamine solution to the point where the IV tubing joins the vascular catheter. Initially a rapid infusion is provided (eg, up to 20 mL/h) until the heart rate increases, indicating response to the arrival of the catecholamine in the patient's circulation. The infusion rate can then be reduced and the dose titrated to produce desired effects. The initial rapid infusion rate will prevent any delay in the delivery of the medication to the patient through the tubing dead space. Alternatively, the catecholamine infusion may be joined ("piggy-backed") to another IV crystalloid infusion that is administered at a rapid rate, resulting in prompt delivery of the drug to the patient. All catecholamines are metabolized rapidly, so titration of the infusion rate based on patient cardiovascular response (including heart rate) should prevent undesirable side effects. Drug tables, charts, or tapes should be readily available. Length-based resuscitation tapes eliminate the need for estimation of weight or age or for calculations.

Resuscitation Medications

Epinephrine

Therapeutic Considerations

Epinephrine (adrenaline) is an endogenous catecholamine with α- and β-adrenergic effects.[30,31] α-Adrenergic action (vasoconstriction) increases systemic vascular resistance and elevates the systolic and diastolic blood pressure. In addition, α-adrenergic vasoconstriction reduces blood flow to the splanchnic, renal, mucosal, and dermal vascular beds. β-Adrenergic receptor action increases myocardial contractility and heart rate and relaxes smooth muscle in the skeletal muscle vascular bed and in bronchi.

Epinephrine has been successfully used in the treatment of cardiac arrest for many years. α-Adrenergic effect (vasoconstriction) is the most important action of epinephrine when used in this setting,[32,33] because blood pressure and coronary perfusion pressure are elevated, enhancing delivery of oxygen to the heart. This appears to be the most important action of sympathomimetics in the treatment of cardiac arrest.[34] In animal models of cardiac arrest, epinephrine administration increases blood supply to the myocardium and the brain.[35]

The following cardiovascular effects can be expected after epinephrine administration in the doses used during resuscitation:

- Increased cardiac automaticity
- Increased heart rate
- Increased myocardial contractility
- Increased systemic vascular resistance
- Increased blood pressure (due to increased myocardial contractility and increased systemic vascular resistance)
- Increased myocardial oxygen requirements (due to increased heart rate, increased myocardial contractility, and increased systemic vascular resistance)

Clinically epinephrine elevates perfusion pressure generated during chest compressions, improves the myocardial contractile state, stimulates spontaneous contraction (eg, in asystole), and increases the vigor of ventricular fibrillation. The latter effect appears to enhance the ability to terminate ventricular fibrillation by electrical defibrillation. In addition, during resuscitation epinephrine directs blood flow to the brain and heart.[36,37]

Indications

- Cardiac arrest
- Symptomatic bradycardia unresponsive to ventilation and oxygen administration
- Hypotension not related to volume depletion

The elevation of coronary perfusion pressure associated with epinephrine administration makes this drug useful in the treatment of almost all forms of cardiac arrest.

The most common presenting rhythms in pediatric patients with cardiac arrest are asystole and brady-arrhythmias.[38] In these settings epinephrine may stimulate electrical and mechanical activity of the heart. Although ventricular fibrillation is uncommon in young children,[39-41] the use of epinephrine in children with ventricular fibrillation may render the rhythm more susceptible to electrical defibrillation.[30,32]

Acidosis may depress the action of catecholamines.[42] Therefore, metabolic acidosis should be corrected with oxygen administration, hyperventilation, and restoration of systemic perfusion. Because sodium bicarbonate inactivates catecholamines, it should not be infused into a line containing catecholamines.

Dose

The recommended initial IV or intraosseous dose of epinephrine for symptomatic bradycardia (with a pulse) unresponsive to oxygen and adequate ventilation is 0.01 mg/kg (0.1 mL/kg of the 1:10 000 solution).

The dismal outcome of prehospital, pulseless, normothermic pediatric cardiac arrest has been documented in several studies.[43,44] Survival is uncommon if the pediatric victim remains pulseless after 10 minutes of BLS and ALS and two doses of epinephrine.[44,45] Consideration of

these outcome data plus information from animal studies and one pediatric study prompted a revision of recommended epinephrine doses for the treatment of pediatric pulseless, normothermic cardiac arrest in the 1992 AHA guidelines.[46]

Animal studies have documented improved cerebral and myocardial perfusion and more frequent return of spontaneous circulation after administration of higher doses of epinephrine than previously recommended.[47] However, adult clinical trials did not confirm the beneficial effect of high-dose epinephrine.[48,49] Use of a high epinephrine dose (0.2 mg/kg) was associated with improved survival and neurological outcome (compared with a historical control population) in a *single* study of 20 children with pulseless cardiac arrest (asystole or electromechanical dissociation).[50] These children experienced *witnessed* cardiac arrest and received ALS within 7 minutes.

Because a beneficial effect of a high epinephrine dose has been documented in only one study, the first IV or intraosseous dose of epinephrine for pulseless arrest remains 0.01 mg/kg (0.1 mL of the 1:10 000 solution). If pulseless cardiac arrest persists, the second and subsequent IV or intraosseous doses of epinephrine should be 0.1 mg/kg (0.1 mL/kg of the 1:1000 solution). Doses as high as 0.2 mg/kg may be beneficial.[50] Epinephrine administration should be repeated every 3 to 5 minutes during resuscitation.

Epinephrine is absorbed from the tracheobronchial tree, although in a human study of adult cardiac arrest, endotracheal delivery produced peak blood levels less than one tenth the peak blood level achieved with IV administration.[20] Similar results have been reported in nonarrest adult animal studies.[51,52] Unfortunately, very little data exists regarding endotracheal drug absorption in pediatric victims of cardiac arrest. The recommended endotracheal epinephrine dose is 0.1 mg/kg (0.1 mL/kg of the 1:1000 solution). This dose of epinephrine should be diluted with normal saline to a volume of 3 to 5 mL and instilled into the endotracheal tube. Alternatively, the drug may be delivered beyond the tip of the endotracheal tube by instillation through a suction catheter followed by a 3- to 5-mL flush of normal saline. Following endotracheal drug administration, several positive-pressure breaths must be provided. Once vascular access is achieved, epinephrine should be administered intravenously (begin with the first intravenous dose — 0.01 mg/kg of 1:10 000).

It is important to note that the *volume* of epinephrine administered is 0.1 mL/kg whether conventional or high-dose epinephrine is provided. The *dose* of epinephrine is determined by the concentration of the drug (conventional dose = 0.1 mL/kg of 1:10 000, and high dose = 0.1 mL/kg of 1:1000). All endotracheal doses of epinephrine are high dose (0.1 mg/kg of 1:1000).

Precautions

Since the new dosing recommendations require the use of two different dilutions of epinephrine, care must be taken to avoid errors in concentration selection and dosing. The patient should be closely monitored during epinephrine therapy for side effects, including postresuscitation hypertension and tachyarrhythmias. Epinephrine should not be added to a bicarbonate infusion since catecholamines are inactivated by an alkaline solution.

Available Preparations

Prefilled syringes of the 1:10 000 solution are recommended for intravenous or intraosseous administration during resuscitation of bradycardia and for the first dose of epinephrine in asystole. These syringes are available in 3-mL (0.1 mg/mL) and 10-mL (0.1 mg/mL) volumes.

Preparations of 1:1000 solutions of epinephrine should be available for epinephrine administered by the endotracheal route and for high-dose intravenous or intraosseous treatment of pulseless arrest. This epinephrine concentration is available in 1-mL and 2-mL syringes and 30-mL (1 mg/mL) vials.

Sodium Bicarbonate

Therapeutic Considerations

During cardiopulmonary arrest, acidosis of mixed metabolic and respiratory origin develops. Hypoxia-induced anaerobic metabolism generates lactic acid and metabolic acidosis. In addition, ventilatory failure causes carbon dioxide retention (hypercarbia) and respiratory acidosis. Arterial oxygen tension (PaO_2), arterial carbon dioxide tension ($PaCO_2$), and hydrogen ion (H^+) concentration (reflected by pH) are directly measured from arterial blood. Although PaO_2 is used to evaluate arterial oxygen content, only pH and $PaCO_2$ are important in determination of acid-base balance.

Metabolic acids, derived from intermediary metabolism of amino acids, fats, and carbohydrates, are normally excreted by the kidney. Renal perfusion is inadequate in the presence of shock or cardiac arrest, so acid excretion is insufficient. In addition, lactic acid produced during anaerobic metabolism cannot be metabolized until oxygen delivery to tissues is restored.

Acidosis detected during resuscitation is ideally corrected through the restoration of effective ventilation and systemic perfusion. Treatment of mild-to-moderate metabolic acidosis usually requires only hyperventilation and treatment of shock to restore effective tissue oxygenation and perfusion.

In Example 2 earlier in the chapter, if hyperventilation reduced the $PaCO_2$ to 30 mm Hg, the pH would rise to 7.26. The administration of bicarbonate could correct the pH to near normal levels, although restoration of perfusion is usually sufficient to correct the acidosis.

Although pH changes are measured in plasma, intracellular changes in pH are likely to affect physiologic homeostasis more significantly. Changes in $PaCO_2$ will alter the pH of cerebrospinal fluid much more rapidly

and profoundly than changes in plasma HCO_3^- concentration.[53] The same phenomenon occurs across cellular membranes: increases in $PaCO_2$ depress cardiac function more than decreases in pH produced by accumulation of fixed acids.[54] Bicarbonate administration may transiently depress cardiac function, presumably on the basis of a transient increase in $PaCO_2$ and intracellular PCO_2 with a depression of intracellular pH.[55] Bicarbonate administration in the presence of lactic acidosis has been shown to depress intracellular pH in hepatocytes.[56] These studies emphasize the importance of ventilation in the acute management of the child with acidosis accompanying cardiac arrest or shock. Sodium bicarbonate is *not* a first-line drug for resuscitation.

Indications

Since respiratory failure is the major cause of cardiac arrest in the pediatric patient,[41,44] prompt and efficient establishment of effective ventilation is essential for the management of acidosis and hypoxemia. The primary treatment of metabolic acidosis includes hyperventilation to reduce the $PaCO_2$ and volume resuscitation and/or vasoactive support to improve systemic perfusion. Sodium bicarbonate administration during resuscitation has not been shown to improve survival.[57] In fact, sodium bicarbonate may reduce coronary artery perfusion pressure.[58]

Administration of sodium bicarbonate results in a reaction in which the HCO_3^- ion combines with H^+ ions in the blood, thereby elevating the plasma pH:

$$HCO_3^- + H^+ \rightarrow H_2CO_3 \rightarrow CO_2 + H_2O$$

Note that carbon dioxide is formed as H^+ is buffered. Since carbon dioxide can cross cell membranes more rapidly than bicarbonate, the administration of sodium bicarbonate does not improve,[59] and may transiently worsen, intracellular acidosis,[60] impairing myocardial performance.[55,59] Sodium bicarbonate administration in hypoxic lactic acidosis has been shown to lower cardiac index and blood pressure and worsen lactic acidosis.[61] Adult patients with congestive heart failure demonstrate a decline in myocardial performance following bicarbonate administration.[62] In addition, animal models suggest that reperfusion of the postarrest heart with an *acidotic* solution improves myocardial function.[63] In view of the potential adverse effects, sodium bicarbonate is not indicated in the treatment of mild-to-moderate metabolic acidosis, especially if associated with hypovolemia. The acidosis is likely to resolve if adequate volume replacement and ventilatory support are provided. Sodium bicarbonate administration for the treatment of severe acidosis remains controversial. When severe acidosis is associated with cardiac arrest, initial therapy should always include establishment of a patent, secure airway, hyperventilation, chest compressions, and administration of epinephrine. Sodium bicarbonate should be considered only for treatment of documented severe acidosis associated with prolonged cardiac arrest or an unstable hemodynamic state, hyperkalemia, or tricyclic antidepressant overdose.

Dose

The optimal dose of sodium bicarbonate remains controversial. The severity of metabolic acidosis is related to the length of the arrest and is likely to be greater in out-of-hospital arrests than in those occurring in the hospital. Even when cardiac arrest is of long duration (eg, out-of-hospital arrest or an unmonitored hospitalized patient), initial therapy should focus on establishment of a patent airway, ventilation, and restoration of circulation. If cardiac arrest continues after the airway is secured and hyperventilation, chest compressions, and epinephrine administration are accomplished, 1 mEq/kg of sodium bicarbonate may be administered via the IV or intraosseous (*not* endotracheal) route. Further doses of sodium bicarbonate are ideally determined following evaluation of arterial pH and $PaCO_2$ after return of spontaneous circulation. These values may be misleading during cardiac arrest, however, because they appear to reflect the effectiveness of *ventilation* rather than *perfusion,* and they correlate poorly with mixed venous pH and PCO_2.[64,65] When arterial pH and PCO_2 measurements are unavailable or unreliable during prolonged cardiac arrest, subsequent doses of sodium bicarbonate (0.5 mEq/kg) may be administered empirically every 10 minutes by slow (1 to 2 minutes) infusion.

Precautions

Excessive administration of sodium bicarbonate may result in metabolic alkalosis, which produces the following detrimental effects:

- Displacement of the oxyhemoglobin dissociation curve to the left with impaired tissue oxygen delivery[66]
- Acute intracellular shift of potassium with a lowering of serum potassium concentration
- Decreased plasma ionized calcium concentration caused by greater binding of calcium to serum proteins
- Decreased fibrillation threshold[67]
- Sodium and water overload (1 mEq of sodium is delivered with each mEq of bicarbonate)

The standard 8.4% solution of sodium bicarbonate is very hyperosmolar (2000 mOsm/L) compared with plasma (280 mOsm/L), and repeated doses can produce symptomatic hypernatremia and hyperosmolarity[68] as well as transient vasodilation and hypotension.[69] In premature infants, this hyperosmolarity has been correlated with an increased risk for periventricular-intraventricular hemorrhage.[70] For this reason, the 4.2% solution (0.5 mEq/mL) should be used in premature infants.

Carbon dioxide production is transiently increased following sodium bicarbonate administration. This newly formed carbon dioxide can cross the blood-brain barrier and cell membranes much more rapidly than HCO_3^-, causing paradoxical cerebrospinal fluid and intracellular acidosis.[53,56] This is particularly problematic when metabolic acidosis is prolonged (eg, diabetic ketoacidosis).

Intravenous and intraosseous tubing must be irrigated with normal saline before and after infusions of sodium bicarbonate. Catecholamines are very slowly inactivated by, and calcium salts precipitate in, bicarbonate solutions. Since sodium bicarbonate is hyperosmolar, it may sclerose small veins and produce a chemical burn if extravasated into the subcutaneous tissues. Sodium bicarbonate should not be administered into the tracheo-bronchial tree for treatment of metabolic acidosis.

Available Preparations

Sodium bicarbonate is available in prefilled syringes in the following volumes and concentrations:

50 mL of 8.4% solution (1 mEq/mL)
10 mL of 8.4% solution (1 mEq/mL)
10 mL of 4.2% solution (0.5 mEq/mL)

The half-strength solution is typically used for infants younger than 3 months.

Atropine

Therapeutic Considerations

Atropine sulfate is a parasympatholytic drug that accelerates sinus or atrial pacemakers and atrioventricular conduction.

Indications

Symptomatic bradycardia requires support of oxygenation and ventilation. Epinephrine therapy is often indicated. Atropine is used to treat symptomatic bradycardia (ie, associated with poor perfusion or hypotension), to prevent or treat vagally mediated bradycardia accompanying intubation attempts, and to treat the uncommon occurrence of symptomatic bradycardia with atrioventricular block. In any young child, cardiac output is heart rate–dependent, and *symptomatic bradycardia* (heart rate less than 60 beats per minute associated with poor perfusion) must be treated even if blood pressure is normal. Since bradycardia usually results from hypoxemia, initial treatment of such bradycardia must include ventilation and oxygenation rather than the administration of atropine. It is uncertain whether atropine is useful in the treatment of asystole; laboratory and clinical studies have failed to demonstrate its efficacy in cardiac arrest.[71,72] Because the efficacy of atropine administration during cardiac arrest in infants and children is unknown, a vagolytic dose of atropine (see below) may be administered during resuscitative efforts.

Dose

When atropine is administered, the dose must be sufficient to produce vagolytic effects and avoid paradoxical bradycardia.[73] The recommended atropine dose is 0.02 mg/kg with a minimum dose of 0.1 mg and a maximum *single* dose of 0.5 mg for a child and 1.0 mg for an adolescent. This dose may be repeated after 5 minutes for a maximum *total* dose of 1.0 mg for a child and 2.0 mg for an adolescent. Atropine may be administered via the IV, intraosseous, or endotracheal route. The optimal atropine dose for endotracheal administration has not been established. The IV dose may be administered endotracheally, although absorption into the circulation may be unreliable. The IV dose should be increased two to three times and either diluted to a volume of 3 to 5 mL for endotracheal administration or administered via suction catheter beyond the tip of the endotracheal tube and flushed into the lower airways using 3 to 5 mL of normal saline. Following administration of any drug by the endotracheal route, several positive-pressure breaths should be provided.

Precautions

Atropine is generally well tolerated by children, but tachycardia may follow its administration. Low doses of atropine may be accompanied by a paradoxical bradycardia in infants,[73] so the minimum dose (0.1 mg) must be administered. If atropine is administered to block vagal-induced bradycardia during intubation, the development of hypoxemia-induced bradycardia may be masked. Pulse oximetry may enable detection of hypoxemia in this situation.

Atropine will produce pupil dilation, so it may be useful to document the effect of atropine administration on pupil size. Atropine will not affect the pupil constrictive response to light, so pupils should constrict briskly even after atropine administration.

Available Preparations

Prefilled syringes: 10 mL (0.1 mg/mL)
  5 mL (0.1 mg/mL)
Vials: 1 mL (1 mg/mL)

A 0.4 mg/mL preparation of atropine is available but is not practical for resuscitation use.

Naloxone

Therapeutic Considerations

Naloxone hydrochloride, a pure narcotic (opiate) antagonist, reverses the effects of narcotic poisoning, including respiratory depression, sedation, hypotension, and hypoperfusion.[74-76] Naloxone acts rapidly (<2 minutes to onset of drug action) with a 45-minute average duration of action. Even at high doses, naloxone is extremely safe.[77] Initial doses may be repeated at 2-minute intervals until the desired degree of narcotic reversal is achieved. A continuous IV infusion of naloxone may be desirable if the narcotic involved has a longer duration of action than naloxone.[78]

Indications

Naloxone may be used to reverse the effects of narcotic poisoning, including respiratory depression, sedation, hypotension, and hypoperfusion. When a narcotic (opiate) or unknown toxic injection is suspected, the intravenous or intratracheal route of naloxone administration is recommended.[79] No well-controlled studies in infants and children directly compare the efficacy of various routes of administration (intravenous and intratracheal versus intramuscular or subcutaneous). Some concern remains that absorption of intramuscular or subcutaneous medications may be erratic in patients with hypotension or hypoperfusion.

Dose

The currently recommended dose of naloxone is 0.1 mg/kg for infants and children from birth to 5 years of age or up to 20 kg of body weight. Children older than 5 years of age or weighing more than 20 kg may be given 2.0 mg.[79] Naloxone doses ranging from 0.005 to 0.4 mg/kg have been reported in the literature. Continuous IV infusions of 0.04 to 0.16 mg/kg per hour have been well tolerated.[78] Therapy should be titrated to produce the desired effect. This dose will generally achieve *total* reversal of narcotic effects. If total reversal is not required, smaller doses may be used.

Precautions

Even at high doses, naloxone is safe. Rare side effects are generally related to abrupt reversal of narcotic depression and include nausea and vomiting, tachycardia, hypertension, tremulousness, seizures, and cardiac dysrhythmias. Naloxone's short duration of action may result in recurrence of symptoms of narcotic intoxication.[74] Naloxone should be administered with caution immediately after birth to infants of addicted mothers, since it may precipitate abrupt narcotic withdrawal and seizures in these infants.

Available Preparations

Vials: 0.4 mg/mL (1 mL, 10 mL)
  1 mg/mL (2 mL)

Glucose

Therapeutic Considerations

Small infants and chronically ill children have limited glycogen stores that may be rapidly depleted during episodes of cardiopulmonary distress, leading to hypoglycemia. Since clinical signs of hypoglycemia may mimic those of hypoxemia (poor perfusion, diaphoresis, tachycardia, hypothermia, irritability or lethargy, and hypotension), the serum glucose concentration of all unstable infants and children must be closely monitored.

Because glucose is the major metabolic substrate for the neonatal myocardium, hypoglycemia may depress neonatal myocardial function. Although fatty acids normally function as the major metabolic substrate for the myocardium of older infants and children, glucose provides a significant energy source during episodes of ischemia. However, whether glucose administration improves the cardiac function or survival of hypoglycemic children with cardiac arrest is unknown. It would seem reasonable to normalize blood glucose levels when documented hypoglycemia is present. But routine administration of glucose without evaluation of the serum or capillary glucose concentration cannot be recommended.

The effects of hypoglycemia and hyperglycemia on the ischemic brain continue to be evaluated. Data from newborn animal models suggest that the ischemic *neonatal* brain may benefit from glucose administration.[80] Data from adult animal models, however, suggest that the *mature* brain may be harmed by glucose administration,[81] particularly if glucose is administered immediately before or during cardiac arrest and resuscitation.[5,6] Clinical studies in children with severe head injury, submersion, and shock have demonstrated an association between hyperglycemia and poor neurological outcome.[7,8] These studies emphasize the need to evaluate the serum glucose concentration and to avoid routine glucose administration.

Indications

A rapid bedside glucose test should be performed to evaluate the serum glucose concentration of any critically ill or injured infant or young child with cardiorespiratory instability. The glucose level determination should be repeated if the child fails to respond to initial resuscitative measures. Glucose administration should be considered if hypoglycemia is present or the infant or child fails to respond to standard resuscitation measures. If a bedside glucose determination is not available and clinically the infant is at risk for hypoglycemia, empiric treatment with glucose (0.5-1.0 g/kg) can be considered.

Dose

Glucose should be administered in a dose of 0.5 to 1.0 g/kg IV. A maximum concentration of 25% dextrose in water ($D_{25}W$) should be infused via a peripheral vein. Since glucose is supplied as $D_{50}W$, it must be diluted 1:1 with sterile water before peripheral venous administration, resulting in a volume of 2 to 4 mL/kg. A $D_{10}W$ solution can be prepared by diluting the $D_{50}W$ 1:4 with sterile water. If this concentration is used, the resulting volume (5 to 10 mL/kg) should be administered over 20 minutes.

A bolus of 10 to 20 mL/kg of 5% dextrose and normal saline or lactated Ringer's will also provide 0.5 to 1.0 g/kg of glucose to treat documented hypoglycemia in the child requiring volume administration (although glucose-containing solutions are not routinely used for bolus therapy).

Precautions

Hypertonic glucose (eg, $D_{25}W$ or $D_{50}W$) is very hyperosmolar and may sclerose peripheral veins. Repeated administration of hypertonic glucose may result in hyperglycemia and an increase in serum osmolality. These changes have been associated with poor outcome in children with severe head injury,[7] submersion,[8] and shock.

In general, the concentration of glucose administered to neonates should not exceed 12.5%.

Available Preparations

Glucose is available in vials and prefilled syringes:
  50 mL of $D_{50}W$ (0.5 g/mL)
  Dilute 1:1 with sterile water to make $D_{25}W$.

Calcium Chloride

Therapeutic Considerations

Calcium is essential to excitation-contraction coupling. When cardiac muscle cells are excited, calcium ions enter the cytoplasm and induce the coupling of actin and myosin. This event is terminated when calcium ions are actively pumped out of the cytoplasm. In normal hearts calcium increases myocardial contractile function. In the presence of myocardial ischemia, energy sources are depleted and this pumping mechanism may be compromised, allowing calcium to accumulate in the cytoplasm. This hypercalcemia may have toxic consequence.

Approximately half of intravascular calcium is ionized. This physiologically active portion must be considered when evaluating the child's calcium balance. The plasma ionized calcium is affected by pH and serum albumin concentration because these factors affect calcium binding to protein. Acidosis increases the plasma ionized calcium, and alkalosis decreases the plasma ionized calcium. Although a fall in serum albumin concentration is associated with a decrease in total calcium, the ionized calcium concentration may remain normal because a smaller amount of calcium is bound to protein. Conversely, although a rise in serum albumin is associated with a rise in total calcium concentration, the ionized calcium concentration may be inadequate because more calcium is bound to protein.[82,83]

Septic shock and blood transfusions have also been linked with alterations in serum ionized calcium. Children with septic shock may demonstrate a decrease in serum ionized calcium despite a normal total serum calcium.[44,84] The serum ionized calcium may also fall after administration of blood preserved with citrate-phosphate-dextran.[82,83,85]

Inotropic effects of calcium following cardiac arrest were initially documented in cardiovascular surgical patients after cardiopulmonary bypass.[86] However, studies have shown that calcium entry into the cell cytoplasm is the final common pathway of cell death,[87] and calcium administration during cardiac arrest may actually cause injury.[88] The deleterious effects of calcium are also suggested by the salutary effects of calcium channel blockers in myocardial preservation during cardiopulmonary bypass.[89]

Indications

Calcium is not recommended for the treatment of either asystole or electromechanical dissociation.[46] No evidence supports its use in asystole, and its value in the treatment of electromechanical dissociation is questionable.[90] Evidence also suggests that administration of an adrenergic drug is much more effective than calcium in the treatment of electromechanical dissociation.[91]

Calcium therapy is indicated for treatment of documented or suspected hypocalcemia, hyperkalemia,[83] hypermagnesemia, and calcium channel blocker overdose.[92]

Dose

Calcium is available as three different salts. Calcium chloride or calcium gluconate will effectively correct hypocalcemia, provided that each delivers an equivalent dose of elemental calcium. Calcium gluconate (10%) contains approximately 9 mg/mL of elemental calcium, and calcium chloride (10%) contains approximately 27.2 mg/mL of elemental calcium. The dose and volume of calcium gluconate must be three times the dose and volume of calcium chloride to provide an equivalent dose of elemental calcium. Calcium chloride is most commonly used in critically ill children[93] and adults[94] and appears to produce consistently higher and more predictable levels of elemental calcium when administered to correct hypocalcemia.[93,94]

The current recommended dose of 5 to 7 mg/kg of elemental calcium for treatment of hypocalcemia is extrapolated from adult data and limited pediatric data.[93,94] Calcium chloride is a 10% solution (100 mg/mL of the calcium salt) that contains 1.36 mEq/mL elemental calcium (27.2 mg/mL elemental calcium). Therefore, a dose of 0.2 to 0.25 mL/kg calcium chloride will deliver 5 to 7 mg/kg elemental calcium (20 to 25 mg/kg calcium salt). The first dose of calcium should be infused *slowly* (no faster than 100 mg/min) and repeated once after 10 minutes, if required. Since repeated doses of calcium increase the risk of morbidity, the dose should be repeated only if *measured* calcium deficiency, particularly plasma ionized calcium deficiency, is present.

Precautions

Rapid calcium administration may induce significant bradycardia and even cardiac asystole, especially if the patient is receiving digoxin. Calcium forms an insoluble precipitate in the presence of sodium bicarbonate. It can sclerose peripheral veins and produce a severe chemical burn if the medication infiltrates into surrounding tissue.

Available Preparations

Prefilled syringes: 10 mL calcium chloride, 10% (100 mg/mL = 27.2 mg elemental calcium/mL)

For drugs used in the treatment of arrhythmias, see chapter 7.

Medications for Postresuscitation Hemodynamic Stabilization

The choice of drugs in the postarrest setting should be individualized for each patient, and there is no consensus about drug selection. It is important to keep in mind the goals of initial therapy — restoration of adequate blood pressure and effective perfusion and correction of hypoxemia and acidosis. These goals are vital to neurologic preservation after a hypoxic-ischemic insult. Therefore, the most potent drugs should be used initially to stabilize the patient. If the patient improves, less potent agents can be substituted. Figure 1 summarizes this approach to stabilization of the postarrest patient in shock.

Postarrest patients are often poorly perfused, hypotensive, and acidotic. After a cardiac arrest, the most common reason for poor perfusion is cardiogenic shock[95] resulting from arrest-associated myocardial ischemia. Some patients may also demonstrate poor lung compliance, which makes positive-pressure ventilation difficult. In all patients, attention should be focused on support of effective ventilation, oxygenation, and perfusion.

The treatment for poor tissue perfusion is determined by the patient's hemodynamic state. In all patients, it is reasonable to consider careful administration of a fluid bolus of 10 to 20 mL/kg over several minutes with close monitoring. If the patient's lung compliance deteriorates or pulmonary edema develops, ventilation must be supported and the need for fluid administration must be reevaluated.

Three inotropic agents are commonly used in the postarrest setting — dopamine, dobutamine, and epinephrine. Although dopamine is often the drug of choice for adults, epinephrine is the drug of choice for pediatric patients during and immediately following resuscitation.

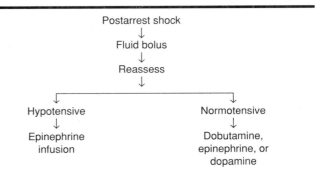

Fig 1. Approach to medications for postresuscitation hemodynamic stabilization.

These medications are administered as continuous infusions following initial resuscitation and return of spontaneous circulation. They are intended to improve blood pressure or systemic perfusion. They should not be mixed for prolonged periods with sodium bicarbonate or other alkaline solutions.

Epinephrine Infusion

Therapeutic Considerations

The actions of epinephrine were summarized earlier in this chapter. Epinephrine is a potent catecholamine that acts directly on the adrenergic receptors rather than through a release of stored norepinephrine. Epinephrine has dose-related actions. Low-dose infusions (less than approximately 0.3 µg/kg per minute) are primarily associated with β-adrenergic effects,[30] including an increase in myocardial contractility, heart rate, pulse pressure, and systolic blood pressure. As the infusion is increased beyond approximately 0.3 µg/kg per minute, α-adrenergic effects predominate and are likely to produce an increase in systolic and diastolic blood pressures and a narrowing of pulse pressure.

Indications

Indications for epinephrine infusion include signs of poor systemic perfusion or hypotension in the patient with adequate intravascular volume and a stable rhythm. Epinephrine infusion may also be indicated for hemodynamically significant bradycardia. An epinephrine infusion may be initiated during resuscitation of a patient with asystolic or pulseless arrest if intermittent bolus therapy fails to restore a perfusing cardiac rhythm. Epinephrine is preferable to other catecholamines for the patient who may have depleted myocardial norepinephrine stores, such as the young infant or the child with chronic congestive heart failure.

Dose

Epinephrine infusions should be delivered through a well-secured peripheral venous catheter or (preferably) a central venous catheter to ensure a reliable route of administration and to minimize the risk of extravasation. The infusion can be prepared by multiplying 0.6 by the patient's weight in kg. The resulting number equals the number of mg of epinephrine to be added to a solution diluted to 100 mL. Infusion of the solution at a rate of 1 mL/h will deliver 0.1 µg/kg per minute of epinephrine. Since epinephrine has a short half-life (approximately 2 minutes), the infusion rate should be adjusted every 5 minutes until the desired clinical effect (eg, increased heart rate or blood pressure or improved systemic perfusion) is achieved. It is generally advisable to begin with an infusion of approximately 20 mL/h until a clinical response in the form of tachycardia is detected. This indicates that the drug has cleared the tubing dead space and has entered the patient's circulation, producing a response. The infusion is then reduced to the desired rate (0.1 to 1.0 µg/kg per minute). Doses as high as 5.0 µg/kg per minute may occasionally be provided, although the patient must be monitored closely for evidence of tachyarrhythmias and other side effects (see below).

Precautions

Epinephrine can produce significant supraventricular or ventricular tachycardia and ventricular ectopy. High-dose infusions (more than 0.5 to 0.6 µg/kg per minute) may produce profound vasoconstriction that compromises extremity and skin perfusion. Even in lower doses, epinephrine may decrease renal and hepatic blood flow,[30] but renal function as assessed by urine output will improve if shock is successfully treated.[96] Infiltration of an epinephrine infusion can cause local ischemia and tissue necrosis.

Available Preparations

Vials: (1:1000) 1 mg/mL
Do not use the prefilled syringes
(1:10 000 dilution) for preparation of infusions.

Dopamine

Therapeutic Considerations

Dopamine is an endogenous catecholamine with complex cardiovascular effects.[30] In low doses (2 to 5 µg/kg per minute) dopamine produces little direct cardiac action but does increase renal, splanchnic, coronary, and cerebral blood flow through stimulation of dopaminergic receptors.[97] At infusion rates greater than 5 µg/kg per minute, dopamine produces both direct stimulation of the cardiac β-adrenergic receptors and indirect cardiac stimulation through the release of norepinephrine stored in cardiac sympathetic nerves.[30,97,98] If norepinephrine stores are depleted, such as in patients with chronic congestive heart failure,[30,99] the inotropic effects of dopamine are diminished. Young infants may demonstrate limited dopamine inotropic effects because sympathetic innervation of the ventricular myocardium may be incomplete.[100]

In the peripheral vascular bed, dopamine also has both direct and indirect actions at α- and β-adrenergic receptors. In low doses, vasodilatory effects predominate[30]; at higher doses, α-adrenergic vasoconstriction occurs. Dopamine infusion rates of 5 to 10 µg/kg per minute are thought to increase cardiac contractility, often without detectable effects on heart rate and blood pressure.[30] At infusion rates of 10 to 20 µg/kg per minute, vasoconstriction increases blood pressure; however, tachycardia may be significant and problematic. A patient may not respond predictably to dopamine infusion because of variability in the patient's own endogenous catecholamine response, pharmacokinetics, organ system function, and available stores of norepinephrine.

Indications

Dopamine may be used for the treatment of hypotension or poor peripheral perfusion in the pediatric patient with adequate intravascular volume and a stable rhythm. Low doses (2.0 to 5.0 μg/kg per minute) may enhance renal and splanchnic blood flow and urine output.

Dose

Dopamine has a short plasma half-life and must be delivered by a constant infusion controlled by an infusion pump. The infusion is prepared by adding 6 mg dopamine × the child's body weight in kilograms to sufficient diluent to create a solution totaling 100 mL. Infusions of 1 mL per hour of this mixture deliver 1.0 μg/kg per minute. An infusion of 10 mL/h or 10 μg/kg per minute is a reasonable starting dose for the child with shock. The infusion can then be adjusted after evaluation of the patient's urine output, systemic perfusion, or blood pressure. Infusion rates greater than 20 μg/kg per minute produce predominantly vasoconstrictive effects without further inotropic effect. If further inotropic effect is needed, epinephrine, with more potent α- and β-adrenergic effects, is probably preferable to infusion of dopamine in excess of 20 μg/kg per minute.

Precautions

Dopamine may produce tachycardia (and secondary increase in myocardial oxygen demand), arrhythmias, and hypertension. Reported dopamine-induced arrhythmias include premature ventricular contractions, supraventricular tachycardia, and ventricular tachycardia.[101] High infusion rates of dopamine (>20 μg/kg per minute) may produce severe peripheral vasoconstriction and ischemia in the child with shock.

Dopamine infusions should be delivered via a secure, large-bore peripheral venous catheter. High concentrations and large volume infusions should be administered via a central venous catheter. Extravasation of the infusion can result in local ischemia and tissue necrosis. Dopamine and other catecholamines cannot be mixed with sodium bicarbonate because they are inactivated by alkaline pH.

Available Preparations

Vials:　　5 mL (40 mg/mL)
　　　　　10 mL (40 mg/mL)

Dobutamine

Therapeutic Considerations

Dobutamine is a synthetic catecholamine possessing relatively selective action at β-adrenergic receptors. Its effects include increased cardiac contractility and heart rate, often with mild dilation of the peripheral vascular bed.[30,102] Unlike dopamine, dobutamine acts directly on β₁ receptors and does not depend on the presence of adequate stores of norepinephrine to produce these effects. In addition, it has no dopaminergic effects, so it does not affect renal or splanchnic blood flow directly. In children with cardiogenic shock, dobutamine increases cardiac output and decreases pulmonary capillary pressure and systemic vascular resistance.[103,104] Dobutamine appears to be less effective than epinephrine in septic shock,[104] particularly if hypotension is present, because it may increase existing systemic vasodilation.

Indications

Dobutamine may be used for the treatment of hypoperfusion, particularly if associated with high systemic vascular resistance. Although comparative clinical studies are lacking, dobutamine appears to have no clear advantages over dopamine in this setting and may not increase blood pressure as effectively. Dobutamine may be most effective in the treatment of severe congestive heart failure or cardiogenic shock, especially if caused by cardiomyopathy.[105] A theoretical advantage of dobutamine is its ability to decrease peripheral vascular resistance in this setting.

Dose

Like other catecholamines, dobutamine has a short plasma half-life and must be administered by a constant infusion via a large-bore venous catheter regulated by an infusion pump. High doses should be administered via a central venous catheter. The infusion is prepared by adding 6 mg dobutamine × the child's body weight in kilograms to sufficient diluent to create a solution totaling 100 mL. Infusions of this solution are begun at 5 to 10 mL per hour, which delivers 5 to 10 μg/kg per minute. The pharmacokinetics of and therapeutic response to dobutamine vary greatly among children.[106] The infusion rate should be adjusted as needed to stabilize the patient's blood pressure and perfusion. Infusion rates greater than 20 μg/kg per minute are usually not required.

Precautions

Dobutamine may produce tachycardia, tachyarrhythmias, or ectopic beats. Nausea, vomiting, hypertension, and hypotension are less frequent side effects. Extravasation of dobutamine may produce tissue ischemia and necrosis; central venous infusion is preferred for this reason. Like other catecholamines, dobutamine is inactivated slowly in alkaline solutions.

Available Preparations

Vials:　　10 mL (25 mg/mL)
　　　　　20 mL (12.5 mg/mL)

Lidocaine Infusion

Therapeutic Considerations

Lidocaine suppresses ventricular arrhythmias predominantly by decreasing automaticity (it reduces the slope of phase 4 diastolic depolarization). It also exerts local anesthetic effects that may help suppress ventricular ectopy.

Indications

Ventricular arrhythmias, including ventricular tachycardia and ventricular fibrillation, are uncommon in children. When they are observed, they are usually associated with metabolic abnormalities, drug intoxication, myocarditis, or structural heart disease. If the ventricular arrhythmias are thought to be caused by metabolic abnormalities or drug intoxication, lidocaine infusion is not warranted — the treatment of choice for the arrhythmia is correction of the causative condition.

Lidocaine infusion may be indicated for the treatment of recurrent ventricular tachycardia, ventricular fibrillation, or significant ventricular ectopy (multiple premature ventricular contractions) of unknown origin following resuscitation. Lidocaine is contraindicated, however, in children with wide-complex ventricular escape beats associated with bradycardia. Lidocaine is indicated during postresuscitation stabilization of children with ventricular arrhythmias associated with suspected myocarditis or structural heart disease.

Dose

The dose is 20 to 50 µg/kg per minute. The infusion should contain 120 mg lidocaine in 100 mL D_5W, administered at a rate of 20 to 50 µg/kg per minute (1 to 2.5 mL/kg per hour). Since the elimination half-life of lidocaine is several hours, a loading dose is required to achieve therapeutic concentration rapidly. Therefore, if a bolus dose of lidocaine has not been administered within the previous 15 minutes, administer a bolus of 1 mg/kg before initiation of the infusion.

Precautions

Excessive plasma concentrations of lidocaine may produce myocardial and circulatory depression and possible central nervous system symptoms, including drowsiness, disorientation, muscle twitching, or seizures.

Lidocaine undergoes hepatic metabolism that is dependent on adequate hepatic blood flow. Therefore, the risk of toxicity is increased when this drug is administered to children with low cardiac output or severe congestive heart failure, compromising hepatic blood flow. In these children, the infusion dose should be reduced to 20 µg/kg per minute or less.

Available Preparations

Prefilled Syringes: 5 mg/mL, 10 mg/mL, 15 mg/mL, 20 mg/mL
Vials: 40 mg/mL, 100 mg/mL, and 200 mg/mL

Isoproterenol

Therapeutic Considerations

Isoproterenol is a pure β-adrenergic agonist. It increases heart rate, atrioventricular conduction velocity, cardiac contractility, and myocardial oxygen consumption. Isoproterenol causes peripheral vasodilation, particularly in skeletal muscle, which contains a high density of β-adrenergic receptors. Cardiac output increases if circulating blood volume is adequate,[107] but pulse pressure increases because diastolic pressure falls. Bronchodilation also occurs with isoproterenol administration.

Indications

Isoproterenol may be used for the treatment of hemodynamically significant bradycardia caused by heart block that is unresponsive to atropine or that recurs shortly after atropine administration. Isoproterenol use may be considered when the heart rate is less than 60 beats per minute in an infant with poor perfusion, even if the measured blood pressure is normal. However, epinephrine infusion is preferable in this setting since it is less likely to decrease diastolic blood pressure (see "Precautions" below).

Dose

Isoproterenol has a very short half-life (1½ minutes) after IV infusion[28] and should be administered as a constant infusion controlled by an infusion pump. The infusion is prepared by adding 0.6 mg (3 mL) isoproterenol × the child's body weight in kilograms to sufficient diluent to create a solution totaling 100 mL (see "Drug Administration"). An infusion rate of 1 mL per hour will deliver 0.1 µg/kg per minute. The infusion should be started at 5 mL/h (0.5 µg/kg per minute), then titrated according to patient response. Titration can be accomplished by adjusting the infusion rate every 5 minutes once a heart rate or blood pressure response is obtained. Infusion rates as high as 1.0 µg/kg per minute may be required, although the dose is often limited by the resulting tachycardia.

Precautions

During CPR catecholamines are administered primarily for their α-adrenergic effects to improve coronary perfusion by increasing blood pressure.[32,34,91] Isoproterenol may actually compromise coronary perfusion because it has no α-adrenergic effects and it decreases diastolic

Table 1. Drugs Used in Pediatric Advanced Life Support

Drugs	Dosage (Pediatric)	Remarks
Adenosine	0.1-0.2 mg/kg Maximum single dose: 12 mg	Rapid IV bolus
Atropine sulfate*	0.02 mg/kg	Minimum dose: 0.1 mg Maximum single dose: 0.5 mg in child, 1.0 mg in adolescent
Bretylium	5 mg/kg; may be increased to 10 mg/kg	Rapid IV
Calcium chloride 10%	20 mg/kg	Give slowly.
Dopamine hydrochloride	2-20 μg/kg per min	α-Adrenergic action dominates at $\geq$15-20 μg/kg per min.
Dobutamine hydrochloride	2-20 μg/kg per min	Titrate to desired effect.
Epinephrine for bradycardia*	IV/IO: 0.01 mg/kg (1:10 000, 0.1 mL/kg) ET: 0.1 mg/kg (1:1000, 0.1 mL/kg)	Be aware of total dose of preservative administered (if preservatives are present in epinephrine preparation) when high doses are used.
Epinephrine for asystolic or pulseless arrest*	**First dose:** IV/IO: 0.01 mg/kg (1:10 000, 0.1 mL/kg) ET: 0.1 mg/kg (1:1000, 0.1 mL/kg) IV/IO doses as high as 0.2 mg/kg of 1:1000 may be effective. **Subsequent doses:** IV/IO/ET: 0.1 mg/kg (1:1000, 0.1 mL/kg) • Repeat every 3-5 min. IV/IO doses as high as 0.2 mg/kg of 1:1000 may be effective.	Be aware of total dose of preservative administered (if preservatives are present in epinephrine preparation) when high doses are used.
Epinephrine infusion	Initial at 0.1 μg/kg per min Higher infusion dose used if asystole present	Titrate to desired effect (0.1-1.0 μg/kg per min).
Lidocaine*	1 mg/kg	
Lidocaine infusion	20-50 μg/kg per min	
Naloxone*	If $\leq$ 5 years old or $\leq$ 20 kg: 0.1 mg/kg If > 5 years old or > 20 kg: 2.0 mg	Titrate to desired effect.
Sodium bicarbonate	1 mEq/kg per dose or 0.3 × kg × base deficit	Infuse slowly and only if ventilation is adequate.

*For ET administration dilute medication with normal saline to a volume of 3 to 5 mL and follow with several positive-pressure ventilations.

blood pressure.[107] Isoproterenol also increases myocardial oxygen demand by increasing myocardial contractility and heart rate. The increase in heart rate may further decrease coronary perfusion by decreasing diastolic filling time. For these reasons, isoproterenol should *not* be used to treat cardiac arrest. Isoproterenol cardiotoxicity has been described following administration to asthmatic children,[108] but the implications of these observations for other pediatric patients are unclear.

Available Preparations

Vials: 5 mL (0.2 mg/mL)

Drugs used in pediatric advanced life support are summarized in Table 1. Preparation of catecholamine infusions is given in Table 2.

Table 2. Preparation of Catecholamine Infusions in Infants and Children*

Medication	Dilution*	Delivery Rate
Isoproterenol Epinephrine	0.6 × body weight (kg) is the mg dose added to sufficient diluent to create a total volume of 100 mL[†]	1 mL/h delivers 0.1 µg/kg/min
Dopamine Dobutamine	6 × body weight (kg) is the mg dose added to sufficient diluent to create a total volume of 100 mL[†]	1 mL/h delivers 1 µg/kg/min

*This provides an initial concentration only. Drug concentration can be adjusted based on the patient's fluid requirements or limitations.

[†]In large patients the amount of drug used to create 100 mL of the drug infusion may deplete the available supply of the drug. To reduce the volume of drug needed to prepare the infusion, decrease the drug concentration by a factor of 10 and increase the hourly infusion rate by a factor of 10. For example, according to the formula above, a 20-kg child would require 12 mg (20 × 0.6) or 60 mL (0.2 mg/mL) of isoproterenol per 100 mL. Instead, dilute 1.2 mg (6 mL) in a solution totaling 100 mL and infuse the final solution at 10 mL/h (instead of 1 mL/h).

If high doses of the drug are required (eg, greater than or equal to 10 µg/kg per minute), the resulting amount of fluid delivered may be excessive for small infants or children. Under these conditions, the concentration of the drug may be *increased* by a factor of 3, 5, or 10 and the rate of infusion *decreased* by the same factor.

References

1. Griffel MI, Kaufman BS. Pharmacology of colloids and crystalloids. *Crit Care Clin.* 1992;8:235-253.
2. Nacht A. The use of blood products in shock. *Crit Care Clin.* 1992;8:255-291.
3. Carcillo JA, Davis AL, Zaritsky A. Role of early fluid resuscitation in pediatric septic shock. *JAMA.* 1991;266:1242-1245.
4. Pulsinelli WA, Waldman S, Rawlinson D, Plum F. Moderate hyperglycemia augments ischemic brain damage: a neuropathologic study in the rat. *Neurology.* 1982;32:1239-1246.
5. Nakakimura K, Fleischer JE, Drummond JC, et al. Glucose administration before cardiac arrest worsens neurologic outcome in cats. *Anesthesiology.* 1990;72:1005-1011.
6. D'Alecy LG, Lundy EF, Barton KJ, Zelenock GB. Dextrose containing intravenous fluid impairs outcome and increases death after eight minutes of cardiac arrest and resuscitation in dogs. *Surgery.* 1986;100:505-511.
7. Michaud LJ, Rivara FP, Longstreth WT Jr, Grady MS. Elevated initial blood glucose levels and poor outcome following severe brain injuries in children. *J Trauma.* 1991;31:1356-1362.
8. Graf W, Brutocao D, Nazar Y, Suczbacher S, Quan L. Admission glucose level as a predictor of survival and neurological outcome in pediatric submersion victims. *Ann Neurol.* 1991;30:473. Abstract.
9. Ditchey RV, Lindenfeld JA. Potential adverse effects of volume loading on perfusion of vital organs during closed-chest resuscitation. *Circulation.* 1984;69:181-189.
10. Voorhees WD, Ralston SH, Kougias C, Schmidtz PMW. Fluid loading with whole blood or Ringer's lactate solution during CPR in dogs. *Resuscitation.* 1987;15:113.
11. Ostrea EM Jr, Odell GB. The influence of bicarbonate administration on blood pH in a 'closed system': clinical implications. *J Pediatr.* 1972; 80:671-680.
12. Rhodes PG, Hall RT, Hellerstein S. The effects of single infusion of hypertonic sodium bicarbonate on body composition in neonates with acidosis. *J Pediatr.* 1977;90:789-795.
13. Rossetti VA, Thompson BM, Aprahamian C, Darin JC, Mateer JR. Difficulty and delay in intravascular access in pediatric arrests. *Ann Emerg Med.* 1984;13:406. Abstract.
14. Lillis KA, Jaffe DM. Prehospital intravenous access in children. *Ann Emerg Med.* 1992;21:1430-1434.
15. Ward JT Jr. Endotracheal drug therapy. *Am J Emerg Med.* 1983;1:71-82.
16. Roberts JR, Greenberg MI, Knaub MA, Kendrick ZV, Baskin SI. Blood levels following intravenous and endotracheal epinephrine administration. *J Am Coll Emerg Phys.* 1979;8:53-56.
17. Roberts JR, Greenberg MI, Knaub M, Baskin SI. Comparison of the pharmacological effects of epinephrine administered by the intravenous and endotracheal routes. *J Am Coll Emerg Phys.* 1978;7:260-264.
18. Mazkereth R, Paret G, Ezra D, et al. Epinephrine blood concentrations after peripheral bronchial versus endotracheal administration of epinephrine in dogs. *Crit Care Med.* 1992;20:1582-1587.
19. Aitkenhead AR. Drug administration during CPR: what route? *Resuscitation.* 1991;22:191-195.
20. Quinton DN, O'Byrne G, Aitkenhead AR. Comparison of endotracheal and peripheral intravenous adrenaline in cardiac arrest: is the endotracheal route reliable? *Lancet.* 1987;1:828-829.
21. Ralston SH, Voorhees WD, Babbs CF. Intrapulmonary epinephrine during prolonged cardiopulmonary resuscitation: improved regional blood flow and resuscitation in dogs. *Ann Emerg Med.* 1984;13:79-86.
22. Jasani MS, Nadkarni VM, Finkelstein MS, Mandell GA, Salzman SK, Norman ME. Endotracheal epinephrine administration technique effects in pediatric porcine hypoxic-hypercarbic arrest. *Crit Care Med.* In press.
23. Hedges JR, Barsan WB, Doan LA, et al. Central versus peripheral intravenous routes in cardiopulmonary resuscitation. *Am J Emerg Med.* 1984;2:385-390.
24. Kuhn GJ, White BC, Swetnam RE, et al. Peripheral versus central circulation times during CPR: a pilot study. *Ann Emerg Med.* 1981;10:417-419.
25. Dalsey WC, Barsan WG, Joyce SM, Hedges JR, Lukes SJ, Doan LA. Comparison of superior vena caval and inferior vena caval access using a radioisotope technique during normal perfusion and cardiopulmonary resuscitation. *Ann Emerg Med.* 1984;13:881-884.
26. Fleisher G, Caputo G, Baskin M. Comparison of external jugular and peripheral venous administration of sodium bicarbonate in puppies. *Crit Care Med.* 1989;17:251-254.
27. Berg RA. Emergency infusion of catecholamines into bone marrow. *Am J Dis Child.* 1984;138:810-811.
28. Thompson BM, Rossetti V, Miller J, et al. Intraosseous administration of sodium bicarbonate: an effective means of pH normalization in the canine model. *Ann Emerg Med.* 1984;13:405. Abstract.
29. Andropoulos DB, Soifer SJ, Schrieber MD. Plasma epinephrine concentrations after intraosseous and central venous injection during cardiopulmonary resuscitation in the lamb. *J Pediatr.* 1990;116:312-315.
30. Zaritsky A, Chernow B. Use of catecholamines in pediatrics. *J Pediatr.* 1985;105:341-350.
31. Paradis NA, Koscove EM. Epinephrine in cardiac arrest: a critical review. *Ann Emerg Med.* 1990;19:1288-1301.
32. Otto CW, Yakaitis RW, Blitt CD. Mechanism of action of epinephrine in resuscitation from asphyxial arrest. *Crit Care Med.* 1981;9:321-324.
33. Paradis NA, Martin GB, Rosenberg J, et al. The effect of standard- and high-dose epinephrine on coronary perfusion pressure during prolonged cardiopulmonary resuscitation. *JAMA.* 1991;265:1139-1144.
34. Otto CW. Cardiovascular pharmacology, II: the use of catecholamines, pressor agents, digitalis, and corticosteroids in CPR and emergency cardiac care. *Circulation.* 1986;74:IV-80-IV-85.
35. Schleien CL, Dean JM, Koehler RC, et al. Effect of epinephrine on cerebral and myocardial perfusion in an infant animal preparation of cardiopulmonary resuscitation. *Circulation.* 1986;73:809-817.
36. Michael JK, Guerci AD, Koehler RC, et al. Mechanisms by which epinephrine augments cerebral and myocardial perfusion during cardiopulmonary resuscitation in dogs. *Circulation.* 1984;69:822-835.
37. Angelos MG, DeBehnke DJ, Leasure JE. Arterial blood gases during cardiac arrest: markers of blood flow in a canine model. *Resuscitation.* 1992;23:101-111.

38. Friesen RM, Duncan P, Tweed WA, Bristow G. Appraisal of pediatric cardiopulmonary resuscitation. *Can Med Assoc J.* 1982;126:1055-1058.

39. Coffing CR, Quan L, Graves JR, et al. Etiologies and outcomes of the pulseless, nonbreathing pediatric patient presenting with ventricular fibrillation. *Ann Emerg Med.* 1992;21:1046. Abstract.

40. Chandra NC, Krischer JP. The demographics of cardiac arrest support 'phone fast' for children. *Circulation.* 1993;88(suppl 1):I193. Abstract.

41. Eisenberg M, Bergner L, Hallstrom A. Epidemiology of cardiac arrest and resuscitation in children. *Ann Emerg Med.* 1983;12: 672-674.

42. Mitchell JH, Wildenthal K, Johnson RL Jr. The effects of acid-base disturbances on cardiovascular and pulmonary function. *Kidney Int.* 1972;1:375-389.

43. O'Rourke PP. Outcome of children who are apneic and pulseless in the emergency room. *Crit Care Med.* 1986;14:466-468.

44. Zaritsky A, Nadkarni V, Getson P, Kuehl K. CPR in children. *Ann Emerg Med.* 1987;16:1107-1111.

45. Nichols DG, Kettrick RG, Swedlow DB, Lee S, Passman R, Ludwig S. Factors influencing outcome of cardiopulmonary resuscitation in children. *Pediatr Emerg Care.* 1986;2:1-5.

46. Emergency Cardiac Care Committee, American Heart Association, Guidelines for cardiopulmonary resuscitation and emergency cardiac care, part VI: pediatric advanced life support. *JAMA.* 1992;268:2262-2275.

47. Brown CG, Werman HA. Adrenergic agonist during cardiopulmonary resuscitation. *Resuscitation.* 1990;19:1-16.

48. Stiell IG, Hebert PC, Weitzman BN, et al. High-dose epinephrine in adult cardiac arrest. *N Engl J Med.* 1992;327:1045-1050.

49. Brown CG, Martin DR, Pepe PE, et al. A comparison of standard-dose and high-dose epinephrine in cardiac arrest outside the hospital. *N Engl J Med.* 1992;327:1051-1055.

50. Goetting MG, Paradis NA. High-dose epinephrine improves outcome from pediatric cardiac arrest. *Ann Emerg Med.* 1991; 20:22-26.

51. Chernow B, Holbrook P, D'Angona DS Jr, et al. Epinephrine absorption after intratracheal administration. *Anesth Analg.* 1984;63:829-832.

52. Roberts JR, Greenberg MI, Knaub MA, Kendrick ZV, Baskin SI. Blood levels following intravenous and endotracheal epinephrine administration. *J Am Coll Emerg Phys.* 1979;8:53-56.

53. Berenyi KJ, Wolk M, Killip T. Cerebrospinal fluid acidosis complicating therapy of experimental cardiopulmonary arrest. *Circulation.* 1975;52:319-324.

54. Steenbergen C, Deleeuw G, Rich T, Williamson JR. Effects of acidosis and ischemia on contractility and intracellular pH of rat heart. *Circ Res.* 1977;41:849-858.

55. Clancy RL, Cingolani HE, Taylor RR, Graham TP Jr, Gilmore JP. Influence of sodium bicarbonate on myocardial performance. *Am J Physiol.* 1967;212:917-923.

56. Arieff AI, Leach W, Park R, Lazarowitz VC. Systemic effects of NaHCO$_3$ in experimental lactic acidosis in dogs. *Am J Physiol.* 1982;242:F586-F591.

57. Gazmuri RJ, von Planta M, Weil MH, Rackow EC. Cardiac effects of carbon dioxide–consuming and carbon dioxide–generating buffers during cardiopulmonary resuscitation. *J Am Coll Cardiol.* 1990;15:482-490.

58. Kette F, Weil M, Gazmuri R, et al. Buffer solutions may compromise cardiac resuscitation by reducing coronary perfusion pressure. *JAMA.* 1991;266:2121-2126.

59. Kette F, Weil MH, von Planta M, Gazmuri RJ, Rackow EC. Buffer agents do not reverse intramyocardial acidosis during cardiac resuscitation. *Circulation.* 1990;81:1660-1666.

60. Cohen RD, Simpson BR, Goodwin FJ, Strunin L. The early effects of infusion of sodium bicarbonate and sodium lactate on intracellular hydrogen ion activity in dogs. *Clin Sci.* 1967;33:233-247.

61. Graf H, Leach W, Arieff AI. Evidence for a detrimental effect of bicarbonate therapy in hypoxic lactic acidosis. *Science.* 1985;227: 754-756.

62. Bersin RM, Chatterjee K, Arieff AI. Metabolic and hemodynamic consequences of sodium bicarbonate administration in patients with heart disease. *Am J Med.* 1989;87:7-14.

63. Kitakaze M, Weisfeldt ML, Marban E. Acidosis during early reperfusion prevents myocardial stunning in perfused ferret hearts. *J Clin Invest.* 1988;82:920-927.

64. Weil MH, Rackow EC, Trevino R, Grundler W, Falk JL, Griffel MI. Difference in acid-base state between venous and arterial blood during cardiopulmonary resuscitation. *N Engl J Med.* 1986;315:153-156.

65. Johnson BA, Weil MH. Redefining ischemia due to circulatory failure on dual defects of oxygen deficits and of carbon dioxide excesses. *Crit Care Med.* 1991;19:1432-1438.

66. Bellingham AJ, Detter JC, Lenfant C. Regulatory mechanisms of hemoglobin oxygen affinity in acidosis and alkalosis. *J Clin Invest.* 1971;50:700-706.

67. Bishop RL, Weisfeldt ML. Sodium bicarbonate administration during cardiac arrest. *JAMA.* 1976;235:506-509.

68. Mättar JA, Weil MH, Shubin H, Stein L. Cardiac arrest in the critically ill, II: hyperosmolal states following cardiac arrest. *Am J Med.* 1974; 56:162-168.

69. Coté CJ, Greenhow DE, Marshall BE. The hypotensive response to rapid intravenous administration of hypertonic solutions in man and in the rabbit. *Anesthesiology.* 1979;50:30-35.

70. Howell J. Sodium bicarbonate in the perinatal setting — revisited. *Clin Perinat.* 1987;14:807-816.

71. Coon GA, Clinton JE, Ruiz E. Use of atropine for brady-asystolic prehospital cardiac arrest. *Ann Emerg Med.* 1981;10:462-467.

72. Redding JS, Haynes RR, Thomas JD. Drug therapy in resuscitation from electromechanical dissociation. *Crit Care Med.* 1983; 11:681-684.

73. Dauchot P, Gravenstein JS. Effects of atropine on the electrocardiogram in different age groups. *Clin Pharmacol Ther.* 1971;12:274-280.

74. Chernow B, ed. *The Pharmacologic Approach to the Critically Ill Patient.* 2nd ed. Baltimore, Md: Williams & Wilkins; 1988:486-487.

75. Sharts-Engel NC. Naloxone review and pediatric dosage update. *J Maternal Child Health Nurs.* 1991;16:182.

76. Drug Evaluation Monograph: Naloxone. Micromedex, Inc., Vol. 78, 1974-1993.

77. Chernick V, Manfreda J, Debooy V, et al. Clinical trial of naloxone in birth asphyxia. *J Pediatr.* 1988;113:519-525.

78. Tenebein M. Continuous naloxone infusion for opiate poisoning in infancy. *J Pediatr.* 1984;105:645-648.

79. AAP Committee on Drugs. Naloxone dosage and route of administration for infants and children: addendum to emergency drug doses for infants and children. *Pediatrics.* 1990;86:484.

80. Voorhies TM, Rawlinson D, Vannucci RC. Glucose and perinatal hypoxic-ischemic brain damage in the rat. *Neurology.* 1986;36:1115-1118.

81. Sieber FE, Traystman RJ. Special issues: glucose and the brain. *Crit Care Med.* 1992;20:104-114.

82. Hazinski MF. Cardiovascular disorders. In: Hazinski MF, ed. *Nursing Care of the Critically Ill Child.* 2nd ed. St Louis, Mo: Mosby Year Book; 1992.

83. Oh MS, Carroll HJ. Electrolyte disorders. In: Chernow B, Lake CR, eds. *The Pharmacologic Approach to the Critically Ill Patient.* Baltimore, Md: Williams & Wilkins; 1983:715.

84. Cardenas-Rivero N, Chernow B, Stoiko MA, Nussbaum SR, Todres ID. Hypocalcemia in critically ill children. *J Pediatr.* 1989; 114:946-951.

85. Coté CJ, Drop LJ, Hoaglin DC, Daniels AL, Young ET. Ionized hypocalcemia after fresh frozen plasma administration to thermally injured children: effects of infusion rate, duration, and treatment with calcium chloride. *Anesth Analg.* 1988;67:152-160.

86. Stulz PM, Scheidegger D, Drop LJ, Lowenstein E, Laver MB. Ventricular pump performance during hypocalcemia: clinical and experimental studies. *J Thorac Cardiovasc Surg.* 1979;78:185-194.

87. Katz AM, Reuter H. Cellular calcium and cardiac cell death. *Am J Cardiol.* 1979;44:188-190.

88. Dembo DH. Calcium in advanced life support. *Crit Care Med.* 1981;9:358-359.

89. Clark RE, Christlieb IY, Ferguson TB, et al. The first American clinical trial of nifedipine in cardioplegia: a report of the first 12 month experience. *J Thorac Cardiovasc Surg.* 1981;82:848-859.

90. Stueven HA, Thompson B, Aprahamian C, Tonsfeldt DJ, Kastenson EH. The effectiveness of calcium chloride in refractory electromechanical dissociation. *Ann Emerg Med.* 1985;14: 626-629.

91. Redding JS, Haynes RR, Thomas JD. Drug therapy in resuscitation from electromechanical dissociation. *Crit Care Med.* 1983; 11:681-684.

92. Henry M, Kay MM, Viccellio P. Cardiogenic shock associated with calcium channel and beta blockers: reversal with intravenous calcium chloride. *Am J Emerg Med.* 1985;3:334-336.

93. Broner CW, Stidham GL, Westen-Kirchner DF, Watson AC. A prospective, randomized double-blind comparison of calcium chloride and calcium gluconate therapies for hypocalcemia in critically ill children. *J Pediatr.* 1990;117:986-989.

94. White RD, Goldsmith RS, Rodriguez R, Moffitt EA, Pluth JR. Plasma ionic calcium levels following injection of chloride, gluconate, and gluceptate salts of calcium. *J Thorac Cardiovasc Surg.* 1976;71:609-613.

95. Lucking SE, Pollack MM, Fields AI. Shock following generalized hypoxic-ischemic injury in previously healthy infants and children. *J Pediatr.* 1986;108:359-364.

96. Coffin LH Jr, Ankeney JL, Beheler EM. Experimental study and clinical use of epinephrine for treatment of low cardiac output syndrome. *Circulation.* 1966;33(suppl 4):I-78-I-85.

97. Notterman DA, Greenwald BM, Moran F, DiMaio-Hunter A, Metakis L, Reidenberg MM. Dopamine clearance in critically ill infants and children: effect of age and organ system dysfunction. *Clin Pharmacol Ther.* 1990;48:138-147.

98. Farmer JB. Indirect sympathomimetic actions of dopamine. *J Pharm Pharmacol.* 1966;18:261-262.

99. Leier CV, Heban PT, Huss P, Bush CA, Lewis RP. Comparative systemic and regional hemodynamic effects of dopamine and dobutamine in patients with cardiomyopathic heart failure. *Circulation.* 1978;58:466-475.

100. Driscoll DJ, Gillette PC, Ezrailson EG, Schwartz A. Inotropic response of the neonatal canine myocardium to dopamine. *Pediatr Res.* 1978;12:42-45.

101. Guller B, Fields AI, Coleman MG, Holbrook PR. Changes in cardiac rhythm in children treated with dopamine. *Crit Care Med.* 1978;6:151-154.

102. Leier CV, Unverferth DV. Drugs five years later: dobutamine. *Ann Intern Med.* 1983;99:490-496.

103. Schranz D, Stopfkuchen H, Jüngst BK, Clemens R, Emmrich P. Hemodynamic effects of dobutamine in children with cardiovascular failure. *Eur J Pediatr.* 1982;139:4-7.

104. Perkin RM, Levin DL, Webb R, Aquino A, Reedy J. Dobutamine: a hemodynamic evaluation in children with shock. *J Pediatr.* 1982;100:977-983.

105. Liang CS, Sherman LG, Doherty JU, Wellington K, Lee VW, Hood WB Jr. Sustained improvement of cardiac function in patients with congestive heart failure after short-term infusion of dobutamine. *Circulation.* 1984;69:113-119.

106. Banner W Jr, Vernon DD, Minton SD, Dean JM. Nonlinear dobutamine pharmacokinetics in a pediatric population. *Crit Care Med.* 1991;19:871-875.

107. Mueller H, Ayres SM, Gregory JJ, Gianelli S Jr, Grace WJ. Hemodynamics, coronary blood flow, and myocardial metabolism in coronary shock: response to L-norepinephrine and isoproterenol. *J Clin Invest.* 1970;49:1885-1902.

108. Maguire JF, O'Rourke PP, Colan SD, Geha RS, Crone R. Cardiotoxicity during treatment of severe childhood asthma. *Pediatrics.* 1991;88:1180-1186.

Cardiac Rhythm Disturbances

Chapter 7

In infants and children, life-threatening cardiac rhythm disturbances are more frequently the result rather than the cause of acute cardiovascular emergencies. Primary cardiac arrest is uncommon in this age group. Typically cardiac arrest is the end result of hypoxemia and acidosis resulting from respiratory insufficiency or shock. Thus, in the pediatric age group attention must first be directed toward establishment of a patent airway, effective ventilation, adequate oxygenation, and circulatory stabilization. This chapter is limited to a discussion of the arrhythmias most commonly associated with emergency situations requiring CPR and is not intended to be a comprehensive review of pediatric cardiac arrhythmias.

The Normal Electrocardiogram

The surface electrocardiogram (ECG) is a graphic representation of the sequence of myocardial depolarization and repolarization, with each normal cardiac cycle consisting of a P, a QRS, and a T wave (Fig 1). Electrical depolarization begins in the sinoatrial node at the junction of the superior vena cava and right atrium and advances via atrial tissue and the internodal pathways to the atrioventricular (AV) junctional tissue, where it slows temporarily. It then progresses via the bundle of His and its divisions to depolarize the ventricular myocardium (Fig 2). The first deflection on the surface ECG (P wave) represents depolarization of both atria. The delay of the impulse in the junctional tissue of the AV node and the time required to spread the impulse through the bundle of His are represented by the PR interval. The QRS represents depolarization of the ventricular myocardium. Ventricular repolarization is characterized on the surface ECG as the ST segment and the T wave (Fig 3).

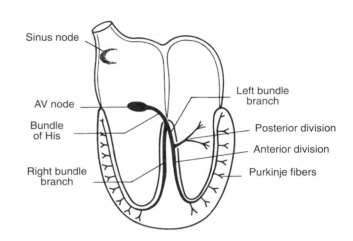

Fig 2. The cardiac conduction system.

The normal heart rate is influenced by the child's age and activity level and such pathologic conditions as fever or hemorrhage. There is a wide variation in the normal heart rate and a gradual decline with age (Table 1).[1-5] The child's clinical condition and sleep-awake state must always be considered when the heart rate is evaluated. A febrile infant with normal cardiovascular function can have a heart rate of 200 beats per minute or higher. This can make differentiation of sinus tachycardia from a tachyarrhythmia (supraventricular tachycardia) difficult.

Monitoring the ECG

The ECG should be continuously monitored in children who have evidence of respiratory or cardiovascular instability, including children who have sustained a cardiopulmonary arrest. The ECG provides no information about the effectiveness of myocardial contractility or quality of tissue perfusion. As a result, therapy must always be based on clinical evaluation of the patient correlated with information derived from the ECG.

Hardware

An ECG monitoring system consists of a display screen and a heart rate tachometer that determines the heart rate from the R-R interval. Ideally the system also includes a printer that provides a paper copy of the tracing. Some monitors also contain a memory that can store rhythm disturbances for later recall and analysis. ECG recorders may be used as monitors, but they waste a great deal of recording paper.

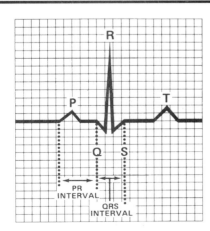

Fig 1. The electrocardiogram.

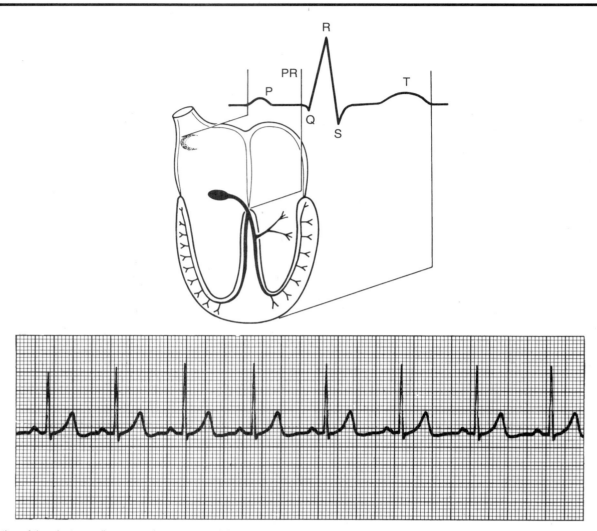

Fig 3. Relation of the electrocardiogram to the anatomy of the conduction system.

The ECG impulse is conducted from the patient to the cardiac monitor through three color-coded cables attached to the patient with disposable adhesive monitoring pads or metal electrodes. Both are available in small sizes convenient for pediatric patients. Large (adult) adhesive monitoring pads may be adapted for pediatric use by trimming excess tape from the electrodes to make them smaller. Metal electrodes are usually attached to the extremities. Disposable adhesive monitoring pads may be applied to either the chest or the extremities. When the disposable adhesive disk electrodes are placed in optimal position, an ECG of good quality will be produced that includes visible P waves, triggering of the tachometer by the R wave but not the T wave, and absence of artifact. Electrodes should be placed at the periphery of the anterior chest to avoid interference with chest compressions if CPR becomes necessary. If electrode placement on the anterior chest is avoided, auscultation of the heart and lungs is facilitated, and chest radiographs will be free of radiopaque artifact. Electrodes are typically placed on the shoulders or the lateral chest surfaces, and the ground electrode is usually placed on the abdomen or thigh (Fig 4).

Artifacts

Healthcare providers who use an ECG monitoring system must become familiar with artifacts commonly observed on an ECG. Four of the most common artifacts are

- A straight line (resembling asystole) or a wavy line (resembling coarse fibrillation), both of which may be caused by a loose wire or monitoring electrode
- A tall T wave that may be mistaken by the tachometer for an R wave, resulting in "double counting" of the heart rate and a digital heart rate display that is twice the actual rate
- Absence of P waves, which can result from lead placement that is perpendicular to the P-wave axis
- 60-cycle interference that is caused by electrical interference

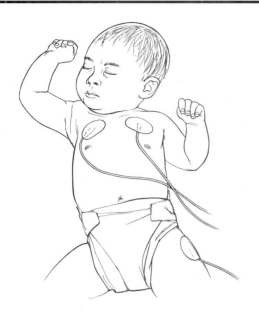

Fig 4. Placement of electrodes for electrocardiographic monitoring.

These and other artifacts may complicate interpretation of the ECG. Clinical assessment of the child must always be correlated with the ECG before therapy is initiated.

Abnormal Rhythms

Principles of Therapy

A rhythm disturbance in a child should be treated as an emergency *only* if it compromises cardiac output or has the potential to degenerate into a lethal (collapse) rhythm. Cardiac output is the product of stroke volume and heart rate. Cardiac output may diminish as a result of very rapid rates, which compromise diastolic filling and therefore stroke volume, and as a result of very slow rates. For assessment of systemic perfusion and signs of shock, see chapter 2.

Specific rhythm disturbances may require evaluation by a pediatric cardiologist, but specialty training is not required to provide emergency treatment for the vast majority of rhythm disturbances associated with hemodynamic collapse in the pediatric age group. In the setting of acute emergencies, cardiac rhythm disturbances should be classified according to their effect on central pulses:

- Fast pulse rate = tachyarrhythmia
- Slow pulse rate = bradyarrhythmia
- Absent pulse = pulseless arrest (collapse rhythm)

Cardiac rhythms that result in excessively fast rates include supraventricular and ventricular tachycardias. If tachyarrhythmias result in cardiovascular instability and signs of shock, the most rapid and effective method of treatment is synchronized cardioversion (see below).

Slow rhythms associated with cardiovascular instability are usually the result of AV block or suppression of normal sinus node impulse generation caused by hypoxemia and acidosis. Initial therapy for these rhythms includes establishment of a patent airway, provision of adequate ventilation and oxygenation, and administration of medications to improve perfusion (ie, sympathomimetics).

The absence of palpable pulses is associated with asystole, ventricular fibrillation, pulseless ventricular tachycardia, or a pulseless electrical activity (PEA), such as electromechanical dissociation.

Tachyarrhythmias

Sinus Tachycardia

Sinus tachycardia is defined as a rate of sinus node discharge higher than normal for age (Table 1). It typically develops in response to a need for increased cardiac output or oxygen delivery. As a result, it is often a nonspecific clinical sign rather than a true arrhythmia. Common causes of sinus tachycardia include anxiety, fever, pain, blood loss, sepsis, or shock.

Table 1. Heart Rates in Normal Children[1-5]*

Age	Awake Rate	Mean	Sleeping Rate
Newborn to 3 mo	85 to 205	140	80 to 160
3 mo to 2 y	100 to 190	130	75 to 160
2 y to 10 y	60 to 140	80	60 to 90
>10 y	60 to 100	75	50 to 90

*From Gillette.[5]

The Electrocardiogram (Fig 5):
- Rate is greater than normal for age.
- Rhythm is regular with normal P wave axis, normal P-QRS-T wave sequence, and normal QRS duration.

Therapy:

Therapy is directed at treating the underlying cause. Since the tachycardia is a symptom, attempts to decrease the heart rate by pharmacologic means are inappropriate.

Supraventricular Tachycardia

Supraventricular tachycardia (SVT) is a rapid, often paroxysmal, regular rhythm most commonly caused by a reentry mechanism that involves an accessory pathway and/or the AV conduction system. Although SVT is usually well tolerated in most infants and older children, it can lead to cardiovascular collapse and clinical evidence of shock in some small infants.[6,7]

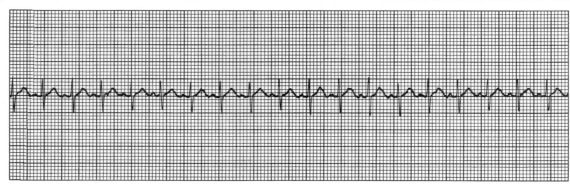

Fig 5. Sinus tachycardia (180 beats per minute) in a febrile 3-year-old.

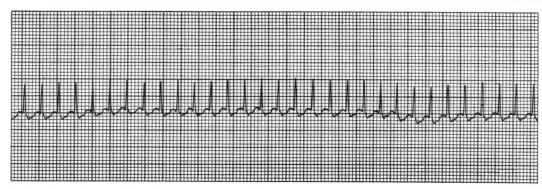

Fig 6. Supraventricular tachycardia in an infant. The heart rate is about 300 beats per minute.

The Electrocardiogram (Fig 6):

- Heart rate associated with SVT varies with age. In infants the heart rate is often approximately 240 beats per minute or higher.
- The rhythm is usually regular since associated AV block is rare.
- P waves may not be identifiable, especially when the ventricular rate is high.
- QRS duration is normal (less than 0.08 second) in most (>90%) children.[8] SVT with aberrant conduction (wide QRS) may be difficult to distinguish from ventricular tachycardia, but this form of SVT is rare in infants and children.
- ST and T wave changes consistent with myocardial ischemia may be observed if tachycardia persists.

Differentiation between extreme sinus tachycardia associated with sepsis or hypovolemia and SVT may be difficult, particularly because either rhythm may be associated with poor systemic perfusion. The following may aid differentiation:

1. *Heart rate*: Sinus tachycardia is usually associated with a heart rate less than 200 beats per minute. In most (60%) infants with SVT, the heart rate is greater than 230 beats per minute.[9]
2. *ECG*: P waves may be difficult to identify in both sinus tachycardia and SVT once the ventricular rate exceeds 200 beats per minute. If the P waves can be identified, the P wave axis is usually abnormal in SVT but normal in sinus tachycardia.
3. *Variability*: In sinus tachycardia the rate may vary from beat to beat, but there is no beat-to-beat variation in SVT. Termination of SVT is abrupt, whereas the heart rate slows gradually in sinus tachycardia.

Therapy:

Synchronized Cardioversion. Synchronized cardioversion is the treatment of choice for patients with tachyarrhythmias (SVT, VT, atrial fibrillation, atrial flutter) who show evidence of cardiovascular compromise. Synchronization of delivered energy with the ECG reduces the possibility of inducing VF, which can occur if an electrical impulse is delivered during the relative refractory period of the ventricle.[10] The initial energy dose is 0.5 J/kg, and if the tachyarrhythmia persists, the dose is doubled. If conversion to sinus rhythm still does not occur, the diagnosis of SVT should be reconsidered; sinus tachycardia may actually be present. The procedure for synchronized cardioversion is the same as that outlined for defibrillation (see below), with the following exceptions:

1. If the paddles are not of the monitoring type, the ECG must be joined to the defibrillator.
2. The synchronizer circuit must be activated (a light blinks, and an indicator flashes on the monitor with each QRS). On some older models, the QRS must be upright for proper activation.

3. The discharge buttons must be pressed and held until the countershock is delivered (often several QRS complexes).

Ideally infants and children should be intubated and ventilated with 100% oxygen before cardioversion, and secure vascular access (venous or intraosseous) should be achieved. Administration of a sedative and an analgesic should also be considered. However, if shock is present, cardioversion should not be delayed while these therapies are instituted.

Adenosine. Adenosine is the drug of choice for the treatment of SVT in symptomatic infants and children. Adenosine[11-13] is an endogenous nucleoside that produces transient AV block to interrupt a reentry circuit that includes AV junctional tissue. The major advantage of adenosine is its extremely short half-life (less than 10 seconds), which minimizes the duration of side effects and makes it relatively safe. Adenosine does not interfere with other cardiac drugs and may be used in children with Wolff-Parkinson-White syndrome or other AV bypass tracts.

In infants with SVT-associated shock, adenosine administration may precede cardioversion if vascular access is available, but *cardioversion should not be delayed* while intravenous access is achieved.

Dose: 0.1 mg/kg as a rapid IV bolus with constant ECG monitoring. Because of the short half-life, the bolus of adenosine must be immediately followed by 2 to 3 mL of normal saline and the injection port used must be the one nearest the hub of the catheter. If there is no effect, the dose may be doubled once. The maximum single dose should not exceed 12 mg.

Verapamil. Verapamil is a calcium channel blocker that exerts its antiarrhythmic effect by slowing conduction and prolonging the effective refractory period in the AV junctional tissue. Its negative inotropic effect may cause serious myocardial depression. Because profound brady-cardia, hypotension, and asystole have been reported following verapamil administration, this drug should not be used to treat SVT in an emergency setting in infants less than 1 year of age, in children with congestive heart failure or myocardial depression, in children receiving β-adrenergic–blocking drugs, or in those who may have a bypass tract.[14,15]

Ventricular Tachycardia

Ventricular tachycardia (VT) is uncommon in the pediatric age group. In the presence of VT, the ventricular rate may vary from near normal to more than 400 beats per minute. Slow ventricular rates may be well tolerated, but rapid ventricular rates compromise stroke volume and cardiac output and may degenerate into ventricular fibrillation. The majority of children who develop VT have underlying structural heart disease or prolonged QT syndrome. Other potential causes include acute hypoxemia, acidosis, electrolyte imbalance, drug toxicity (eg, tricyclic antidepressants), and poisons.

The Electrocardiogram (Fig 7):
- Ventricular rate is at least 120 beats per minute and regular.
- The QRS is wide (greater than 0.08 second).
- P waves are often not identifiable. When present, they may not be related to the QRS (AV dissociation). At slower rates atria may be depolarized in a retrograde manner, and therefore there will be a 1:1 VA association.
- T waves are usually opposite in polarity to the QRS.
- It may be difficult to differentiate SVT with aberrant conduction from VT. Fortunately, aberrant conduction is present in less than 10% of children with SVT. Previously undiagnosed wide QRS tachycardia in an infant or child should be treated as VT until proven otherwise.

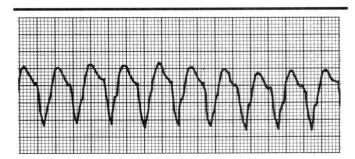

Fig 7. Ventricular tachycardia. The ventricular rhythm is regular at a rate of 158 beats per minute, the QRS is wide, and there is no evidence of atrial depolarization.

Therapy:

VT without palpable pulses is treated like ventricular fibrillation. If VT is associated with signs of shock (low cardiac output, poor perfusion) but pulses are palpable, the indicated treatment is synchronized cardioversion. Ideally the patient is intubated and ventilated with 100% oxygen, secure vascular access (intravenous or intraosseous) is established, and adequate sedation and analgesia are provided. If the underlying cause of the VT is determined (eg, electrolyte imbalance or drug toxicity), it must be treated.

Lidocaine is useful to raise the threshold for ventricular fibrillation and to suppress postcardioversion ventricular ectopy, so it should be administered before cardioversion if vascular access has been established and the drug is readily available. A loading dose of 1 mg/kg of lidocaine is administered, followed by an infusion at 20 to 50 µg/kg per minute. However, cardioversion should *not* be delayed in an unstable child if the drug is not readily available or if vascular access has not been achieved. Lidocaine infusion should be considered following return of spontaneous circulation if the ventricular arrhythmias are thought to be associated with myocarditis or structural heart disease (see chapter 6).

A lidocaine infusion is prepared by adding 120 mg of lidocaine to 5% dextrose in water to bring the total volume of medication plus diluent to 100 mL (concentration of 1.2 mg/mL). An infusion rate of 1.0 to 2.5 mL/kg per hour will deliver 20 to 50 µg/kg per minute. An alternative concentration is prepared by multiplying 60 by the kilogram body weight to determine the amount of lidocaine (in milligrams) to be added to a solution of 5% dextrose in water for a total volume of 100 mL. Infusion of 2 to 5 mL per hour of this solution will provide 20 to 50 µg/kg per minute. To ensure adequate plasma concentration, a bolus of 1 mg/kg is administered before the infusion is initiated.

Excessive plasma concentrations of lidocaine may produce myocardial and circulatory depression and possible central nervous system symptoms, including drowsiness, disorientation, muscle twitching, or seizures. If reduced lidocaine clearance is suspected, such as might occur in patients with shock or chronic congestive heart failure, lidocaine infusions should be reduced to a maximum of 20 µg/kg per minute.

Bretylium Tosylate. There are no data on the usefulness of bretylium tosylate in the pediatric age group. It may be administered if defibrillation and lidocaine are ineffective in correcting pediatric VF. The recommended dose is 5 mg/kg by rapid IV infusion. If VF persists after an additional defibrillation attempt, a dose of 10 mg/kg may be given.

Bradyarrhythmias

Hypoxemia, hypotension, and acidosis interfere with normal function of the sinus node and AV junctional tissue and slow conduction through normal pathways. Sinus bradycardia, sinus node arrest with a slow junctional or ventricular escape rhythm, and various degrees of AV block are the most common terminal rhythms in children.[16]

The Electrocardiogram:

• Rate is slow.
• P waves may or may not be visible.
• QRS duration may be normal or prolonged, depending on the pacemaker focus.
• The P and QRS are often unrelated (AV dissociation).

Therapy:

When CPR is required, a precise diagnosis of the specific bradyarrhythmia is not important. Therapy can be initiated once the rhythm is determined to be too slow for age and clinical condition.

Bradycardia (heart rate less than 60 beats per minute) associated with poor systemic perfusion should be treated in any infant or child, even if the blood pressure is normal. Adequate ventilation with 100% oxygen must be ensured, chest compressions performed, and epinephrine and atropine are administered as necessary (Fig 8).

Epinephrine (see also chapter 6) is a catecholamine with both α- and β-adrenergic receptor–stimulating action. β-Adrenergic receptor action increases myocardial contractility and heart rate. The recommended initial intravenous or intraosseous dose of epinephrine for the treatment of symptomatic bradycardia unresponsive to ventilation and oxygen administration is 0.01 mg/kg of the 1:10 000 solution (0.1 mL/kg). The dose given via the endotracheal tube is 0.1 mg/kg of the 1:1000 solution (0.1 mL/kg), diluted to a volume of 3 to 5 mL prior to instillation.

Atropine sulfate is a parasympatholytic drug that accelerates sinus or atrial pacemakers and enhances AV conduction. It should be used to treat bradycardia only after adequate ventilation and oxygenation have been ensured, since hypoxemia is a common cause of bradycardia. Atropine may be used to treat vagally mediated bradycardia during intubation if effective oxygenation is documented. Although atropine may be used to treat bradycardia associated with clinical evidence of shock (poor perfusion or hypotension), in this setting epinephrine may be more effective. Symptomatic bradycardia with AV block may be treated with atropine.

A vagolytic dose of atropine must be administered since smaller doses may produce paradoxical bradycardia.[17] The recommended dose is 0.02 mg/kg, with a minimum dose of 0.1 mg and a maximum single dose of 0.5 mg for a child and 1 mg for an adolescent. The dose may be repeated in 5 minutes to a maximum total dose of 1.0 mg for a child and 2.0 mg for an adolescent. The intravenous dose may be administered endotracheally, although absorption into the circulation by this route may be unreliable. The intravenous dose should be increased by two to three times and diluted to a minimum volume of 3 to 5 mL for endotracheal instillation. Tachycardia that follows atropine administration is usually sinus tachycardia and is usually well tolerated in the pediatric patient.

Pulseless Arrest

Pulseless arrest is clinically diagnosed by the absence of a palpable central pulse accompanied by apnea. The cardiac mechanism may be due to asystole, ventricular fibrillation, or a form of pulseless electrical activity (including electromechanical dissociation).

Asystole

Asystole is a form of pulseless arrest associated with absent cardiac electrical activity. Clinical confirmation (absent pulse, absent spontaneous respirations, poor perfusion) is mandatory since a straight line can also be caused by a loose ECG monitoring lead.

The Electrocardiogram (Fig 9):

• Straight line appears on the ECG monitor.
• P waves are occasionally observed.

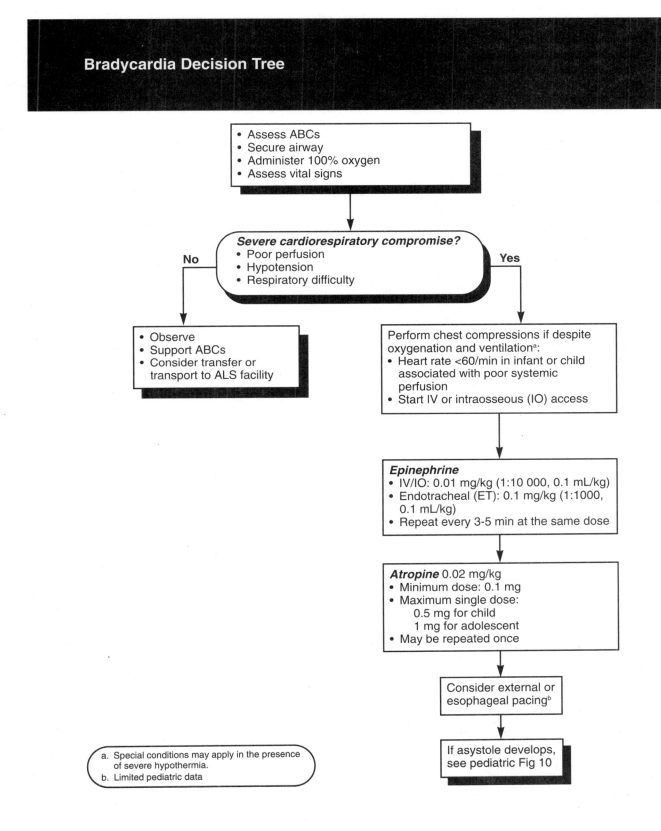

Bradycardia Decision Tree

- Assess ABCs
- Secure airway
- Administer 100% oxygen
- Assess vital signs

Severe cardiorespiratory compromise?
- Poor perfusion
- Hypotension
- Respiratory difficulty

No

Yes

- Observe
- Support ABCs
- Consider transfer or transport to ALS facility

Perform chest compressions if despite oxygenation and ventilation[a]:
- Heart rate <60/min in infant or child associated with poor systemic perfusion
- Start IV or intraosseous (IO) access

Epinephrine
- IV/IO: 0.01 mg/kg (1:10 000, 0.1 mL/kg)
- Endotracheal (ET): 0.1 mg/kg (1:1000, 0.1 mL/kg)
- Repeat every 3-5 min at the same dose

Atropine 0.02 mg/kg
- Minimum dose: 0.1 mg
- Maximum single dose:
    0.5 mg for child
    1 mg for adolescent
- May be repeated once

Consider external or esophageal pacing[b]

If asystole develops, see pediatric Fig 10

a. Special conditions may apply in the presence of severe hypothermia.
b. Limited pediatric data

Fig 8. The bradycardia decision tree.

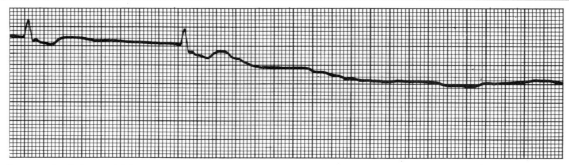

Fig 9. Ventricular asystole. Only two QRS complexes, probably representing ventricular escape beats, are seen. These complexes are followed by the absence of organized electrical activity.

Therapy:

Resuscitation for cardiac arrest should be provided (Fig 10).

Ventricular Fibrillation

Ventricular fibrillation (VF) is a chaotic, disorganized series of depolarizations that results in a quivering myocardium without organized contraction. Ventricular systole does not occur, so pulses are not palpable. VF is an uncommon terminal event in the pediatric age group and is documented in only about 10% of children in whom a terminal rhythm is recorded.[18] Resuscitation outcome, however, appears to be considerably better if VF rather than asystole or electromechanical dissociation is the underlying rhythm on initial presentation.[19] When an infant or child is pulseless, initial therapy includes establishment of adequate ventilation and oxygenation and provision of manual external chest compressions. Defibrillation should be attempted *only* if VF is confirmed by ECG monitoring. Pulseless VT is treated in the same manner as VF.

The Electrocardiogram (Fig 11):

- There are no identifiable P, QRS, or T waves.
- VF waves are chaotic and can be classified as coarse or fine by the height of the waves (however, treatment is identical for all classifications of VF).

Therapy:

Defibrillation. The definitive treatment for VF or pulseless VT is prompt defibrillation, but defibrillation is not indicated for treatment of asystole.[20] Ventilation with 100% oxygen and chest compressions should be continued until the moment of defibrillation. Ideally, vascular access is secured, but defibrillation should not be delayed to achieve this access.

Defibrillation is the untimed (asynchronous) depolarization of a critical mass of myocardial cells to allow spontaneous organized myocardial depolarization to resume. If organized depolarization does not resume, VF will continue or will progress to electrical silence. At this point restoration of spontaneous cardiac activity may be impossible. Synchronized cardioversion also results in depolarization of the myocardium, but cardioversion provides depolarization that is timed (synchronous) with the patient's intrinsic electrical activity. Since the patient with VF has no organized cardiac electrical activity, defibrillation must be provided.

Successful defibrillation requires the passage of sufficient electric current (amperes) through the heart. This current flow depends on the energy (joules) provided and the transthoracic impedance (ohms), which is the resistance to current flow. If transthoracic impedance is high, more energy is required to achieve sufficient current for successful defibrillation or cardioversion. Factors that determine transthoracic impedance include energy selected, electrode size, paddle-skin coupling material, number of shocks, time intervals between shocks, phase of ventilation, size of chest, and paddle electrode pressure.[21-26]

Energy Dose. The optimal energy dose for defibrillation in infants and children has not been established. Although available information does not demonstrate a relation between energy dose and weight, a starting dose of 2 J/kg for defibrillation is recommended[27,28] until further data are available. To minimize transthoracic impedance, the operator should press firmly on the electrode paddles during defibrillation. If VF continues after defibrillation with 2 J/kg, the energy level should be doubled (4 J/kg), since the initial energy level may have been too small. If the second attempt at defibrillation is delivered rapidly after the first, the current delivered to the heart will be increased because the initial attempt reduces transthoracic impedance. The third attempt, if it is necessary, should again use an energy level of 4 J/kg. When three shocks are required, they should be delivered rapidly and consecutively. Time between shocks should be just brief enough to check the rhythm with the electrode paddles in place. If VF continues, the second and third attempts at defibrillation should be made without pausing to perform CPR or check the pulse. If VF continues despite the three defibrillation attempts, energy levels may need to be increased further, but ventilation with 100% oxygen, chest compressions, and epinephrine administration should precede further defibrillation attempts. Continued VF may necessitate additional therapy with epinephrine, lidocaine, or bretylium. Whenever epinephrine, lidocaine, or

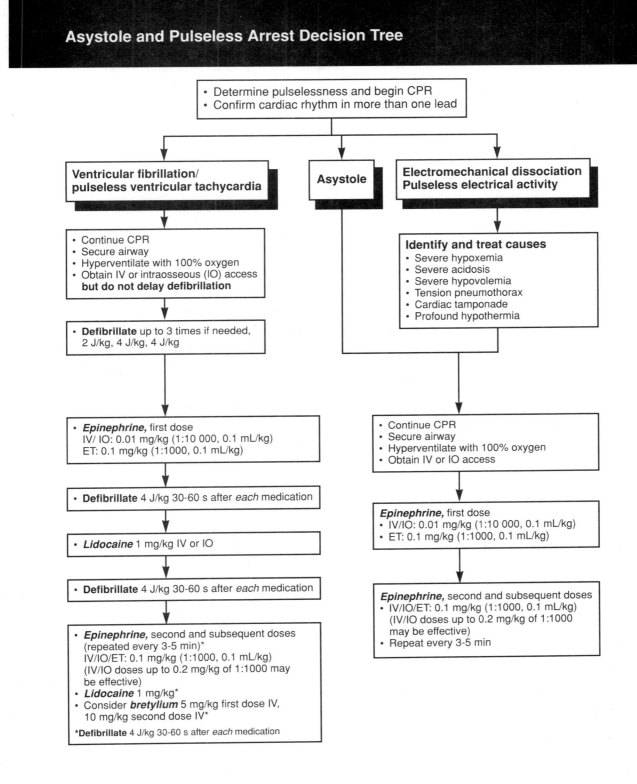

Fig 10. Asystole and pulseless arrest decision tree.

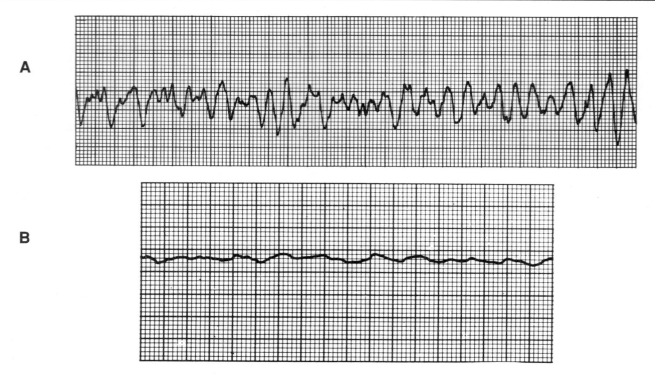

Fig 11. Ventricular fibrillation. A, Coarse VF. Note high-amplitude waveforms that vary in size, shape, and rhythm, representing chaotic ventricular electrical activity. B, Fine VF. Electrical activity is much reduced.

bretylium is administered to the patient with VF, *each dose should be followed within 30 to 60 seconds by defibrillation (4 J/kg)*. If VF is terminated but then recurs, defibrillation should be repeated at the energy level that previously resulted in successful defibrillation.

Paddle Size. Paddle size is one determinant of transthoracic impedance — the larger the size, the lower the impedance.[27,29,30] The paddle selected should be the largest size that allows good chest contact over the entire paddle surface area and good separation between the two paddles. "Infant" paddles (4.5 cm) should generally be used for infants up to approximately 1 year of age or 10 kg. "Adult" paddles (8 to 13 cm) should generally be used for patients older than 1 year or weighing more than 10 kg.

Electrode Interface. Since the skin acts as a resistor between the electrode paddles and the heart, a low-impedance interface medium (such as electrode cream or paste, saline-soaked gauze pads, or self-adhesive defibrillation pads) is recommended. Sonographic gels are unacceptable, alcohol pads represent a fire hazard and can produce serious chest burns, and bare paddles result in very high chest impedance.[23] The interface medium under one electrode paddle (eg, saline from a saline-soaked pad) must not come in contact with the medium under the other electrode, or bridging will occur. If bridging occurs, a short circuit will be created and an inadequate amount of current will traverse the heart.

Electrode Position. Electrode paddles must be placed so that the heart is between them. Anterior-posterior electrode position, with one electrode on the anterior chest over the heart and the other on the back, is theoretically superior but impractical during CPR. In standard electrode position, one paddle is placed on the upper right chest below the clavicle and the other to the left of the left nipple in the anterior axillary line. A mirror-image electrode placement is used if dextrocardia is present. Anterior-posterior paddle placement may be necessary for an infant if only adult paddles are available.

Safety. Defibrillation is potentially dangerous to the operator and other personnel who might come in conducting contact with the electrical current.[31] The person performing defibrillation must therefore always announce that the defibrillator will be discharged. Before each defibrillation attempt, the person who controls the defibrillator discharge buttons should state clearly, "I am going to shock on three. One — I am clear." The operator checks to make sure that there is no contact with the patient, stretcher, or equipment other than the paddle handles. The operator then states, "Two — you are clear," and checks to make sure that no other personnel are in contact with the patient, including healthcare providers performing ventilations and compressions. All hands must be removed from all equipment in contact with the patient, including the endotracheal tube, ventilation bag, and intravenous solutions. Finally, the operator states, "Three — everybody is clear," and discharges the defibrillator. The person operating the defibrillator need not use this exact wording but should use wording that is similar.

Defibrillator Testing. At the very low defibrillation dose settings required for infants, the stored and delivered energies of the defibrillator may vary significantly. All defibrillators should be checked periodically for safety and accuracy. It is especially important that defibrillators used for infants and children be checked at very low energy doses and that any variations between set and delivered energies be prominently posted on the machine.

Defibrillation Sequence. If VF is observed on the ECG monitor:

1. Continue ventilation with 100% oxygen and chest compressions without interruption (except during defibrillation).
2. Apply conductive medium to infant paddles (patient younger than approximately 1 year) or adult paddles (patient older than 1 year).
3. Turn on the defibrillator power; the synchronous mode should *not* be activated.
4. Select the energy dose and charge the capacitor.
5. Stop chest compressions and place paddles in the proper position on the chest.
6. Recheck the rhythm on the monitor.
7. Clear the area to ensure that no personnel are in contact with the patient, the bed, or the equipment ("one — I am clear; two — you are clear; three — everybody is clear").
8. Apply firm pressure to the paddles while simultaneously depressing the discharge buttons.
9. Evaluate ECG.

Electromechanical Dissociation

Electromechanical dissociation (EMD) is a form of pulseless electrical activity (PEA) characterized by organized electrical activity on ECG but with inadequate cardiac output and absent pulses. Causes include hypoxemia, severe acidosis, hypovolemia, tension pneumothorax, and pericardial tamponade. Other potential causes are hyperkalemia, profound hypothermia, and drug overdose (including overdose of tricyclic antidepressants, β blockers, and calcium channel blocking medications).

Outcome after EMD is poor unless the specific cause can be promptly identified and treated. Chest compressions, hyperventilation using 100% oxygen, intubation, and administration of epinephrine should be accomplished while the cause of EMD is sought (Fig 10).

Noninvasive (Transcutaneous) Pacing

Noninvasive transcutaneous pacing has been used for several years to treat adults with bradycardia and asystole,[32,33] but experience with children is limited.[33-36] Since this form of pacing is very uncomfortable, its use is reserved for children with profound symptomatic bradycardia refractory to BLS and ALS. Transcutaneous pacing has not been effective in improving the survival rate of children with out-of-hospital unwitnessed cardiac arrest.[34]

Noninvasive pacing requires the use of an external pacing unit and two large adhesive-backed electrodes. If the child weighs less than 15 kg, pediatric small or medium electrodes are recommended.[37] If the child weighs more than 15 kg, adult electrodes are used. The negative electrode is placed over the heart on the anterior chest and the positive electrode behind the heart on the back. If the back cannot be used, the positive electrode is placed on the right side of the anterior chest beneath the clavicle and the negative electrode on the left side of the chest over the fourth intercostal space, in the midaxillary area. Precise placement of electrodes does not appear to be necessary provided that the negative electrode is placed near the apex of the heart.[38]

Either ventricular fixed-rate or ventricular-inhibited pacing may be provided noninvasively. Pacemaker output usually will require adjustment to ensure that every impulse results in ventricular depolarization (capture). If smaller electrodes are used, the pacemaker output required to produce capture generally will be lower than if larger electrodes are used.[32] If ventricular-inhibited pacing is performed, the sensitivity of the pacemaker must be adjusted so that intrinsic ventricular electrical activity is appropriately sensed by the pacemaker. Because of the large pacing artifact that often occurs with transcutaneous pacing, it may be difficult to determine whether ventricular depolarization and contraction is taking place. This determination may be made by palpation of a pulse or from the pressure wave of an indwelling arterial cannula.

References

1. Alimurung MM, Joseph LG, Nadas AS, Massell BF. Unipolar precordial and extremity electrocardiogram in normal infants and children. *Circulation.* 1951;4:420-429.
2. Ziegler RF. *Electrocardiographic Studies in Normal Infants and Children.* Springfield, Ill: Charles C Thomas Publishing; 1951.
3. Furman RA, Halloran WR. Electrocardiogram in the first two months of life. *J Pediatr.* 1951;39:307-319.
4. Tudbury PB, Atkinson DW. Electrocardiograms of 100 normal infants and young children. *J Pediatr.* 1950;34:466-481.
5. Gillette PC, Garson A Jr, Porter CJ, McNamara DG. Dysrhythmias. In: Adams FH, Emmanouilides GC, Riemenschneider TA, eds. *Moss' Heart Disease in Infants, Children, and Adolescents.* 4th ed. Baltimore, Md: Williams & Wilkins; 1989:725-741.
6. Olley PH. Cardiac arrhythmias. In: Keith JD, Rowe RD, Vlad P, eds. *Heart Disease in Infancy and Childhood.* 3rd ed. New York, NY: Macmillan Publishing Co Inc; 1978:279-280.
7. Gikonyo BM, Dunnigan A, Benson DW Jr. Cardiovascular collapse in infants: association with paroxysmal atrial tachycardia. *Pediatrics.* 1985;76:922-926.
8. Garson A Jr. Supraventricular tachycardia. In: Gillette PC, Garson A Jr, eds. *Pediatric Cardiac Dysrhythmias.* New York, NY: Grune & Stratton Inc; 1981.
9. Fisher DJ, Gross DM, Garson A Jr. Rapid sinus tachycardia: differentiation from supraventricular tachycardia. *Am J Dis Child.* 1983;137:164-166.

10. Lown B. Electrical reversion of cardiac arrhythmias. *Br Heart J.* 1967;29:469-489.

11. Overholt ED, Rheuban KS, Gutgesell HP, Lerman BB, DiMarco JP. Usefulness of adenosine for arrhythmias in infants and children. *Am J Cardiol.* 1988;61:336-340.

12. Rossi AF, Burton DA. Adenosine in altering short- and long-term treatment of supraventricular tachycardia in infants. *Am J Cardiol.* 1989;64:685-686.

13. Till J, Shinebourne EA, Rigby ML, Clarke B, Ward DE, Rowland E. Efficacy and safety of adenosine in the treatment of supraventricular tachycardia in infants and children. *Br Heart J.* 1989;62: 204-211.

14. Radford D. Side effects of verapamil in infants. *Arch Dis Child.* 1983;58:465-466.

15. Epstein ML, Kiel EA, Victorica BE. Cardiac decompensation following verapamil therapy in infants with supraventricular tachycardia. *Pediatrics.* 1985;75:737-740.

16. Walsh CK, Krongrad E. Terminal cardiac electrical activity in pediatric patients. *Am J Cardiol.* 1983;51:557-561.

17. Dauchot P, Gravenstein JS. Effects of atropine on the electrocardiogram in different age groups. *Clin Pharmacol Ther.* 1971; 12:274-280.

18. Eisenberg M, Bergner L, Hallstrom A. Epidemiology of cardiac arrest and resuscitation in children. *Ann Emerg Med.* 1983;12: 672-674.

19. Coffing CR, Quan L, Graves JR, et al. Etiologies and outcomes of the pulseless, nonbreathing pediatric patient presenting with ventricular fibrillation. *Ann Emerg Med.* 1992;21:1046. Abstract.

20. Losek JD, Hennes H, Glaeser PW, Smith DS, Hendley G. Prehospital countershock treatment of pediatric asystole. *Am J Emerg Med.* 1989;7:571-575.

21. Kerber RE, Kouba C, Martins J, et al. Advance prediction of transthoracic impedance in human defibrillation and cardioversion: importance of impedance in determining the success of low-energy shocks. *Circulation.* 1984;70:303-308.

22. Kerber RE, Grayzel J, Hoyt R, Marcus M, Kennedy J. Transthoracic resistance in human defibrillation: influence of body weight, chest size, serial shocks, paddle size, and paddle contact pressure. *Circulation.* 1981;63:676-682.

23. Sirna SJ, Ferguson DW, Charbonnier F, Kerber RE. Factors affecting transthoracic impedance during electrical cardioversion. *Am J Cardiol.* 1988;62:1048-1052.

24. Lerman BB, DiMarco JP, Haines DE. Current-based versus energy-based ventricular defibrillation: a prospective study. *J Am Coll Cardiol.* 1988;12:1259-1264.

25. Dalzell GW, Cunningham SR, Anderson J, Adgey AA. Initial experience with a microprocessor controlled current-based defibrillator. *Br Heart J.* 1989;61:502-505.

26. Kerber RE, Martins JB, Kelly KJ, et al. Self-adhesive preapplied electrode pads for defibrillation and cardioversion. *J Am Coll Cardiol.* 1984;3:815-820.

27. Chameides L, Brown GE, Raye JR, Todres DI, Viles PH. Guidelines for defibrillation in infants and children: report of the American Heart Association Target Activity Group: cardiopulmonary resuscitation in the young. *Circulation.* 1977;56(suppl): 502A-503A.

28. Gutgesell HP, Tacker HA, Geddes LA, Davis JS, Lie JT, McNamara DG. Energy dose for ventricular defibrillation of children. *Pediatrics.* 1976;58:898-901.

29. Atkins DL, Sirna S, Kieso R, Charbonnier F, Kerber RE. Pediatric defibrillation: importance of paddle size in determining transthoracic impedance. *Pediatrics.* 1988;82:914-918.

30. Atkins DL, Kerber RE. Pediatric defibrillation: current flow is improved by using 'adult' paddle electrodes. *Circulation.* 1992;86(suppl I):I235. Abstract.

31. Gibbs W, Eisenberg M, Damon SK. Dangers of defibrillation: injuries to emergency personnel during patient resuscitation. *Am J Emerg Med.* 1990;8:101-104.

32. Zoll PM, Zoll RH, Falk RH, Clinton JE, Eitel DR, Antman EM. External noninvasive temporary cardiac pacing: clinical trials. *Circulation.* 1985;71:937-944.

33. Dalsey WC, Syverud SA, Hedges JR. Emergency department use of transcutaneous pacing for cardiac arrests. *Crit Care Med.* 1985;13:399-401.

34. Quan L, Graves JR, Kinder DR, Horan S, Cummins RO. Transcutaneous cardiac pacing in the treatment of out-of-hospital pediatric cardiac arrests. *Ann Emerg Med.* 1992;21:905-909.

35. Cummins RO, Haulman J, Quan L, Graves JR, Peterson D, Horan S. Near-fatal yew berry intoxication treated with external cardiac pacing and digoxin-specific FAB antibody fragments. *Ann Emerg Med.* 1990;19:38-43.

36. Kissoon N, Rosenberg HC, Kronick JB. Role of transcutaneous pacing in the setting of a failing permanent pacemaker. *Pediatr Emerg Care.* 1989;5:178-180.

37. Beland MJ, Hesslein PS, Finlay CD, Faerron-Angel JE, Williams WG, Rowe RD. Noninvasive transcutaneous cardiac pacing in children. *PACE Pacing Clin Electrophysiol.* 1987;10:1262-1270.

38. Falk RH, Ngai ST. External cardiac pacing: influence of electrode placement on pacing threshold. *Crit Care Med.* 1986;14:931-932.

Trauma Resuscitation

Chapter 8

Rapid cardiorespiratory assessment and prompt establishment of effective ventilation, oxygenation, and perfusion are the keys to the successful treatment of a child with a life-threatening illness or injury. The purpose of this chapter is to present those principles of care that impact the integrity of the airway, breathing, and circulation or influence the priorities of advanced life support (ALS) for the pediatric trauma patient. For information about the fundamentals of pediatric trauma management, the provider is referred to structured educational opportunities such as the Advanced Trauma Life Support Course (ATLS)[1] of the American College of Surgeons or the Advanced Pediatric Life Support Course (APLS)[2] of the American Academy of Pediatrics and the American College of Emergency Physicians. Both courses specifically address the early care of the injured child and use the same assessment-based approach to recognition of cardiopulmonary failure and support of ventilation, oxygenation, and perfusion emphasized throughout the Pediatric Advanced Life Support Course. Information about injury prevention is contained in the Pediatric Basic Life Support Course.

Approach to Pediatric Trauma Resuscitation

Trauma remains the leading cause of death and disability in the pediatric age group.[3] Because the injured child has significant potential for full recovery,[4-7] resuscitation must begin as soon as possible after injury, preferably at the scene. The principles of resuscitation of the seriously injured child are the same as for any other pediatric patient. However, some aspects of initial stabilization of the pediatric trauma patient are unique and require special emphasis.

The child with multisystem trauma may have both respiratory failure and shock, so both must be treated rapidly and effectively. Assessment and support of cardiopulmonary function are fundamental aspects of the primary survey performed during the initial minutes of trauma care. At the same time that cardiopulmonary function is assessed, a rapid thoracoabdominal examination must be performed to detect life-threatening chest injuries or conditions that may interfere with successful resuscitation. For example, ventilation, oxygenation, and perfusion may be ineffective until a tension pneumothorax is treated or a major source of external bleeding is controlled.

The treatment of most abnormalities found during the primary survey, including needle decompression of tension pneumothorax, direct pressure control of external hemorrhage, or nasogastric tube decompression of

gastric distention, is described later in this chapter or elsewhere in the course. These lifesaving measures should precede other treatments that may be required for multisystem trauma. Definitive evaluation and initial treatment of most other injuries can be safely undertaken after ventilation, oxygenation, and perfusion have been restored. Such definitive care is provided upon completion of the *secondary survey*, a detailed head-to-toe examination for detection of specific injuries. This secondary survey is unique to trauma care and is not included in this course.

Improper resuscitation has been identified as a major cause of preventable pediatric trauma death.[8] Common errors in pediatric trauma resuscitation include failure to (1) open and maintain the airway, (2) provide appropriate fluid resuscitation to children with head injury, and (3) recognize and treat internal hemorrhage.[9] A qualified surgeon should be involved as early as possible in the course of resuscitation. Children with multisystem trauma or significant mortality risk (Pediatric Trauma Score[10] of 8 or less or Revised Trauma Score[11] of 11 or less [Table 1]) should, if possible, be transported to trauma centers with expertise in treating pediatric patients.[12-14]

Table 1. Pediatric Trauma Score and Revised Trauma Score

	Pediatric Trauma Score*		
	Coded Value		
Patient Characteristics	+2	+1	−1
Weight (kg)	>20	10-20	<10
Airway	Normal	Maintained	Unmaintained
Systolic blood pressure (mm Hg)	>90	50-90	<50
Central nervous system	Awake	Obtunded	Coma
Open wound	None	Minor	Major
Skeletal trauma	None	Closed	Open, multiple

	Revised Trauma Score†		
Glasgow Coma Scale Score‡	Systolic Blood Pressure (mm Hg)	Respiratory Rate (breaths/minute)	Coded Value
13-15	>89	10-29	4
9-12	76-89	>29	3
6-8	50-75	6-9	2
4-5	1-49	1-5	1
3	0	0	0

*From Tepas.[10]
†From Champion.[11]
‡Refer to Table 2.

Airway

Establishment of a patent airway with simultaneous control of the cervical spine is particularly difficult in the pediatric victim of multisystem trauma. The child's narrow airway is easily obstructed by foreign matter such as blood, mucus, and dental fragments and must be cleared by suctioning with a rigid, large-bore device, such as a Yankauer suction. Occasionally, direct foreign-body retrieval with Rovenstein (pediatric Magill) forceps is necessary.

Cervical spine injury is less common in pediatric than in adult trauma,[15] because the child's spine is more elastic and mobile than that of the adult and the softer pediatric vertebrae are less likely to fracture with minor stress.[16] Although the short but mobile pediatric cervical spine may be less likely to sustain damage during minor injury, the risk of cervical spine injury is increased whenever the child is subjected to the inertial forces applied to the neck during acceleration-deceleration, eg, those involving motor vehicles or falls from a height.[16] The risk of such injury is increased because the child's head is proportionally larger than the head of an adult and is more likely to "lead" if the child falls or is propelled through or out of an automobile. Thus, serious head injury and concomitant cervical spine injury may occur. Associated spinal cord damage is usually the result of subluxation, most often at the atlanto-occipital (base of skull – C1) or atlantoaxial (C1-C2) joints in infants and toddlers or the lower (C5-C7) cervical spine in school-age children.[17]

Cervical spine injury may be anatomic or functional. Anatomic injury is associated with bony vertebral abnormality, while functional injury consists of spinal cord injury without radiographic abnormality (SCIWORA).[18] The increased elasticity and mobility of the pediatric spine that permits SCIWORA is attributable to the relative laxity of cervical spine ligaments, incomplete development of cervical musculature, and the shallow orientation of facet joints in young children.

SCIWORA is now recognized as an important cause of pediatric spinal cord injury[19,20] and accounts for a large number of prehospital deaths that previously were attributed to head trauma.[21] By definition, this form of spinal cord injury cannot be excluded by radiographic examination. Thus, the lateral cervical spine x-ray commonly used to rule out injury to the cervical spine in adult blunt trauma victims cannot rule out such an injury in young children. Cervical spinal cord injury must therefore be assumed to be present in all children with multiple injuries, especially those who are apneic, and appropriate precautions must be taken to avoid potential exacerbation of injury during each phase of airway management and control.

Immediate airway obstruction or respiratory arrest may develop in the child with severe closed head injury through three mechanisms:

- Upper airway closure due to soft tissue obstruction by the tongue and epiglottis, which occurs when the child loses consciousness[22,23]

- Cervical spine transection with subsequent respiratory arrest
- Midbrain or medullary contusion

The airway of the pediatric trauma victim must therefore be fully opened and maintained while the cervical spine is manually immobilized in a neutral position. This is best accomplished using the combined jaw-thrust/spinal-stabilization maneuver[24] (Fig 1). *Traction on or movement of the neck must be avoided.* Instead, the head and neck must be held firmly in a neutral position to prevent cervical motion. Note that the head tilt–chin lift maneuver to open the airway is contraindicated in trauma patients, because manipulation of the head may result in conversion of an incomplete to a complete spinal cord injury.

After the airway has been effectively opened and the cervical spine has been simultaneously stabilized, an oral airway may be used. A semirigid extrication collar should be applied (Fig 2), but it must fit perfectly because excessively large collars may allow neck flexion or hyperextension. Soft collars do not immobilize the cervical spine effectively and have no role in initial stabilization of the child with multiple injuries.[25]

Optimal immobilization of the cervical spine is achieved with a long spine board, commercial head immobilizers, foam blocks or linen rolls, and tape, in addition to the

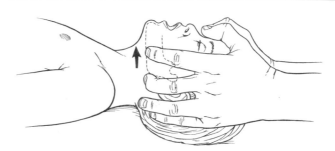

Fig 1. Proper method of simultaneous cervical spine stabilization during airway opening in the child with multiple injuries.

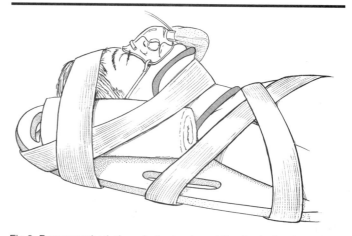

Fig 2. Proper method of cervical spine immobilization in the child with multiple injuries.

cervical collar. This is accomplished after immobilization of the upper torso with shoulder straps (Fig 2). The prominent occiput of the child predisposes the neck to slight flexion when the child is placed on a completely flat spine board.[26] Pediatric spine boards with shallow head wells may facilitate maintenance of a neutral position.[25] If such a board is unavailable, a thin layer of firm padding is placed on a flat board under the child's torso to elevate the torso approximately 2 cm, allowing the head to assume a neutral position.

Indications for endotracheal intubation of the child trauma victim are

- Respiratory arrest
- Respiratory failure (hypoventilation, arterial hypoxemia despite supplemental oxygen therapy, and/or respiratory acidosis)
- Airway obstruction
- Coma — Glasgow Coma[27] or modified Pediatric Coma Score[28-30] of 8 or less (see Table 2)
- Need for prolonged ventilatory support (eg, thoracic injuries or need for diagnostic studies)

Table 2. Glasgow Coma Scale and Pediatric Coma Scale

Glasgow Coma Scale[27]	Coded Value	Adelaide Pediatric Coma Scale[30]	Coded Value
Eye Opening		Eye Opening	
Spontaneous	4	Spontaneous	4
To speech	3	To speech	3
To pain	2	To pain	2
None	1	None	1
Best Verbal Response		Best Verbal Response	
Oriented	5	Oriented	5
Confused	4	Words	4
Inappropriate words	3	Vocal sounds	3
Incomprehensible sounds	2	Cries	2
None	1	None	1
Best Motor Response*		Best Motor Response*	
Obeys	6	Obeys commands	5
Localizes	5	Localizes pain	4
Withdraws	4	Flexion to pain	3
Abnormal flexion	3	Extension to pain	2
Extensor response	2	None	1
None	1	Total‡	3-14
Total	3-15	‡Normal Aggregate Score	
		0-6 months	9
		6-12 months	11
		1-2 years	12
		2-5 years	13
		>5 years	14

Modified Glasgow Coma Scale for Infants and Children†			
	Child	Infant	Score
Eye opening	Spontaneous	Spontaneous	4
	To verbal stimuli	To verbal stimuli	3
	To pain only	To pain only	2
	No response	No response	1
Verbal response	Oriented, appropriate	Coos and babbles	5
	Confused	Irritable cries	4
	Inappropriate words	Cries to pain	3
	Incomprehensible words or nonspecific sounds	Moans to pain	2
	No response	No response	1
Motor response*	Obeys commands	Moves spontaneously and purposefully	6
	Localizes painful stimulus	Withdraws to touch	5
	Withdraws in response to pain	Withdraws in response to pain	4
	Flexion in response to pain	Decorticate posturing (abnormal flexion) in response to pain	3
	Extension in response to pain	Decerebrate posturing (abnormal extension) in response to pain	2
	No response	No response	1

*If the patient is intubated, unconscious, or preverbal, the most important part of this scale is motor response. This section should be carefully evaluated.

†Modified from Davis RJ, et al. Head and spinal cord injury. In: Rogers MC, ed. *Textbook of Pediatric Intensive Care*. Baltimore, Md: Williams & Wilkins; 1987. James H, Anas N, Perkin RM. *Brain Insults in Infants and Children*. New York, NY: Grune & Stratton; 1985. Morray JP, et al. Coma scale for use in brain-injured children. *Crit Care Med*. 1984;12:1018. Reproduced from Hazinski MF. Neurologic disorders. In: Hazinski MF, ed. *Nursing Care of the Critically Ill Child*. 2nd ed. St Louis, Mo: Mosby Year Book; 1992.

Endotracheal intubation of the pediatric trauma victim may be difficult because the neck *must* remain in a neutral position and cannot be hyperextended during the procedure. The orotracheal route is the preferred approach for endotracheal intubation of children 8 years old or younger. The nasotracheal route is contraindicated because it is extremely difficult to direct the tube anteriorly through the vocal cords in young children without direct visualization. In addition, adenoid tissue is much more prominent and susceptible to injury during emergent intubation.

If the child is properly immobilized on a spine board and a semirigid cervical collar is in place, endotracheal intubation can occasionally be accomplished by one person. If this is impossible, if the child is agitated, or if there is any doubt about the effectiveness of cervical spine immobilization, one rescuer must stabilize the neck while the second rescuer performs the endotracheal intubation (Fig 3). Endotracheal intubation should always be preceded by bag-valve–mask ventilation and oxygenation. If the child is conscious, administration of a short-acting neuromuscular blocking agent, such as succinylcholine, followed immediately by a sedative or anesthetic, such as thiopental, may be necessary to avoid a concomitant increase in intracranial pressure. Sedatives or narcotics should not be administered until the child's neurologic and cardiovascular status is carefully evaluated. *These drugs should be used only by personnel who are familiar with their use and complications* and are properly trained in the technique of rapid sequence induction.[31] Sedative or narcotic use is contraindicated if the patient is hypotensive.

Though rarely necessary in pediatric trauma victims, cricothyrotomy may be required in the presence of severe orofacial trauma, although the increasing availability of fiberoptic laryngoscopy has mitigated this need in recent years. Most children with cervical spine fractures or dislocations have stable injuries that can be managed successfully with spinal immobilization and endotracheal intubation.[32] However, cricothyrotomy may occasionally be useful in the care of the patient with an unstable cervical spine injury. For a detailed description of cricothyrotomy, see chapter 4.

Breathing

Effectiveness of ventilation and oxygenation must be continuously evaluated. If the airway is patent and respiratory effort is effective (adequate bilateral, symmetrical chest rise and air entry with no central cyanosis), the injured child should receive supplemental oxygen in the highest available concentration through a nonrebreathing mask. If respiratory effort is ineffective, ventilatory assistance with a bag-valve–mask device and reservoir delivering 100% oxygen is required. This assistance must eventually be followed by endotracheal intubation.

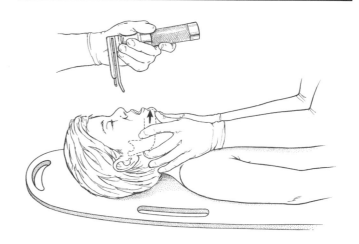

Fig 3. Proper method of cervical spine stabilization during endotracheal intubation of the child with multiple injuries.

Hyperventilation is often necessary during initial stabilization of the pediatric trauma patient to eliminate excess carbon dioxide and to maintain moderate hypocarbia ($Paco_2$ 22 to 29 mm Hg). Such hyperventilation corrects any respiratory acidosis associated with alveolar hypoventilation and temporarily buffers metabolic acidosis caused by persistent hypovolemia and shock. In addition, hyperventilation and resultant hypocarbia should reduce the excessive cerebral blood flow thought to be present immediately following head trauma.[33,34] Such hyperventilation may reduce the increased intracranial pressure associated with excessive cerebral blood flow if cerebral carbon dioxide vascular reactivity is preserved.[35,36] Extreme hyperventilation probably should be avoided, since it may reduce cerebral blood flow to levels associated with ischemia.

In the absence of blood gas analysis, the amount of hyperventilation required to produce moderate hypocarbia and respiratory alkalosis may be difficult to judge. A tidal volume that produces visible chest expansion is approximately 1 to 1.5 times the normal tidal volume. If the child's normal ventilatory rate for age is doubled and only short pauses are allowed between breaths, the minute ventilation provided will be approximately twice normal. Such hyperventilation should quickly reduce the $Paco_2$ below 30 mm Hg unless preexistent hypercarbia is present.

Ventilation of the injured child may be compromised by gastric distention caused by swallowed air, overzealous ventilatory assistance via a bag-valve–mask device, or a leak around an uncuffed endotracheal tube.[37] Significant gastric distention limits diaphragm motion and increases the risk of vomiting and aspiration. A nasogastric tube should therefore be inserted as soon as the airway is controlled. However, *orogastric* tubes should be used in children with severe craniofacial trauma with maxillofacial or basilar skull fracture to avoid potential intracranial migration of nasogastric tubes in such conditions.[38]

Circulation

Circulatory support of the pediatric trauma victim requires simultaneous control of external hemorrhage, assessment and support of cardiovascular function and systemic perfusion, and restoration and maintenance of adequate blood volume. Surgical intervention may be required to control internal bleeding. Blood transfusion is of paramount importance in the initial stabilization of the pediatric trauma patient who has sustained significant blood loss, to restore oxygen delivery as well as intravascular volume. In fact, failure to recognize and control internal bleeding is thought to be a leading cause of preventable death in children with multiple injuries.[9] For this reason, evaluation and stabilization of the child's systemic perfusion must be accomplished quickly, with the early involvement of a surgeon.

Control of external hemorrhage must be accomplished immediately by application of direct pressure over the wound(s). Sterile gauze dressings and latex gloves should be used to protect both the patient and rescuer from infection. Thin dressings applied with pressure are more effective than bulky dressings, which may absorb large quantities of blood and may also dissipate the amount of pressure actually applied to the wound. Blind application of hemostatic clamps is contraindicated, and tourniquets should not be used except in cases of traumatic amputation associated with uncontrolled bleeding from a major vessel. Open or closed long bone fractures may also bleed extensively and should be immobilized in an anatomic position using appropriate splints.

Signs of shock may be observed immediately or may evolve gradually following trauma. If acute hemorrhage totals more than 15% of blood volume, signs of circulatory failure (tachycardia, decrease in intensity of peripheral pulses, delayed capillary refill, and cool extremities) will be observed. *Hypotension will not be present until 25% to 30% or more of the child's blood volume is lost acutely.*[39] Therefore, careful observation of the child's systemic perfusion is required at all times, and rapid resuscitation must be provided if compromise in systemic perfusion is detected. Signs of shock may initially be subtle in the child and may be difficult to differentiate from signs of pain or fear.

Reliable vascular access in the pediatric trauma patient must be obtained quickly. Two short, large-bore catheters are placed at peripheral sites, preferably in the upper extremities because injuries to the lower extremities are more common in young children. The efficacy of fluid resuscitation in young subjects may be unrelated to the site of venous access[40] but will be determined by the fluid volume, fluid type, and speed of delivery. The intraosseous route is an acceptable form of vascular access in the child younger than 6 years if an intravenous route cannot be established rapidly.[41-49] If these methods of access are unsuccessful, percutaneous cannulation of the femoral vein at the groin or saphenous vein cutdown

at the ankle should be attempted if skilled personnel are available. Healthcare providers should attempt to secure the largest catheter in the largest vein possible at the sites with which they are most experienced (see chapter 5).

If systemic perfusion is inadequate but blood pressure is normal (compensated shock), mild to moderate hypovolemia (class I-II hemorrhage) is present (see Table 3), and rapid volume replacement with a bolus of 20 mL/kg of isotonic crystalloid (lactated Ringer's or normal saline) solution should be provided. Additional boluses of 20 mL/kg isotonic crystalloid solution may be required if systemic perfusion does not improve. Administration of blood should be considered if signs of shock persist after two boluses of crystalloid solution. The presence of frank hypotension (uncompensated shock) indicates a 25% to 30% or greater blood volume loss (class III-IV hemorrhage) and the need for immediate volume replacement and blood transfusion. The use of a pressure infusion system or a "wide open" intravenous system may be necessary to administer fluids quickly in these patients. Urgent transfusion is also necessary if the child fails to respond to administration of a total of 50 mL/kg of isotonic crystalloid solution, and surgical intervention may also be necessary. If perfusion and blood pressure are adequate, large volume infusions may be detrimental and should be avoided.

Blood should be administered in boluses of 10 mL/kg of packed red blood cells mixed with normal saline solution warmed to body temperature. Warming of blood products will help increase the speed of transfusion and help rewarm the patient. Alternatively, boluses of 20 mL/kg of whole blood may be administered. These boluses should be repeated until systemic perfusion is adequate. Under ideal circumstances, administered blood should be type specific and crossmatched. However, transfusion must not be delayed to await compatibility studies if shock continues despite crystalloid therapy. Instead, O-negative blood should be administered immediately.

If shock persists despite control of external hemorrhage and volume resuscitation, internal bleeding is likely. Such bleeding requires continued transfusion therapy, surgical assessment, and probable urgent surgical exploration. For this reason, a qualified surgeon should be notified before the arrival of any child with multiple injuries in the emergency department and should be involved in initial evaluation and stabilization. Blood samples for type and crossmatch should also be obtained immediately upon the arrival of a child in the emergency department.

Volume resuscitation and blood transfusion should continue as long as signs of shock are present in a child with head injury. In fact, ischemia may complicate traumatic brain injury unless intravascular volume is effectively restored. Once intravascular volume and systemic perfusion have been restored, excessive fluid administration should be avoided, since it may produce complications of hypervolemia or extravascular fluid

Table 3. Classification of Hemorrhagic Shock in Pediatric Trauma Patients Based on Systemic Signs

System	Class I Very mild hemorrhage (<15% blood volume loss)	Class II Mild hemorrhage (15% to 25% blood volume loss)	Class III Moderate hemorrhage (26% to 39% blood volume loss)	Class IV Severe hemorrhage (≥40% blood volume loss)
Cardiovascular	Heart rate normal or mildly increased	Tachycardia	Significant tachycardia	Severe tachycardia
	Normal pulses	Peripheral pulses may be diminished	Thready peripheral pulses	Thready central pulses
	Normal blood pressure	Normal blood pressure	Hypotension	Significant hypotension
	Normal pH	Normal pH	Metabolic acidosis	Significant acidosis
Respiratory	Rate normal	Tachypnea	Moderate tachypnea	Severe tachypnea
Central nervous system	Slightly anxious	Irritable, confused	Irritable or lethargic	Lethargic
		Combative	Diminished pain response	Coma
Skin	Warm, pink	Cool extremities, mottling	Cool extremities, mottling or pallor	Cold extremities, pallor or cyanosis
	Capillary refill brisk	Delayed capillary refill	Prolonged capillary refill	
Kidneys	Normal urine output	Oliguria, increased specific gravity	Oliguria, increased BUN	Anuria

Modified from American College of Surgeons. *Advanced Trauma Life Support Course.* 4th ed. Chicago, Ill: American College of Surgeons; 1992, and Fleisher GR, Ludwig S. *Textbook of Pediatric Emergency Medicine.* 2nd ed. Baltimore, Md: Williams & Wilkins; 1988. Reproduced with permission from Soud T, Pieper P, Hazinski MF. Pediatric trauma. In: Hazinski MF, ed. *Nursing Care of the Critically Ill Child.* 2nd ed. St Louis, Mo: Mosby Year Book; 1992.

shifts. Isolated head injury rarely causes sufficient blood loss to produce shock, although scalp lacerations may produce significant blood loss. If shock *is* present in a child with head injury and no external bleeding site can be identified, an internal bleeding source is likely and intra-abdominal hemorrhage must be ruled out.

Signs of intra-abdominal bleeding caused by organ rupture include abdominal tenderness, distention that does not improve following nasogastric decompression, and signs of shock. Nasogastric aspirate that is blood- or bile-stained also suggests the possibility of injury to intra-abdominal organs. Intra-abdominal bleeding, particularly if associated with shock, is a life-threatening surgical emergency that must be expeditiously evaluated and treated by qualified personnel. Isolated long bone or pelvic fractures may also cause significant blood loss in children, but these fractures rarely produce a sufficient volume deficit to result in hypotensive shock[50] and therefore usually do not pose an immediate threat to the integrity of vital organs or functions.

Medical antishock trousers (MAST) have not been effective in the treatment of hemorrhagic shock associated with major pediatric trauma (with the exception of pelvic fractures[51,52]). Furthermore, serious complications, including lower extremity compartment syndromes[53] and ischemic events,[54] may result from their use. The rise in blood pressure observed following MAST inflation in hemorrhagic shock results less from augmented venous return than from increased systemic vascular resistance produced by obstruction of lower extremity blood flow.[55-59] For this reason there is concern that MAST may increase

the rate of bleeding in areas above the garment and worsen survival, particularly in penetrating trauma.[60,61] While anecdotal reports suggest that MAST may occasionally be useful in the management of shock associated with pediatric blunt trauma if vascular access is delayed,[45,62] recent evidence indicates that the trousers offer no demonstrable survival benefit for most children with profound hypotension and may actually worsen outcome in children with mild to moderate hypotension.[63] Thus, MAST cannot be recommended for use in the treatment of hemorrhagic shock associated with major pediatric trauma, except in cases involving unstable pelvic fractures.

If used in children with unstable pelvic fractures, MAST should be inflated to a minimum pressure of 40 to 50 mm Hg. Lower pressures are ineffective in increasing blood pressure, and significantly higher pressures predispose tissue to ischemia.[64,65] If the patient's condition deteriorates suddenly after MAST inflation, the device should be immediately deflated. The abdominal compartment should never be inflated, because it may compress abdominal contents against the diaphragm and compromise ventilation.[66] Infusion of fluid and drugs from more distal sites does not appear to be hindered by MAST inflation,[67-69] but MAST application eliminates the femoral and intraosseous routes of vascular access. Severe head injury is no longer considered a contraindication to MAST, since the trousers produce minimal increase in intracranial pressure.[70]

Life-Threatening Chest Injuries

Although serious chest injuries are uncommon in pediatric trauma, some intrathoracic injuries, including tension pneumothorax, open pneumothorax, massive hemothorax, cardiac tamponade, and flail chest, may constitute an immediate threat to life and must be treated to establish effective ventilation, oxygenation, and perfusion. The pediatric chest wall is extremely compliant, so severe blunt chest trauma may be sustained without associated rib fractures or other overt evidence of trauma.[71] For this reason intrathoracic injuries must be suspected and ruled out whenever there is a significant history of blunt trauma. The presence of rib fractures indicates that severe chest trauma has occurred, and injury to underlying organs, such as the liver, spleen, and lungs, is likely to be present.[71]

The two injuries most likely to impede initial stabilization of the pediatric trauma victim are tension pneumothorax and open pneumothorax. Flail chest and massive hemothorax are also problematic but are best managed initially by aggressive treatment of the respiratory failure and shock they produce. Flail chest is usually treated with prolonged positive-pressure ventilation. Massive hemothorax requires urgent placement of a chest tube. Cardiac tamponade may occur with penetrating chest trauma but is extremely rare in childhood blunt trauma. It requires emergent surgical drainage and repair.

Tension pneumothorax is caused by the trapping of air behind a one-way "flap-valve" defect in the lung and results from penetrating chest trauma or acute barotrauma sustained at the moment of blunt injury. The child with tension pneumothorax demonstrates severe respiratory distress, distended neck veins, and contralateral tracheal deviation. Hyperresonance to percussion, decreased chest expansion, and diminished breath sounds will be found on the side of the injury and will be particularly evident during positive-pressure ventilation. Systemic perfusion will be severely compromised as the mediastinum shifts to the contralateral side, twisting the superior and inferior vena cavae and obstructing venous return.

Urgent treatment of tension pneumothorax requires needle decompression followed by placement of a chest tube. Decompression must precede confirmatory chest x-ray if signs of respiratory distress or shock are present. Needle decompression is accomplished using an over-the-needle catheter, which is inserted through the second intercostal space on the midclavicular line, just above the third rib. The pneumothorax may be vented to the atmosphere until the chest tube is inserted.

Open pneumothorax, or "sucking chest wound," results from a penetrating chest wound that allows free, bidirectional flow of air between the affected hemithorax and the surrounding atmosphere. It prevents effective ventilation by causing equilibration of intrathoracic and extrathoracic pressure. This results in paradoxical shifting of the mediastinum to the contralateral side with each spontaneous breath. Because the mediastinum is particularly mobile during childhood, sucking chest wounds may be lethal. Fortunately they are rare.[72]

Treatment of a respiratory decompensation associated with an open pneumothorax consists of positive-pressure ventilation. In addition, the wound should be covered using an occlusive dressing such as Vaseline® gauze. This dressing should be taped on three sides to allow egress of entrapped air during exhalation. Dressing application should be followed by insertion of a chest tube, unless the defect is so large that it requires immediate surgical repair.

Summary

Most pediatric trauma-related mortality occurs before admission to the hospital,[73] either in the field or in the emergency department. The initial stabilization of the pediatric trauma victim therefore requires immediate treatment of respiratory failure, shock, and life-threatening chest injuries to ensure effectiveness of ventilation, oxygenation, and perfusion until definitive trauma care becomes available. Simultaneously the cervical spine must be protected from possible injury or reinjury. Rapid cardiopulmonary assessment, basic airway maneuvers, and vascular access skills are all that will be required for the majority of patients. Occasionally needle decompression of a tension pneumothorax or establishment of a needle cricothyrotomy will be necessary.

The approach to the initial evaluation and stabilization of the child with multiple injuries and respiratory failure or shock is depicted in Table 4. This approach is fundamentally the same as that taken for the child with respiratory failure or shock of nontraumatic cause, with the addition of assessment and treatment of injuries that may impede successful resuscitation. The importance of early blood

Table 4. Approach to the Child With Multiple Injuries

1. Open airway with modified jaw thrust while maintaining manual in-line cervical spine stabilization.
2. Clear oropharynx with rigid suction device and pediatric Magill forceps as indicated.
3. Administer 100% oxygen via nonrebreathing mask if child is awake and breathes spontaneously.
4. Hyperventilate with 100% oxygen using bag-valve mask if child has altered mental status or respiratory distress.
5. Perform Sellick maneuver followed by orotracheal intubation if child is unresponsive or has signs of respiratory failure.
6. Maintain airway patency using appropriate suction device and oropharyngeal airway as necessary.
7. Initiate CPR and control external bleeding as indicated.
8. Examine chest for tension/open pneumothorax; treat if found.
9. Establish venous access; obtain type and crossmatch.
10. Rapidly infuse 20 mL/kg isotonic crystalloid solution if signs of inadequate systemic perfusion are present.
11. Immobilize neck with semirigid collar or head immobilizer and tape.
12. Insert nasal or orogastric tube and decompress stomach.
13. Infuse second crystalloid bolus and give blood as necessary if signs of shock or major hemorrhage are present.
14. Ensure that *pediatric trauma surgeon* has been notified.

replacement and early consultation with a surgeon cannot be overemphasized. Finally, the airway must be maintained while every effort is made to protect the cervical spine. A far greater number of preventable deaths have been attributed to failure to secure the airway in cases of suspected cervical spine injury than have ever been attributed to spinal cord injury itself.

References

1. American College of Surgeons Committee on Trauma. Pediatric trauma. In: *Advanced Trauma Life Support Course Student Manual*. 4th ed. Chicago, Ill: American College of Surgeons; 1992.

2. Bushore MS, ed. *Advanced Pediatric Life Support*. Elk Grove Village, Ill, and Dallas, Tex: American Academy of Pediatrics and American College of Emergency Physicians; 1990.

3. National Research Council Commission on Life Sciences Committee on Trauma Research, Institute of Medicine. *Injury in America: A Continuing Public Health Problem*. Washington, DC: National Academy Press; 1985:19.

4. Kraus JF, Fife D, Cox P, Ramstein K, Conroy C. Incidence, severity, and external causes of pediatric brain injury. *Am J Dis Child*. 1986;140:687-693.

5. Kraus JF, Fife D, Conroy C. Pediatric brain injuries: the nature, clinical course, and early outcomes in a defined United States' population. *Pediatrics*. 1987;79:501-507.

6. Luerssen TG, Klauber MR, Marshall LF. Outcome from head injury related to patient's age: a longitudinal prospective study of adult and pediatric head injury. *J Neurosurg*. 1988;68:409-416.

7. Tepas JJ III, DiScala C, Ramenofsky ML, Barlow B. Mortality and head injury: the pediatric perspective. *J Pediatr Surg*. 1990;25:92-96.

8. McKoy C, Bell MJ. Preventable traumatic deaths in children. *J Pediatr Surg*. 1983;18:505-508.

9. Dykes EH, Spence LJ, Young JG, Bohn DJ, Filler RM, Wesson DE. Preventable pediatric trauma deaths in a metropolitan region. *J Pediatr Surg*. 1989;24:107-110.

10. Tepas JJ III, Mollitt DL, Talbert JL, Bryant M. The pediatric trauma score as a predictor of injury severity in the injured child. *J Pediatr Surg*. 1987;22:14-18.

11. Champion HR, Sacco WJ, Copes WS, Gann DS, Gennarelli TA, Flanagan ME. A revision of the Trauma Score. *J Trauma*. 1989;29:623-629.

12. Pollack MM, Alexander SR, Clarke N, Ruttimann UE, Tesselaar HM, Bachulis AC. Improved outcomes from tertiary center pediatric intensive care: a statewide comparison of tertiary and nontertiary care facilities. *Crit Care Med*. 1991;19:150-159.

13. Nakayama DK, Copes WS, Sacco W. Differences in trauma care among pediatric and nonpediatric trauma centers. *J Pediatr Surg*. 1992;27:427-431.

14. Cooper A, Barlow B, DiScala C, String D, Ray K, Mottley L. Efficacy of pediatric trauma care: results of a population-based study. *J Pediatr Surg*. 1993;28:299-305.

15. Kewalramani LS, Kraus JF, Sterling HM. Acute spinal-cord lesions in a pediatric population: epidemiological and clinical features. *Paraplegia*. 1980;18:206-219.

16. Ruge JR, Sinson GP, McLone DG, Cerullo LJ. Pediatric spinal injury: the very young. *J Neurosurg*. 1988;68:25-30.

17. Hill SA, Miller CA, Kosnik EJ, Hunt WE. Pediatric neck injuries: a clinical study. *J Neurosurg*. 1984;60:700-706.

18. Pang D, Wilberger JE Jr. Spinal cord injury without radiographic abnormalities in children. *J Neurosurg*. 1982;57:114-129.

19. Sneed RC, Stover SL. Undiagnosed spinal cord injuries in brain-injured children. *Am J Dis Child*. 1988;142:965-967.

20. Pang D, Pollack IF. Spinal cord injury without radiographic abnormality in children: the SCIWORA syndrome. *J Trauma*. 1989;29:654-664.

21. Bohn D, Armstrong D, Becker L, Humphreys R. Cervical spine injuries in children. *J Trauma*. 1990;30:463-469.

22. Boidin MP. Airway patency in the unconscious patient. *Br J Anaesth*. 1985;57:306-310.

23. Safar P, Escarraga LA, Chang F. Upper airway obstruction in the unconscious patient. *J Appl Physiol*. 1959;14:760-764.

24. Cooper A, Foltin G, Tunik M. Airway control in the unconscious child victim: description of a new maneuver. *Pediatr Emerg Care*. In press.

25. Huerta C, Griffith R, Joyce SM. Cervical spine stabilization in pediatric patients: evaluation of current techniques. *Ann Emerg Med*. 1987;16:1121-1126.

26. Herzenberg JE, Hensinger RN, Dedrick DK, Phillips WA. Emergency transport and positioning of young children who have an injury of the cervical spine: the standard backboard may be hazardous. *J Bone Joint Surg Am*. 1989;71:15-22.

27. Teasdale G, Jennett B. Assessment of coma and impaired consciousness: a practical scale. *Lancet*. 1974;2:81-84.

28. Simpson D, Reilly P. Pediatric coma scale. *Lancet*. 1982;2:450. Letter.

29. Yager JY, Johnston B, Seshia SS. Coma scales in pediatric practice. *Am J Dis Child*. 1990;144:1088-1091.

30. Simpson DA, Cockington RA, Hanieh A, Raftos J, Reilly PL. Head injuries in infants and young children: the value of the Paediatric Coma Scale. *Childs Nerv Syst*. 1991;7:183-190.

31. Yamamoto LG, Kim GK, Britten AG. Rapid sequence anesthesia induction for emergency intubation. *Pediatr Emerg Care*. 1990;6:200-213.

32. Bivins HG, Ford S, Bezmalinovic Z, Price HM, Williams JL. The effect of axial traction during orotracheal intubation of the trauma victim with an unstable cervical spine. *Ann Emerg Med*. 1988;17:25-29.

33. Lewelt W, Jenkins LW, Miller JD. Autoregulation of cerebral blood flow after experimental fluid percussion injury of the brain. *J Neurosurg*. 1980;53:500-511.

34. Bruce DA, Alavi A, Bilaniuk L, Dolinskas C, Obrist W, Uzzell B. Diffuse cerebral swelling following head injuries in children: the syndrome of 'malignant brain edema.' *J Neurosurg*. 1981;54:170-178.

35. Langfitt TW, Weinstein JD, Kassell NF. Cerebral vasomotor paralysis produced by intracranial hypertension. *Neurology*. 1965;15:622-641.

36. Grubb RL Jr, Raichle ME, Eichling JO, Ter-Pogossian MM. The effects of changes in $PaCO_2$ on cerebral blood volume, blood flow, and vascular mean transit time. *Stroke*. 1974;5:630-639.

37. Cogbill TH, Bintz M, Johnson JA, Strutt PJ. Acute gastric dilatation after trauma. *J Trauma*. 1987;27:1113-1117.

38. Fletcher SA, Henderson LT, Miner ME, Jones JM. The successful surgical removal of intracranial nasogastric tubes. *J Trauma*. 1987;27:948-952.

39. Schwaitzberg SD, Bergman KS, Harris BH. A pediatric trauma model of continuous hemorrhage. *J Pediatr Surg*. 1988;23:605-609.

40. Stylianos S, Jacir NN, Hoffman MA, et al. Optimal intravenous site for volume replacement. *J Trauma*. 1992;33:947. Abstract.

41. Harte FA, Chalmers PC, Walsh RF, Danker PR, Sheikh FM. Intraosseous fluid administration: a parenteral alternative in pediatric resuscitation. *Anesth Analg*. 1987;66:687-689.

42. Goldstein B, Doody D, Briggs S. Emergency intraosseous infusion in severely burned children. *Pediatr Emerg Care*. 1990;6:195-197.

43. Hodge D III, Delgado-Paredes C, Fleisher G. Intraosseous infusion flow rates in hypovolemic 'pediatric' dogs. *Ann Emerg Med*. 1987;16:305-307.

44. Morris RE, Schonfeld N, Haftel AJ. Treatment of hemorrhagic shock with intraosseous administration of crystalloid fluid in the rabbit model. *Ann Emerg Med*. 1987;16:1321-1324.

45. Velasco AL, Delgado-Paredes C, Templeton J, Steigman CK, Templeton JM Jr. Intraosseous infusion of fluids in the initial management of hypovolemic shock in young subjects. *J Pediatr Surg*. 1991;26:2-8.

46. Schoffstall JM, Spivey WH, Davidheiser S, Lathers CM. Intraosseous crystalloid and blood infusion in a swine model. *J Trauma*. 1989;29:384-387.

47. Kramer GC, Walsh JC, Hands RD, et al. Resuscitation of hemorrhage with intraosseous infusion of hypertonic saline/dextran. *Braz J Med Biol Res*. 1989;22:283-286.

48. Halvorsen L, Bay BK, Perron PR, et al. Evaluation of an intraosseous infusion device for the resuscitation of hypovolemic shock. *J Trauma*. 1990;30:652-659.

49. Guy J, Haley K, Zuspan SJ. Use of intraosseous infusion in the pediatric trauma patient. *J Pediatr Surg*. 1993;28:158-161.

50. Barlow B, Niemirska M, Gandhi R, Shelton M. Response to injury in children with closed femur fractures. *J Trauma*. 1987;27:429-430.
51. Garcia V, Eichelberger M, Ziegler M, Templeton JM, Koop CE. Use of military antishock trouser in a child. *J Pediatr Surg*. 1981; 16(suppl 1):544-546.
52. Brunette DD, Fifield G, Ruiz E. Use of pneumatic antishock trousers in the management of pediatric pelvic hemorrhage. *Pediatr Emerg Care*. 1987;3:86-90.
53. Aprahamian C, Gessert G, Bandyk DF, Sell L, Stiehl J, Olson DW. MAST-associated compartment syndrome (MACS): a review. *J Trauma*. 1989;29:549-555.
54. Frampton MW. Lower extremity ischemia associated with use of military antishock trousers. *Ann Emerg Med*. 1984;13:1155-1157.
55. Gaffney FA, Thal ER, Taylor WF, et al. Hemodynamic effects of Medical Anti-Shock Trousers (MAST garment). *J Trauma*. 1981;21:931-937.
56. Abraham E, Cobo JC, Bland RD, Shoemaker WC. Cardiorespiratory effects of pneumatic trousers in critically ill patients. *Arch Surg*. 1984;119:912-916.
57. Mannering D, Bennett ED, Mehta N, Davis AL. Application of the medical anti-shock trouser (MAST) increases cardiac output and tissue perfusion in simulated, mild hypovolaemia. *Intensive Care Med*. 1986;12:143-146.
58. Rubal BJ, Geer MR, Bickell WH. Effects of pneumatic antishock garment inflation in normovolemic subjects. *J Appl Physiol*. 1989;67:339-345.
59. Terai C, Oryuh T, Kimura S, Mizuno K, Okada Y, Mimura K. The autotransfusion effect of external leg counterpressure in simulated mild hypovolemia. *J Trauma*. 1991;31:1165-1168.
60. Mackersie RC, Christensen JM, Lewis FR. The prehospital use of external counterpressure: does MAST make a difference? *J Trauma*. 1984;24:882-888.
61. Mattox KL, Bickell W, Pepe PE, Burch J, Feliciano D. Prospective MAST study in 911 patients. *J Trauma*. 1989;29:1104-1111.
62. Concannon JE, Matre WM, Verhagen AD. Antishock trousers in pediatrics: a case management report. *Clin Pediatr*. 1984;23:78-80.
63. Cooper A, Barlow B, DiScala C, String D. Efficacy of MAST use in children who present in hypotensive shock. *J Trauma*. 1992;33: 151. Abstract.
64. Wayne MA, Macdonald SC. Clinical evaluation of the antishock trouser: prospective study of low-pressure inflation. *Ann Emerg Med*. 1983;12:285-289.
65. Hanke BK, Bivins HG, Knopp R, dos Santos PA. Antishock trousers: a comparison of inflation techniques and inflation pressures. *Ann Emerg Med*. 985;14:636-640.
66. McCabe JB, Seidel DR, Jagger JA. Antishock trouser inflation and pulmonary vital capacity. *Ann Emerg Med*. 1983;12:290-293.
67. Tucker JF, Danzl DF, Teague E, Trujillo J, Bisker J. Infusion of intravenous fluids distal to pneumatic antishock trousers. *J Emerg Med*. 1984;2:79-83.
68. Joyce SM, Barsan WG, Hedges JR, Lukes SJ. Effect of a pneumatic antishock garment on drug delivery via distal venous access. *Ann Emerg Med*. 1984;13:885-890.
69. Mullin MJ, Krohmer JR, McCabe JB. Intravenous fluid flow beneath inflated antishock trousers in a canine hemorrhagic shock model. *Ann Emerg Med*. 1987;16:153-155.
70. Gardner SR, Maull KI, Swensson EE, Ward JD. The effects of the pneumatic antishock garment on intracranial pressure in man: a prospective study of 12 patients with severe head injury. *J Trauma*. 1984;24:896-900.
71. Garcia VF, Gotschall CS, Eichelberger MR, Bowman LM. Rib fractures in children: a marker of severe trauma. *J Trauma*. 1990;30: 695-700.
72. Cooper A, Barlow B, DiScala C, String D. Mortality and truncal injury: the pediatric perspective. *J Pediatr Surg*. 1994;29:33-38.
73. Cooper A, Barlow B, Davidson L, Relethford J, O'Meara J, Mottley L. Epidemiology of pediatric trauma: importance of population-based statistics. *J Pediatr Surg*. 1992;27:149-154.

Newborn Resuscitation

Chapter 9

Ideally, newborn resuscitation should take place in the delivery room or the neonatal ICU, because trained personnel and appropriate equipment should always be readily available in these settings. Resuscitation in the delivery room is addressed in depth in the Neonatal Resuscitation Program (NRP), a separate course that should be completed by all delivery room, newborn nursery, and neonatal intensive care personnel.[1]

Unfortunately, many deliveries occur outside the delivery room — in the home, en route to the hospital, or in the emergency department — where conditions for resuscitation may be suboptimal. This chapter offers a practical approach to resuscitation of the neonate in settings other than the delivery room, so recommendations vary slightly from those contained in the NRP. This approach is based on guidelines established by the American Heart Association and the American Academy of Pediatrics.[2] Since these guidelines are intended for resuscitation of newborns immediately after birth, they differ in minor ways from guidelines for resuscitation of infants and children presented in the remainder of this text.

Triage

Marked changes in the cardiovascular and respiratory systems occur at birth. The cardiovascular system undergoes a transition from fetal to neonatal circulation. The respiratory system, essentially nonfunctional in utero, must suddenly initiate and maintain oxygenation and ventilation. Antepartum events that cause asphyxia may preclude a smooth neonatal cardiopulmonary transition. The aim of resuscitation is to restore and support cardiopulmonary function.

The vast majority of term newborns require no resuscitation beyond maintenance of temperature, suctioning of the airway, and mild stimulation. Only a small number of newborns require further intervention, and most of these infants respond to administration of a high concentration of inspired oxygen and ventilation with bag and mask. A few newborns who are severely asphyxiated may require chest compressions, and even fewer need resuscitative medications.

An inverted pyramid (Fig 1) illustrates the relative frequencies and priorities of neonatal resuscitation. Resuscitation should proceed in an orderly fashion, and reassessment should follow each step to prevent unnecessary intervention and potential complications.

Since the best resuscitation results are obtained in a well-equipped and well-staffed delivery room, every reasonable and safe effort should be made to delay birth until the mother can be transported to a delivery room. Prehospital delays and stops in the emergency department or admitting office are inappropriate.

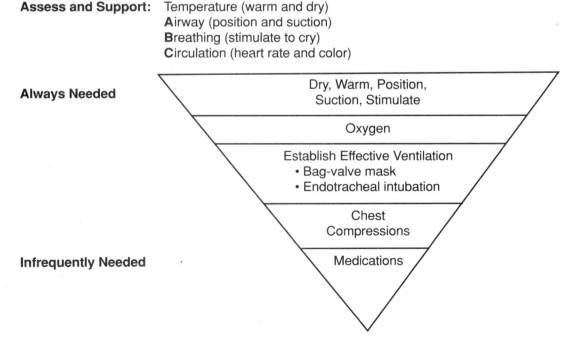

Assess and Support: Temperature (warm and dry)
Airway (position and suction)
Breathing (stimulate to cry)
Circulation (heart rate and color)

Always Needed

Dry, Warm, Position, Suction, Stimulate

Oxygen

Establish Effective Ventilation
• Bag-valve mask
• Endotracheal intubation

Chest Compressions

Infrequently Needed

Medications

Fig 1. Inverted pyramid reflecting relative frequencies of neonatal resuscitation efforts for the newborn who does not have meconium-stained amniotic fluid. Note that a majority of newborns respond to simple measures.

Preparation

Most neonatal resuscitations in the emergency department occur without prior notice. Resuscitation is more likely to be successful if advance preparation of equipment and training of personnel, determination of a brief resuscitation-related history, and assignment of personnel can be accomplished before or during admission of the newborn or mother in active labor.

Advance Preparation

In addition to a standard obstetrical tray, every emergency department should maintain a neonatal resuscitation tray that is readily accessible and regularly checked and replenished. The tray should contain appropriate equipment (Table 1) as well as charts listing correct medication doses for neonates of various weights (Table 2). Ideally a radiant warmer should be kept in the emergency department and personnel oriented to its use. Unless equipment is meticulously organized and maintained and is readily available, even the most knowledgeable and experienced emergency personnel will have difficulty performing successful neonatal resuscitation.

Immediate Preparation

As soon as the need for neonatal resuscitation becomes evident, a prearranged plan should be activated to organize personnel according to levels of competence. There is usually little time to obtain an in-depth obstetrical

Table 1. Newborn Resuscitation Equipment for the Emergency Department (in addition to OB kit)

Gowns, gloves, goggles (for universal precautions)
Towels
Heat source (radiant warmer or heating lamps)
Warmed blankets
Suction with manometer
Self-inflating bag (450 mL to 750 mL)
Face masks (premature, newborn, and infant sizes)
Laryngoscope handles (two) with extra batteries and bulbs
Laryngoscope blades (straight 0 and 1)
Medications and fluids
    Epinephrine 1:10 000
    Volume expanders (5% albumin, normal saline, lactated Ringer's solution)
    Naloxone hydrochloride (1 mg/mL or 0.4 mg/mL)
    Sodium bicarbonate (0.5 mEq/mL — 4.2% solution)*
Bulb syringe
Meconium aspirator (for attachment to mechanical suction)
Endotracheal tubes (2.5, 3.0, 3.5), two of each
Endotracheal tube stylets
Suction catheters (5F, 8F, and 10F), two of each
Umbilical catheters (3.5F and 5F)
Syringes (1, 3, 10, and 20 mL)
Three-way stopcocks
Feeding tubes (8F and 10F)
Sterile umbilical vessel catheterization tray

*If an 8.4% solution is the only one available, it should be diluted 1:1 with sterile water.

history, but a brief history may reveal key information that can assist in the preparation for and performance of resuscitation. For example, if there is a history of particulate meconium in the amniotic fluid, the resuscitation team must be prepared to suction the trachea under direct visualization. If the labor is premature, the need for assisted ventilation may be anticipated. If twins are expected, the team must be prepared to resuscitate two infants. If narcotics have been administered to the mother or if the mother is a known drug addict, the need for assisted ventilation can be anticipated. Additional factors associated with an increased risk for neonatal resuscitation are included in Table 3.

When a newborn is delivered outside the hospital, it may be difficult to maintain body temperature, the airway, and vascular access during transport. On arrival in the emergency department it is necessary to verify airway placement (or reintubate the newborn) and evaluate the patency and placement of vascular catheters. For this reason, preparation for admission and stabilization of any newborn infant in the emergency department is identical to that required for a full resuscitation.

Resuscitation Procedure

Universal Precautions

The US Centers for Disease Control and Prevention has recommended that universal precautions be taken whenever risk of exposure to blood or body fluids is high and the infectious status of the patient is unknown. This high risk is certainly present during delivery of a newborn in the emergency department. All personnel involved in a delivery and newborn resuscitation should use universal precautions.[4]

Gloves and other appropriate protective barriers (including gowns and goggles) should be worn when handling the newborn or contaminated equipment. The rescuer should not perform direct mouth suctioning of the neonatal trachea. Suction equipment (portable or wall suction) should always be available for this procedure.

Temperature

All newborns have difficulty tolerating a cold environment.[5] Depressed infants are especially at risk for complications of cold stress, and recovery from acidosis is delayed by hypothermia.[6] Hypothermia is a special problem for the infant born outside the hospital. Heat loss may be prevented by (1) quickly drying the amniotic fluid covering the infant; (2) placing the infant under a preheated warmer or heat lamps; and (3) removing wet linens from contact with the baby. Radiant warmers are ideal for warming infants but may not be readily available in the emergency department. Heating lamps become very hot and may be hazardous to both infant and personnel unless precautions are taken to maintain the heating bulb

Table 2. Neonatal Resuscitation Card

Initial cardiopulmonary resuscitation

Ventilation rate: 40-60/min when performed without compression
Compression rate: 120/min (performed with ventilations)
Compression:ventilation ratio: 3:1 (pause for ventilation)
Medications: Indicated if heart rate remains <80 bpm despite adequate ventilations with 100% O_2 and chest compressions

Term neonatal vital signs (first 12 h of life)[3]

Heart rate (awake): 100-180 bpm
Respiratory rate: 30-60/min
Systolic blood pressure: 39-59 mm Hg
Diastolic blood pressure: 16-36 mm Hg

Intubation Equipment

Weight	ET Tube Size (mm)/Catheter Size	Laryngoscope Blade
1 kg	2.5/5F	0
2 kg	3.0/6F	0
3 kg	3.5/8F	0-1
4 kg	3.5/8F	1

Medications

Medications	Dose/Route	Concentration	Wt (kg)	Total (mL)	Precautions
Epinephrine	0.01-0.03 mg/kg IV or ET*	1:10 000	1	0.1-0.3	Give rapidly
			2	0.2-0.6	Repeat every
			3	0.3-0.9	3-5 min
			4	0.4-1.2	
Volume Expanders	10 mL/kg IV				Reassess after
— 5% Albumin			1	10	each bolus
— Blood			2	20	
— Normal saline			3	30	
— Ringer's lactate			4	40	
Naloxone	0.1 mg/kg IV, IM, SQ, ET	0.4 mg/mL	1	0.25	Give rapidly
			2	0.50	Repeat every
			3	0.75	2-3 min
			4	1.0	
		1.0 mg/mL	1	0.1	
			2	0.2	
			3	0.3	
			4	0.4	

IM indicates intramuscular; ET, endotracheal tube; IV, intravenous; SQ, subcutaneous.
*Note: ET dose may not result in effective plasma concentration of drug, so IV access should be established as soon as possible. ET drugs should be diluted to volume of 3 to 5 mL before instillation.

at the recommended distance from the baby. Alternative methods of warming infants include warm blankets, warming mattresses, warm towels, and placement of towel-wrapped latex gloves filled with warm water around the infant. The mother may also help warm the infant. If initial evaluation indicates the infant is stable, the infant may be placed naked against the mother's body, with covers placed over both mother and child.

Airway Positioning

The newborn should be placed on his or her back or side with the neck in a neutral position. Hyperextension or flexion of the neck may produce airway obstruction and thus should be avoided. To help maintain correct position, a rolled blanket or towel may be placed under the back and shoulders of the supine infant, thus elevating the torso ¾ or 1 inch off the mattress to extend the neck slightly. If copious secretions are present, the newborn should be placed on his or her side with the neck slightly extended to allow secretions to collect in the mouth rather than in the posterior pharynx.

Airway Suctioning

If meconium stain is observed, the trachea should be suctioned *before* other resuscitative steps are taken (see below). If meconium is absent but suctioning is required to ensure a patent airway, the mouth should be suctioned before the nose. A bulb suction may be adequate. Mechanical suction with an 8F or 10F suction catheter may also be used. If mechanical suction is used,

Table 3. Factors Associated With an Increased Risk for Neonatal Resuscitation

Antepartum Maternal Factors
- Age >35 y or <16 y
- Diabetes
- Hemorrhage
- Drug therapy (eg, magnesium, adrenergic-blocking drugs, lithium carbonate)
- Substance abuse
- Previous fetal or neonatal death
- No prenatal care
- Chronic or pregnancy-induced hypertension
- Anemia or isoimmunization
- Maternal illness (eg, cardiovascular, thyroid, neurologic)
- Multifetal gestation
- Small fetus for maternal dates
- Post-term fetus
- Preterm labor or premature rupture of membranes
- Immature pulmonary studies
- Oligohydramnios
- Diminished fetal activity
- Fetal malformation identified by ultrasound

Intrapartum Maternal or Fetal Factors
- Breech or other abnormal presentation
- Infection
- Prolonged labor
- Prolonged rupture of membranes
- Prolapsed cord
- Maternal sedation
- Operative delivery
- Meconium-stained amniotic fluid
- Indexes of fetal distress (eg, fetal heart rate abnormalities)

negative pressure should not exceed –100 mm Hg (–136 cm H_2O). Deep suctioning of the oropharynx may produce a vagal response and cause bradycardia and/or apnea.[7] Gentle suctioning is usually adequate to remove secretions and should continue for no longer than 3 to 5 seconds per attempt. The infant's heart rate should be monitored during suctioning, and time should be allowed between suction attempts for spontaneous ventilation or assisted ventilation with 100% oxygen.

Stimulation

Most newborns will begin to breathe effectively in response to mild stimulation (drying, warming, and suctioning). Two additional safe methods of tactile stimulation are slapping or flicking the soles of the feet and rubbing the infant's back. More vigorous methods of stimulation should be avoided. If spontaneous and effective respirations are not established after a brief period (5 to 10 seconds) of stimulation, positive-pressure ventilation is required.

Assessment

Assessment of an infant born in the emergency department is performed after the infant is dried and placed in a warm environment, the airway is cleared, and stimulation is provided. These interventions should be accomplished virtually simultaneously. If delivery occurs before arrival in the emergency department, assessment should be performed immediately after the infant is placed in a warmed environment.

Respiratory Effort

The initial assessment includes an evaluation of the presence and quality of respirations. If respirations are adequate, the heart rate is then evaluated. If respirations are inadequate or gasping is present, positive-pressure ventilation should be initiated immediately. If respirations are shallow or slow, a brief period of stimulation may be attempted while 100% oxygen is administered. The rate and depth of respirations should increase after a few seconds of stimulation and administration of oxygen. If no response is noted after 5 to 10 seconds of stimulation and oxygen administration, positive-pressure ventilation with 100% oxygen should be initiated. Continued stimulation of an obviously depressed, cyanotic, and unresponsive infant increases hypoxemia and delays initiation of ventilation.

The mere presence of respirations does not guarantee adequate ventilation. Shallow respirations may primarily ventilate airway dead space and thus provide inadequate alveolar ventilation, resulting in hypoxemia, hypercarbia, and slowing of the heart rate. The heart rate is a reliable indicator of the newborn's degree of distress.

Heart Rate

Heart rate is a critical determinant of the resuscitation sequence and should be evaluated as soon as respiratory effort has been assessed and appropriate corrective action taken. The heart rate may be evaluated by one of the following:

- Palpation of the pulse at the base of the umbilical cord
- Palpation of the brachial or femoral pulse
- Auscultation of the apical heart sounds with a stethoscope.

A cardiotachometer monitoring system can also be used, but time is required to set up the system and electrodes may not stick well while vernix still covers the newborn's body.

If the heart rate is greater than 100 beats per minute and spontaneous respirations are present, assessment continues. If the heart rate is less than 100 beats per minute, positive-pressure ventilation with 100% oxygen should be initiated immediately. If the heart rate is less than 60 beats per minute or 60 to 80 beats per minute and not increasing rapidly despite effective ventilation with 100% oxygen, chest compressions should be initiated.

Color

An infant may be cyanotic despite adequate ventilation and a heart rate greater than 100 beats per minute. If central cyanosis is present in a newborn with spontaneous respirations and an adequate heart rate, 100% oxygen should be administered until the cause of the cyanosis can be determined. Oxygen administration is not indicated for infants with peripheral cyanosis (acrocyanosis), a condition that is common in the first few minutes of life and is not indicative of hypoxemia.

Apgar Score

The Apgar scoring system[8] (Table 4) enables rapid evaluation of a newborn's condition at specific intervals after birth. Five objective signs (heart rate, respirations, muscle tone, reflex irritability, and color) are routinely assessed at 1 and 5 minutes of age. If the 5-minute Apgar score is less than 7, additional scores are obtained every 5 minutes for a total of 20 minutes. The Apgar score cannot, however, be used to determine the need for resuscitation. If resuscitative efforts are required, they should be initiated promptly and should not be delayed while the Apgar score is obtained. In preterm infants the Apgar score is more likely to be affected by gestational age than asphyxia.[9]

Table 4. Apgar Score[8]

Sign	0	1	2
Heart rate per minute	Absent	Slow (less than 100)	Greater than 100
Respirations	Absent	Slow, irregular	Good, crying
Muscle tone	Limp	Some flexion	Active motion
Reflex irritability (catheter in nares)	No response	Grimace	Cough or sneeze
Color	Blue or pale	Pink body with blue extremities	Completely pink

Oxygen

If oxygen is needed during the resuscitation of a newborn, 100% oxygen should be used without concern for its potential hazards. Ideally oxygen should be warmed and humidified, but this may not be possible in an emergency department. Free-flow oxygen may be delivered by a head hood, by a face mask attached to a non–self-inflating ("anesthesia") bag, or by a simple mask held firmly to the infant's face with at least 5 L/min oxygen flow.

Ventilation

Indications for positive-pressure ventilation include

- Apnea or gasping respirations
- Heart rate less than 100 beats per minute
- Persistent central cyanosis despite administration of 100% oxygen

Effective ventilation can usually be provided with a bag and mask.

An assisted ventilatory rate of 40 to 60 breaths per minute should provide adequate ventilation. The tidal volumes required by neonates (especially preterm infants) are smaller than those used for children. To minimize the chance of possible iatrogenic complications (eg, barotrauma), begin bag-valve–mask ventilations carefully and determine visually the volume and force required to produce adequate chest expansions. For effective ventilation the mask must be the appropriate size, and a tight seal must be made between the mask and face. The initial lung inflation requires pressures of 30 to 40 cm H_2O for most newborns, although some require initial pressures as high as 50 cm H_2O. Less pressure (20 cm H_2O) is usually required for succeeding breaths. Observation of adequate chest wall movement is the best indicator of appropriate inflation pressure. If adequate chest expansion is not achieved with initial assisted ventilation, the head and the face mask should be repositioned. Further suctioning of the airway or increased inflation pressures are required if assisted ventilation, provided after repositioning, fails to produce effective chest expansion. If adequate ventilation (as indicated by effective chest expansion and improvement in color and heart rate) cannot be achieved by bag and mask, immediate intubation of the trachea and ventilation via an endotracheal tube are required.

If bag-valve–mask positive-pressure ventilation is required for more than approximately 2 minutes or if gastric distention develops, an orogastric tube (8F or 10F) should be inserted, left open to air, and periodically aspirated with a syringe.

After adequate ventilation has been established for 15 to 30 seconds, the heart rate should be reassessed. If the heart rate is 100 beats per minute or higher and spontaneous respirations are present, positive-pressure ventilation may be gradually discontinued. Gradual reduction in the rate and pressure of assisted ventilation will increase the stimulus for the newborn to resume spontaneous breathing. If spontaneous respirations are inadequate, assisted ventilation must continue.

If, despite adequate ventilation with 100% oxygen, the heart rate is less than 60 beats per minute or between 60 and 80 beats per minute and not rapidly increasing, positive-pressure ventilation should be continued and chest compressions initiated.

Ventilation Bags

Self-inflating Bag. Self-inflating bags do not require a gas source to operate, but they must be used with an oxygen source and reservoir to deliver a high concentration of oxygen. Many self-inflating bags are equipped with a pressure-limiting pop-off valve that is usually preset at 30 to 45 cm H_2O. Since the initial inflation of a newborn's lungs may require higher inspiratory pressures, the pop-off valve may prevent effective inflation unless the valve is occluded. Such bags should therefore have a pop-off valve that is easily bypassed. A resuscitation bag volume greater than 750 mL makes it difficult to judge the small tidal volumes (6 to 8 mL/kg) administered to neonates and may increase the risk of hyperinflation and potential barotrauma. A 450-mL bag may be optimal.

Non–self-inflating ("Anesthesia") Bag. The "anesthesia" bag inflates only when air or oxygen from a compressed gas source is forced into it and a tight seal exists between the mask and face. This bag requires a well-modulated flow of gas into the inlet port and correct adjustment of pop-off or flow-control valves. Since an anesthesia bag can deliver very high pressures, a pressure gauge must be joined to the bag to monitor peak ventilatory pressures generated during ventilation. Proper use of an anesthesia bag requires training and practice but enables provision of a wide range of peak inspiratory pressures and more reliable delivery of high inspired oxygen concentrations than a self-inflating bag.

Face Masks

Face masks for preterm, term, and large newborns (usually called premature, newborn, and infant masks) should be available in the emergency department. Although a tight seal between the mask and face is required to achieve effective ventilation, excessive pressure on the face must be avoided. The most effective masks are designed to fit the contours of the newborn's face and have a low dead space volume (less than 5 mL). Face masks with cushioned rims are recommended because they facilitate creation of an effective seal between face and mask. A correctly positioned mask should cover the infant's nose and mouth but not the eyes.

Endotracheal Intubation

Endotracheal intubation is indicated if (1) bag-valve–mask ventilation is ineffective, (2) tracheal suctioning is required for aspiration of thick, particulate meconium, or (3) prolonged positive-pressure ventilation is necessary.

Supplies and equipment for endotracheal intubation should be assembled and readily available on the neonatal resuscitation tray. Tubes with a uniform internal diameter are recommended; tapered tubes should not be used. Most endotracheal tubes intended for use in newborns have a black vocal cord line guide near the tip. When this guide is placed at the level of the vocal cords, the tip of the tube is likely to be positioned properly in the trachea, above the carina. Endotracheal tube size can be estimated using the infant's weight (Table 2), length, or postconceptual age:

$$\text{ET tube size in mm} = \frac{\text{Postconceptual age in weeks}}{10}$$

After intubation, proper position of the endotracheal tube must be verified by

- Observation of symmetrical chest movement
- Auscultation of equal breath sounds, heard best in the axillae, and absent breath sounds over the stomach
- Observation of improvement in the neonate's color, heart rate, and activity
- Detection of exhaled carbon dioxide

Once proper endotracheal tube position is verified, it should be taped in position. A chest x-ray should be obtained for final confirmation of endotracheal tube placement if the tube is to remain in place after resuscitation.

Chest Compressions

Asphyxia causes peripheral vasoconstriction, tissue hypoxia, acidosis, poor myocardial contractility, bradycardia, and eventual cardiac arrest. This critical state can usually be avoided by prompt initiation of effective ventilation and oxygenation. If a newborn's heart rate is less than 60 beats per minute or is 60 to 80 beats per minute and not rapidly increasing despite effective positive-pressure ventilation with 100% oxygen for approximately 30 seconds, chest compressions should be initiated.

Effective ventilation can occur only if the airway is patent. Patency is assessed by observing bilateral chest expansion. Ventilation with a bag-valve mask may be acceptable, but endotracheal intubation is often required. The experienced healthcare provider will usually elect to intubate the neonate shortly after chest compressions are initiated. A provider inexperienced in neonatal intubation should not delay provision of chest compressions when profound bradycardia is observed if effective ventilation has been achieved with bag and mask. If ventilation is achieved via a bag-valve mask, chest compressions must be briefly interrupted to allow interposition of effective ventilation in a 3:1 compression-ventilation ratio.

Two techniques are acceptable for performing chest compressions in the neonate and small infant. In the preferred technique, the two thumbs are placed on the middle third of the sternum, with the fingers encircling the chest and supporting the back (Fig 2).[10,11] The thumbs should be positioned side by side on the sternum just below the nipple line. If the infant is extremely small or the rescuer's thumbs are extremely large, the thumbs may have to be superimposed one on top of the other. The xiphoid portion of the sternum should *not* be compressed because such compression may damage the neonate's liver.

If the resuscitator's hands are too small to encircle the chest, two-finger compression may be performed, with the ring and middle fingers of one hand on the sternum just below the nipple line. The other hand should support the newborn's back (see chapter 3).

- The sternum is compressed approximately ½ to ¾ inch at a rate of 120 times per minute.
- The compression phase should be smooth, not jerky, and equal to the relaxation phase.

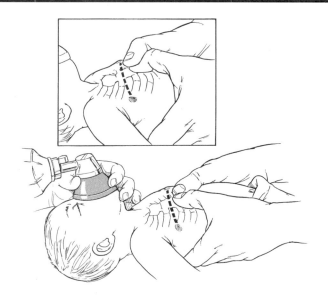

Fig 2. Hand position for chest encirclement technique for external chest compressions in neonates. Thumbs are side by side over the midsternum. In the small newborn, thumbs may need to be superimposed (inset). Gloves should be worn during resuscitation.

- The thumbs or fingers should not be lifted off the sternum during the relaxation phase.
- The spontaneous pulse rate should be checked periodically, and compressions should be discontinued when the heart rate reaches 80 or more beats per minute.
- Compressions must always be accompanied by positive-pressure ventilation with 100% oxygen, since ventilation is of primary importance in newborn resuscitation.

Simultaneous delivery of chest compressions and positive-pressure ventilations will often decrease the efficiency of ventilation; chest compressions interposed with ventilations in a 3:1 ratio may be more effective than simultaneous ventilations and compressions. For this reason

- Three compressions are followed by a brief pause to allow delivery of an effective breath.
- The rate of compressions (120 per minute) will thus result in provision of 90 compressions and 30 breaths each minute.

Medications and Fluids

Bradycardia and shock in the neonatal period usually result from profound hypoxemia. Medications should be administered if, despite adequate ventilation with 100% oxygen and chest compressions, the heart rate remains less than 80 beats per minute.

Routes of Administration

The umbilical vein is the preferred site for vascular access during neonatal resuscitation because it is easily located and cannulated. Special training is required to safely perform umbilical vein catheterization and to maintain the catheter.

The cord is prepped, draped appropriately, and trimmed with a scalpel blade 1 cm above the skin attachment and held firmly with a ligature to prevent bleeding. The umbilical vein is identified as a thin-walled single vessel. In contrast, the umbilical arteries are paired, have thicker walls, and are often constricted. The lumen of the vein is larger than that of the artery; thus, the vessel that continues to bleed after the cord is cut is usually the vein. A 3.5F or a 5F umbilical catheter with a radiopaque marker is prepared for insertion. The catheter is flushed with heparinized saline (0.5 to 1.0 U/mL), attached to a three-way stopcock, and inserted so that the tip is just below the skin and blood can be readily aspirated and any air bubbles evacuated. The umbilical venous catheter is inserted only until a good blood return is obtained. This should correspond to a depth of insertion of 1 to 4 cm and should avoid advancement of the catheter tip into the portal vein or hepatic circulation. Neonatal liver injury (including hemorrhage) has been linked with the administration of hypertonic and alkaline solution (eg, THAM or sodium bicarbonate) into the portal vein, so this position of the catheter tip is avoided. If the catheter tip remains in the distal umbilical vein, any drugs administered by this route can be diluted by the patient's blood before they reach the neonate's liver.

A wedged hepatic position should be suspected if free blood return is absent. If such wedging is suspected, the catheter should be withdrawn to a position where blood can be freely aspirated. The catheter should be withdrawn as soon as possible after resuscitation to minimize the danger of infection or portal vein thrombosis.

Vascular access may also be obtained by other routes. Cannulation of the umbilical artery is time-consuming and more difficult than umbilical vein catheterization but enables monitoring of blood pressure and blood sampling for blood gas analysis and evaluation of acid-base balance. Peripheral veins in the extremities and scalp are difficult to access in neonates during resuscitation but may be used if cannulated.

If fluid and medications are required but umbilical venous or arterial access cannot be obtained, an intraosseous cannula can provide access to a noncollapsible venous plexus. The intraosseous cannula is inserted in the medial aspect of the tibia, just below the tibial tuberosity. Although extensive experience with intraosseous technique has been reported in infants,[12,13] experience in neonates is extremely limited.[14] This method of vascular access should be used only when other routes cannot be established (see chapter 5).

When vascular access *cannot* be achieved, the endotracheal route can be used for delivery of epinephrine[15,16] and naloxone. Since optimal drug doses have not been established for endotracheal administration,[17-19] the intravenous dose should be used.[20,21] Drugs administered via the endotracheal route should be diluted to a volume of

3 to 5 mL of normal saline (use smallest volume for smallest babies), followed by several positive-pressure ventilations. Thus, the medication is ultimately delivered into the distal tracheobronchial tree. Intracardiac injections should never be performed.

Epinephrine (see also chapter 6)

Indications. Asystole or spontaneous heart rate less than 80 beats per minute despite adequate ventilation with 100% oxygen and chest compressions.[22]

Dose. 0.01 to 0.03 mg/kg (0.1 to 0.3 mL/kg of the 1:10 000 solution) may be repeated every 3 to 5 minutes if required.[22] Some patients who do not respond to standard doses of epinephrine may respond to higher doses.[23,24] However, data are inadequate to evaluate the efficacy of high doses of epinephrine in newborns, and the safety of these doses has not been established. High doses of epinephrine may lead to prolonged hypertension, which may in turn lead to complications such as intracranial hemorrhage in preterm infants. In summary, a dose of 0.01 to 0.03 mg/kg of epinephrine is recommended for IV or endotracheal administration. If the neonate has no intravascular access and fails to respond to positive-pressure ventilation with 100% oxygen, and a standard dose of epinephrine by the endotracheal route, administration of a higher epinephrine dose (0.1 mg/kg of 1:1000 solution) by the endotracheal route may be considered. (See the preceding section for information about endotracheal drug administration.)

Route: Intravenous (including intraosseous) or via endotracheal tube.

Volume Expanders

Volume expanders are indicated for treatment of hypovolemia.

Indications: Evidence of acute bleeding from the fetal-maternal unit, including (1) pallor that persists despite oxygenation, (2) faint pulses with a good heart rate, and (3) poor response to resuscitation, including effective ventilation.

Dose: Administer one of the following over 5 to 10 minutes:

- 10 mL/kg O-negative blood crossmatched with the mother's blood
- 10 mL/kg 5% albumin/saline solution or other plasma substitute
- 10 mL/kg normal saline or Ringer's lactate.

Reassess and administer additional boluses as needed.

Route: Intravenous (including intraosseous).

Naloxone Hydrochloride

Naloxone hydrochloride is a narcotic antagonist that does not produce respiratory depression.[25]

Indications: For the reversal of neonatal respiratory depression induced by narcotics administered to the mother within 4 hours of delivery. Prompt and adequate ventilatory support must always be provided before administration of naloxone. Since the duration of action of narcotics may exceed that of naloxone, continued surveillance of the infant is necessary, and repeat administration of naloxone is often needed. Naloxone can induce a withdrawal reaction in an infant of a narcotic-addicted mother and should be used with caution if this condition is suspected.[26] Prolonged ventilatory support may be required by these patients.

Dose: Administer one of the following:

- 0.1 mg/kg (0.1 mL/kg of 1 mg/mL concentration
- 0.25 mL/kg of 0.4 mg/mL concentration). The initial dose may be repeated every 2 to 3 minutes as needed.[27]

Route: Intravenous, intraosseous, via the endotracheal tube, subcutaneous, or intramuscular (if perfusion is adequate).

Other Medications

There is no evidence that atropine, calcium, or sodium bicarbonate is beneficial in the acute phase of neonatal resuscitation at delivery. Sodium bicarbonate should not be used during brief resuscitation episodes but may be beneficial when other therapies are ineffective and resuscitation is prolonged.[28-32]

Meconium

Meconium aspiration syndrome is a significant cause of neonatal morbidity and mortality. This clinical syndrome produces respiratory distress and hypoxemia and is associated with aspiration pneumonia, pneumothorax, and (in severe cases) persistent pulmonary hypertension. Approximately 12% of all deliveries are complicated by the presence of meconium in the amniotic fluid.[33]

Amniotic fluid containing meconium may be thin and watery or thick and particulate (resembling pea soup). Newborns delivered through thick meconium are at greatest risk for meconium aspiration syndrome, although a milder form may be observed when the meconium-stained fluid is thin.[34]

When meconium staining is detected during delivery, delivery should occur in stages to enable suctioning of the newborn's pharynx before the first breath. As soon as the head is delivered, the newborn's mouth, nose, and posterior pharynx should be thoroughly suctioned using a large-bore (12F or 14F) suction catheter. If a large catheter is unavailable, a bulb syringe may be used.[35] Suctioning must be performed before delivery of the shoulders and thorax in order to decrease the risk of meconium aspiration syndrome.[36] Despite suctioning, however, meconium is present in the trachea of approximately 20% to 30% of newborns with meconium staining before the infant's first extrauterine breath. These data suggest a significant incidence of intrauterine aspiration.[37]

When thick meconium is present, suctioning is performed, as described above, before delivery. After delivery the infant is placed in the prepared warmed environment and the following actions are performed immediately (before usual initial steps):

- The hypopharynx is visualized with a laryngoscope and any residual meconium is removed with suctioning.
- The trachea is intubated and the lower airway is suctioned. These interventions should not be delayed while the infant is dried.

Since meconium is viscous, suction should be applied directly to the endotracheal tube. A special adapter (meconium aspirator) to control suction is placed between the endotracheal tube and the suction tubing (Fig 3). As suction is applied directly to the endotracheal tube, the tube is slowly withdrawn. Mechanical suction should be set no higher than −100 mm Hg. In the presence of a significant amount of meconium (demonstrated by a large return), it may be necessary to repeat the intubation and suction until the aspirated material is clear.

When the infant's condition is unstable, it may not be possible to clear the trachea of all meconium before positive-pressure ventilation must be initiated. After initial stabilization is achieved, an orogastric tube should be placed to empty the newborn's stomach since it may contain meconium that could later be regurgitated and aspirated.

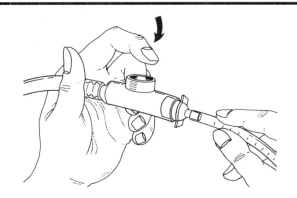

Fig 3. One form of adapter (meconium aspirator) is placed between the endotracheal tube and the suction tubing. Gloves should be worn.

Preterm Newborns

Resuscitation of preterm newborns is associated with a number of additional risks:

- Preterm infants are likely to develop respiratory depression requiring assisted ventilation immediately after birth (the incidence of respiratory depression increases sharply with decreasing gestational age).
- Preterm infants cool at a more rapid rate than full-term newborns when exposed to similar environmental conditions because their ratio of body surface area to volume is higher than that of full-term neonates. For this reason heat loss should be a major concern when caring for preterm infants.[38]

- The brain of the preterm infant has a fragile subependymal germinal matrix that is vulnerable to bleeding when injured by hypoxemia, rapid changes in blood pressure, or wide fluctuations in serum osmolality.[39] Administration of hyperosmolar solutions or large boluses of volume expanders should be avoided, if possible, for this reason.

Postresuscitation Care

The three most common complications of the postresuscitation period include endotracheal tube migration (including dislodgment), tube occlusion by mucus or meconium, and pneumothorax. Endotracheal tube migration can be caused by changes in head position; the endotracheal tube is advanced by neck flexion and is withdrawn by neck extension.[40] Endotracheal tube malposition or obstruction is suggested by decreased chest wall movement, diminished breath sounds, or the return of bradycardia and decreased arterial oxygen saturation. Unexplained hypercarbia should be assumed to result from endotracheal tube obstruction until this complication has been ruled out. Pneumothorax may complicate positive-pressure ventilation and may be difficult to diagnose by auscultation, because breath sounds in the newborn are transmitted from all areas of the lung through the thin chest wall. Pneumothorax should be suspected if a newborn deteriorates after an initial good response to ventilation or fails to respond to resuscitative efforts. Additional signs of pneumothorax include unilateral decrease in chest expansion, altered intensity or pitch of breath sounds, and increased resistance to hand ventilation.

Once ventilation and heart rate are adequate, additional postresuscitation goals of care include

- Provision of a warm environment and frequent assessment of the newborn's temperature
- Bedside determination of blood glucose level and treatment of hypoglycemia
- Arterial blood gas determination and correction of documented severe acidosis
- Achievement of vascular access
- Assessment of perfusion and treatment of hypoperfusion with volume expanders, inotropic agents, or both
- Evaluation of a chest roentgenogram to assess placement of tubes and catheters and to evaluate lung expansion

Communication with a neonatal ICU should be established and transport arrangements made as soon as the need for neonatal resuscitation is evident. Critically ill newborns should ideally be transported by a neonatal transport team specifically trained in the care of sick newborns. Such teams have the expertise and equipment to deliver a high level of neonatal intensive care during transport.

No resuscitation is complete without thorough documentation. The written record of evaluation and therapy must be sent with the newborn and should include copies of all laboratory results and roentgenograms.

References

1. Bloom RS, Cropley CS, Chameides L, ed. *Textbook of Neonatal Resuscitation*. Elk Grove Village, Ill: American Academy of Pediatrics; 1990.
2. Emergency Cardiac Care Committee and Subcommittees, American Heart Association. Guidelines for cardiopulmonary resuscitation and emergency cardiac care, VII: neonatal resuscitation. *JAMA*. 1992;268:2276-2281.
3. Hazinski MF. Children are different. In: Hazinski MF, ed. *Nursing Care of the Critically Ill Child*. 2nd ed. St Louis, Mo: Mosby Year Book; 1992.
4. Centers for Disease Control. Guidelines for prevention of transmission of human immunodeficiency virus and hepatitis B virus to health-care and public-safety workers. *MMWR*. 1989;38(suppl 6): 1-37.
5. Scopes JW, Ahmed I. Range of critical temperatures in sick and premature newborn babies. *Arch Dis Child*. 1966;41:417-419.
6. Adamsons K Jr, Gandy GM, James LS. The influence of thermal factors upon oxygen consumption of the newborn human infant. *J Pediatr*. 1965;66:495-508.
7. Cordero L Jr, Hon EH. Neonatal bradycardia following nasopharyngeal stimulation. *J Pediatr*. 1971;78:441-447.
8. Apgar V. A proposal for a new method of evaluation of the newborn infant. *Anesth Analg*. 1953;32:260-267.
9. Catlin EA, Carpenter MW, Brann BS IV, et al. The Apgar score revisited: influence of gestational age. *J Pediatr*. 1986;109:865-868.
10. Todres ID, Rogers MC. Methods of external cardiac massage in the newborn infant. *J Pediatr*. 1975;86:781-782.
11. David R. Closed chest cardiac massage in the newborn infant. *Pediatrics*. 1988;81:552-554.
12. Arbeiter HI, Greengard J. Tibial bone marrow infusions in infancy. *J Pediatr*. 1944;25:1-12.
13. Fiser D. Intraosseous infusion. *N Engl J Med*. 1990;322:1579-1581.
14. Kelsall AW. Resuscitation with intraosseous lines in neonatal units. *Arch Dis Child*. 1993;68:324-325.
15. Greenberg MI, Roberts JR, Baskin SI, Wagner DK. The use of endotracheal medication for cardiac arrest. *Topics in Emergency Medicine*. 1979;1:29-40.
16. Ward JT Jr. Endotracheal drug therapy. *Am J Emerg Med*. 1983;1:71-82.
17. Lindemann R. Endotracheal administration of epinephrine during cardiopulmonary resuscitation. *Am J Dis Child*. 1982;136:753-754. Letter.
18. Orlowski JP, Gallagher JM, Porembka DT. Endotracheal epinephrine is unreliable. *Resuscitation*. 1990;19:103-113.
19. Quinton DN, O'Byrne G, Aitkenhead AR. Comparison of endotracheal and peripheral intravenous adrenaline in cardiac arrest: is the endotracheal route reliable? *Lancet*. 1987;1:828-829.
20. Roberts JR, Greenberg MI, Knaub MA, Baskin SI. Comparison of the pharmacological effects of epinephrine administered by the intravenous and endotracheal routes. *J Am Coll Emerg Phys*. 1978;7:260-264.
21. Roberts JR, Greenberg MI, Knaub MA, Kendrick ZV, Baskin SI. Blood levels following intravenous and endotracheal epinephrine administration. *J Am Coll Emerg Phys*. 1979;8:53-56.
22. Berkowitz ID, Gervais H, Schleien CL, Koehler RC, Dean JM, Traystman RJ. Epinephrine dosage effects on cerebral and myocardial blood flow in an infant swine model of cardiopulmonary resuscitation. *Anesthesiology*. 1991;75:1041-1050.
23. Goetting MG, Paradis NA. High-dose epinephrine improves outcome from pediatric cardiac arrest. *Ann Emerg Med*. 1991;20:22-26.
24. Paradis NA, Martin GB, Rosenberg J, et al. The effect of standard- and high-dose epinephrine on coronary perfusion pressure during prolonged cardiopulmonary resuscitation. *JAMA*. 1991;265:1139-1144.
25. Handal KA, Schauben JL, Salamone FR. Naloxone. *Ann Emerg Med*. 1983;12:438-445.
26. Cloherty JP, Stark AR, eds. *Manual of Neonatal Care*. 3rd ed. Boston, Mass: Little, Brown and Co; 1991:64.
27. American Academy of Pediatrics Committee on Drugs. Emergency drug doses for infants and children and naloxone use in newborns: clarification. *Pediatrics*. 1989;83:803.
28. Ostrea EM Jr, Odell GB. The influence of bicarbonate administration on blood pH in a 'closed system': clinical implications. *J Pediatr*. 1972;80:671-680.
29. Simmons MA, Adcock EW III, Bard H, Battaglia FC. Hypernatremia and intracranial hemorrhage in neonates. *N Engl J Med*. 1974; 291:6-10.
30. Finberg L. The relationship of intravenous infusions and intracranial hemorrhage: a commentary. *J Pediatr*. 1977;91:777-778.
31. Papile LA, Burstein J, Burstein R, Koffler H, Koops B. Relationship of intravenous sodium bicarbonate infusions and cerebral intraventricular hemorrhage. *J Pediatr*. 1978;93:834-836.
32. Graf H, Leach W, Arieff AI. Evidence for a detrimental effect of bicarbonate therapy in hypoxic lactic acidosis. *Science*. 1985; 227:754-756.
33. Wiswell TE, Tuggle JM, Turner BS. Meconium aspiration syndrome: have we made a difference? *Pediatrics*. 1990;85:715-721.
34. Rossi EM, Philipson EH, Williams TG, Kalhan SC. Meconium aspiration syndrome: intrapartum and neonatal attributes. *Am J Obstet Gynecol*. 1989;161:1106-1110.
35. Locus P, Yeomans E, Crosby U. Efficacy of bulb versus DeLee suction at deliveries complicated by meconium stained amniotic fluid. *Am J Perinatol*. 1990;7:87-91.
36. Carson BS, Losey RW, Bowes WA Jr, Simmons MA. Combined obstetric and pediatric approach to prevent meconium aspiration syndrome. *Am J Obstet Gynecol*. 1976;126:712-715.
37. Falciglia HS. Failure to prevent meconium aspiration syndrome. *Obstet Gynecol*. 1988;71:349-353.
38. Day RL, Caliguiri L, Kamenski C, et al. Body temperature and survival of premature infants. *Pediatrics*. 1964;34:171-181.
39. Hambleton G, Wigglesworth JS. Origin of intraventricular hemorrhage in the preterm infant. *Arch Dis Child*. 1976;51:651-659.
40. Donn SM, Kuhns LR. Mechanism of endotracheal tube movement with change of head position in the neonate. *Pediatr Radiol*. 1980;9:37-40.

Immediate Postarrest Stabilization and Secondary Transport

Chapter 10

Postresuscitation care involves patient stabilization, transport to a tertiary care facility, and ongoing care within that facility. This chapter discusses immediate postarrest stabilization and the care needed during transport.

The goals of postarrest stabilization and transport are prevention of secondary organ injury and delivery of the patient in optimal condition to a tertiary care setting. Successful resuscitation of the infant or child must be followed by continued evaluation of cardiopulmonary function, even if the child's condition initially appears stable. Because infants and children often suffer recurrent hypoxemia or hypercapnia, hemodynamic instability, and an altered sensorium during the immediate postresuscitation period, they should be transferred to a pediatric ICU for further observation, evaluation, and care.[1] Good communication between the referring and receiving hospitals is essential to ensure optimal patient outcome.

Stabilization

General Care

General postresuscitation care is required before and during transport and includes

- Frequent assessment of cardiopulmonary function:
  — Evaluation of ventilation. Signs of effective ventilation include adequate bilateral chest expansion, equal bilateral breath sounds, and absence of nasal flaring or respiratory effort (eg, use of accessory muscles of respiration). In contrast, signs of inadequate ventilation include minimal or unequal chest expansion bilaterally, inadequate or unequal breath sounds, nasal flaring, paradoxical movement of the chest indicating upper airway obstruction, and use of accessory muscles of respiration. Measurement of arterial blood gases confirms adequate oxygenation and effective carbon dioxide elimination. Oxygenation should be monitored continuously with a pulse oximeter or skin surface (transcutaneous) oxygen ($P_{tc}O_2$) monitor.
  — Continuous ECG monitoring of heart rate and rhythm.
  — Evaluation of peripheral circulation and end-organ perfusion, including assessment of skin temperature, capillary refill, quality of distal pulses, level of consciousness, and urine output. An indwelling urinary catheter facilitates continuous evaluation of urine output.
  — Blood pressure recording using an intra-arterial cannula for direct measurement or a Doppler device, sphygmomanometer, or automated blood pressure measurement device for indirect measurement. Blood pressure should be evaluated at least every 5 minutes until stable and every 15 minutes thereafter. Cycled indirect oscillometric blood pressure measurement may be inaccurate in the presence of a compromised circulation.
  — Serial neurologic examinations to detect signs of intracranial hypertension or seizures.
- Administration of humidified oxygen at the highest possible concentration until objective assessment by arterial blood gas analysis or noninvasive monitoring indicates satisfactory arterial oxygenation.
- Insertion and maintenance of two large-bore, functional vascular catheters. The initial theoretical estimated maintenance fluid requirements may be calculated according to the formulas in Table 1. The actual fluid administration rate should be determined for each patient, and special circumstances may require alteration of the content or rate of fluid administration.
- Laboratory evaluation including measurement of serum electrolytes, calcium, and glucose; measurement of hematocrit; and analysis of arterial blood gases. Arterial blood gas analysis should be performed approximately 10 to 15 minutes after initiation of ventilatory support with the ventilating system that will be used during transport. This analysis should be repeated just before transport begins.
- Insertion of a nasogastric tube for gravity drainage. The tube prevents gastric distention caused by air and is particularly useful during positive-pressure ventilation. Insertion of a tube is almost always indicated in the presence of cardiorespiratory distress or a diminished level of consciousness.
- A search for the precipitating cause of the arrest and initiation of the appropriate therapy (eg, antibiotics if the cause is sepsis).
- Careful attention to preservation of core temperature. This is especially, but not exclusively, important in infants. Before transport, overhead heating units can be used for infants and heating lamps for children. During transport, portable incubators are useful for infants; older children and infants not in transport incubators should be covered to maintain warmth. The head represents a relatively large portion of the body surface throughout childhood. Covering the head of the infant or child may help prevent significant heat loss. Warm blankets or thermal reflective or crushable heat packs may facilitate the warming of an infant or child.

Table 1. Calculation of Initial Maintenance Fluid Requirements in Infants and Children

Infants smaller than 10 kg: Infusion of ¼% NS in D_5W at a rate of 4 mL/kg per hour (eg, the maintenance rate for an 8-kg baby is 4 mL x 8 kg = 32 mL/h).

Children 10 to 20 kg: Infusion of ¼% NS in D_5W at a rate of 40 mL/h plus 2 mL/kg per hour for each kilogram between 10 and 20 kg (eg, the maintenance rate for a 15-kg child is 40 mL/h + [2 mL/kg per hour x 5 kg] = 50 mL/h).

Children larger than 20 kg: Infusion of ¼% NS in D_5W at a rate of 60 mL/h plus 1 mL/kg per hour for each kg between 20 and 30 kg (eg, the maintenance rate for a 30-kg child is 60 mL/h + [1 mL/kg per hour x 10 kg] = 70 mL/h).

Special Care for Patients With Organ Failure

Respiratory System

Respiratory failure can be a cause or a result of cardiopulmonary arrest. When hemodynamic stability permits cessation of chest compressions, manual ventilation may be replaced by mechanical ventilation. If mechanical ventilation is unavailable, however, manual ventilation with a bag and endotracheal tube may be continued throughout transport.

Elective intubation is indicated for any infant or child at risk for respiratory or cardiovascular deterioration. The endotracheal tube must be securely taped and proper endotracheal position confirmed by auscultation and chest radiograph. Proper endotracheal tube position must be verified immediately before transport, because recognition of tube displacement may be difficult during transport[2] and reintubation is often impossible. Agitated children may require sedation and administration of muscle relaxants to minimize the risk of endotracheal tube displacement during transport. Diazepam (0.1 to 0.2 mg/kg IV) or morphine sulfate (0.1 mg/kg IV) is frequently used. Muscle paralysis may be achieved with pancuronium bromide (0.1 mg/kg IV) but should not be attempted unless effective ventilation via endotracheal tube is ensured and analgesics or sedatives are administered. Mechanical or manual ventilation must be provided if narcotics, sedatives, or muscle relaxants are used, because these drugs reduce or ablate the ventilatory drive. Infants and children should not receive muscle relaxants unless transport personnel have the equipment, skill, and experience to reintubate the patient.

During mechanical ventilation the effectiveness of ventilation and oxygenation must be verified by arterial blood gas analysis. An arterial blood sample for gas analysis should be obtained after 10 to 15 minutes at the initial ventilatory settings, and ventilatory control should be adjusted accordingly just before transport begins. Arterial blood gas analysis should be repeated approximately 10 to 15 minutes after any significant change in ventilatory support.

Initial Ventilator Settings (Table 2)

Oxygen. Low cardiac output promotes intrapulmonary shunting. Since the risk of hyperoxia during a brief period is negligible compared with the risk of tissue hypoxia, the initial FIO_2 should be 1.0, even in the presence of a high arterial oxygen tension.

Tidal Volume. When a volume-cycled ventilator is used, initial delivered tidal volume should be 10 to 15 mL/kg. Higher volumes are required if a large air leak is present around the endotracheal tube. If a substantial air leak compromises ventilation, it may be necessary to replace the endotracheal tube with a larger one. If there is the potential for difficulties in changing the endotracheal tube, high flows should be used to compensate for the air leak. If the delivered tidal volume is adequate, chest expansion and breath sounds should be equal and adequate bilaterally and the $PaCO_2$ should be normal. Inspiratory time should be a minimum of 0.5 second if possible.

Peak Inspiratory Pressure. When a time-cycled, pressure-limited ventilator is used, the peak inspiratory pressure should be adjusted according to the patient's size and lung compliance to ensure adequate ventilation and chest expansion. When lung compliance is normal, effective ventilation may be achieved at peak inspiratory pressures of 20 to 30 cm H_2O and an inspiratory time of 0.5 to 1.0 second. Higher inspiratory pressures are required in the presence of lung disease or decreased lung compliance. Initial peak inspiratory pressure should be set at the lowest level that provides adequate chest expansion and good breath sounds.

Volume-cycled ventilation is generally preferred because the preset tidal volume may be delivered even if the endotracheal tube is partially occluded. If a volume

Table 2. Initial Ventilator Settings*

Oxygen	100%
Tidal volume†	10-15 mL/kg
Inspiratory time†‡	0.5-1.0 second
Peak inspiratory pressure‡	20-30 cm H_2O if lung compliance normal (lowest level that results in adequate chest expansion)
Respiratory rate	Infants (normal lungs): 20-30 breaths per minute Children (normal lungs): 16-20 breaths per minute (adjust as needed)
PEEP	2-4 cm H_2O (adjust to maximize oxygen delivery)

PEEP indicates positive end-expiratory pressure.
*These settings should be adjusted based on clinical state and arterial blood gas analysis.
†For volume ventilators.
‡For time-cycled, pressure-limited ventilators.

ventilator is used to deliver a tidal volume of 10 to 15 mL/kg, the peak inspiratory pressure is likely to be 20 to 30 cm H_2O. When a volume-limited ventilator is used, the pressure-limit alarm should be set about 10 cm H_2O higher than the peak inspiratory pressure to reduce the risk of barotrauma and to indicate a sudden increase in airway resistance, ie, endotracheal tube occlusion, pneumothorax, or tube migration to the right or left main bronchus.

Respiratory Rate. When mechanical ventilatory support is provided for the patient with normal lungs, a respiratory rate of 20 to 30 breaths per minute is typically required for infants and a rate of 16 to 20 breaths per minute for children. When lung disease is present, higher respiratory rates often must be provided to ensure adequate ventilation.

Rapid respiratory rates reduce the time available for exhalation. In the presence of asthma, bronchiolitis, or other conditions causing air trapping, mechanical ventilation at a rapid rate may result in "stacking" of breaths and high risk of barotrauma, including pneumothorax. When these conditions are present, a tidal volume of 15 mL/kg is delivered at a relatively slow ventilation rate (20 to 25 breaths per minute for infants, 12 to 20 breaths per minute for children, and 8 to 12 breaths per minute for adolescents), and persistent mild or moderate hypercarbia is acceptable. The use of neuromuscular blocking agents is advisable during mechanical ventilation of the child with air trapping, because the child's spontaneous respiratory effort often contributes to further airway obstruction.

Positive End-expiratory Pressure. Intubation bypasses glottic function and eliminates the physiologic positive end-expiratory pressure (PEEP) created during normal coughing, talking, and crying. To maintain adequate functional residual capacity, a PEEP of 2 to 4 cm H_2O should be provided when mechanical ventilation is initiated. Higher levels of PEEP may be required if diffuse alveolar disease or marked ventilation-perfusion mismatch causes inadequate oxygenation. PEEP increases functional residual capacity, reduces intrapulmonary shunting, and can increase lung compliance. High levels of PEEP, however, can produce barotrauma, impede systemic venous return, and distort the geometry of the left ventricle. If systemic venous return and left ventricular function are compromised, the associated fall in cardiac output is likely to reduce oxygen delivery (Oxygen Delivery = Cardiac Output x Arterial Oxygen Content). Optimal PEEP must be determined for each patient: optimal PEEP is characterized as the lowest PEEP necessary for satisfactory oxygen delivery.

Assessment of Ventilation and Oxygenation After Intubation

The effectiveness of ventilation should be clinically assessed frequently (almost continuously) during mechanical ventilation. Tachypnea, head bobbing, nasal flaring, intercostal retractions, and the use of accessory neck and abdominal muscles are signs of increased work of breathing, suggesting that ventilatory support is inadequate. Agitation or lethargy may indicate inadequate oxygenation or ventilation. Cyanosis of the mucous membranes is a clear indication of hypoxemia, although significant hypoxemia may be present even in the absence of cyanosis.

Chest wall movement and breath sounds should be equal bilaterally. Auscultation should be performed over the lateral lung fields (axillary areas). If the tube is in the proper tracheal position, breath sounds should be easily auscultated in these areas but absent over the abdomen.[3] Unilateral breath sounds may indicate main bronchus intubation or may be caused by a mucus plug, foreign-body obstruction, pneumothorax, pleural effusion, or lung consolidation. Rales (crackles), rhonchi, or wheezing may be heard in the presence of pulmonary edema, infection, aspiration, or bronchospasm. Endotracheal tube position can be confirmed by a chest radiograph, although head and neck positioning can affect the location of the tip of the endotracheal tube. The tip should be 1 to 2 cm above the carina and below the clavicles.

Effectiveness of ventilation may be determined by patient observation, evaluation of arterial or capillary blood gases, and end-tidal CO_2 monitoring. End-tidal CO_2 monitors may be used only as "trend" monitors in patients with significant ventilation-perfusion mismatch. Effectiveness of oxygenation is determined by observation of the patient, pulse oximetry, and evaluation of arterial blood gases. Resolution of cyanosis and return of pink color in mucous membranes reflect improved oxygenation. Visible chest rise and good breath sounds with positive-pressure ventilation suggest an adequate tidal volume. Continued efforts by the patient to breathe against the ventilator may indicate inadequate minute ventilation.

Blood for gas analysis should be obtained 10 to 15 minutes after mechanical ventilation is initiated. Samples may be obtained from the radial, posterior tibial, dorsalis pedis, or femoral arteries (see chapter 5). If arterial puncture is unsuccessful, a capillary sample may be obtained from the heel, toe, or finger after the extremity has been warmed for 15 minutes. If blood flows freely and directly into the capillary sampling tube, a reasonably accurate reflection of acid-base status and arterial carbon dioxide tension can be obtained, although the arterial oxygen tension may be underestimated. However, if blood flow is sluggish, all aspects of the gas analysis are potentially unreliable. Noninvasive monitoring devices such as pulse oximeters, transcutaneous O_2 and CO_2 monitors, and exhaled CO_2 monitors are useful because they allow continuous assessment of oxygenation, ventilation, or both. However, these monitors may provide inaccurate results in the presence of hypothermia, poor peripheral perfusion, or endotracheal tube obstruction or displacement — problems may develop in the postresuscitation state.

Cardiovascular System

Circulatory failure may be either the cause or the result of cardiopulmonary arrest. Persistent circulatory dysfunction is likely to develop in the postresuscitation phase, and cardiac output must be supported to ensure adequate delivery of oxygen to tissues.

When hemodynamic stability permits cessation of chest compressions, cardiovascular function should be assessed rapidly (see chapter 2). Recurrent cardiopulmonary arrest can be prevented by improving hemodynamic status. Frequent cardiovascular assessments allow appropriate therapeutic interventions to be initiated before irreversible changes occur. Decreased cardiac output or shock may be caused by insufficient volume resuscitation, loss of peripheral vascular tone (eg, in septic, anaphylactic, or neurogenic shock), myocardial dysfunction, or inadequate or premature withdrawal of cardiovascular support (see chapters 2 and 6).

Whenever the infant or child demonstrates circulatory or respiratory instability, heart rate and rhythm must be monitored continuously until the child's condition is stable (see chapter 7). Blood pressure must be evaluated frequently. Normotension does not ensure adequate cardiac output in children because it may be observed despite the presence of shock. Hypotension is a *late* sign of shock and requires urgent and rapid therapy (see chapter 2). When intense vasoconstriction is present, Korotkoff sounds may be difficult to hear, so blood pressure evaluation by cuff is difficult. Under these conditions, systolic blood pressure may be better estimated by palpation or by use of a Doppler device. In patients with compromised cardiovascular function, direct intra-arterial monitoring should be instituted as soon as practical (see chapter 5).

If central venous access has been established, continuous or intermittent measurement of right heart filling pressure may help guide fluid administration and titration of vasoactive support. Urine output often correlates with effectiveness of renal and systemic perfusion and should be monitored with an indwelling catheter. Although renal failure may result in oliguria, prerenal causes (especially shock) must be ruled out whenever urine output is inadequate.

Laboratory evaluation of the circulatory state includes arterial blood gas and pH analysis and evaluation of serum electrolytes, lactic acid, calcium, glucose, urea nitrogen, and creatinine levels. The presence of metabolic (lactic) acidosis suggests that cardiac output and oxygen delivery are inadequate. Radiographic evaluation of heart size may aid in the assessment of intravascular volume. A small heart is consistent with hypovolemia, and a large heart, in the absence of cardiac disease or dysfunction, is consistent with volume overload.

Central Nervous System

Central nervous system dysfunction may be either the cause or result of cardiopulmonary arrest. The child's responsiveness should be evaluated as alert, responsive to voice, responsive to pain, or unresponsive. A brief neurologic assessment (including evaluation of pupil size and response to light, spontaneous movement and movement in response to painful stimuli, and ability to follow commands) should be performed and documented with each measurement of vital signs, with special attention to any changes in level of consciousness. If significant central nervous system depression is evident, the patient should be intubated and hyperventilated with the $PaCO_2$ maintained at 22 to 29 mm Hg until intracranial pressure can be evaluated more thoroughly. Adequate cerebral perfusion requires support of optimal cardiac output and systemic oxygen delivery.

Renal System

Decreased urine output (less than 1.0 mL/kg per hour for patients up to 30 kg) may result from prerenal causes, inadequate systemic perfusion, renal ischemic damage, or a combination of these conditions. Baseline serum creatinine and blood urea nitrogen and creatinine values should be determined as soon as possible. Evidence of volume depletion requires the administration of additional fluids, and myocardial dysfunction should be treated with vasoactive drugs (see chapter 6). Nephrotoxic drugs and medications excreted by the renal route should be avoided or administered cautiously until renal status can be fully evaluated.

Gastrointestinal System

If bowel sounds are absent, abdominal distention is present, or the patient requires mechanical ventilation, an orogastric or nasogastric tube should be inserted to prevent or treat gastric distention. Blind nasogastric tube placement is contraindicated in the patient with serious facial trauma because intracranial tube migration may result.[4] However, orogastric tubes usually can be passed safely in these patients.

Secondary (Interhospital) Transport

Advances in initial stabilization and intensive care of pediatric patients have improved outcomes of critical illness and injury.[1,5] However, serious illnesses and injuries often do not occur close to a pediatric tertiary care center, and many children must undergo lengthy interhospital transport before reaching a tertiary pediatric ICU.

Pediatric Transport System

Every pediatric tertiary care facility should have an organized pediatric transport system.[5] Ideally the system is regional, with central control by the pediatric tertiary care facility under the direction of a physician trained in pediatric emergency medicine or critical care. Transport of the critically ill or injured infant or child is best performed by a team experienced in such care, even if this results in the delay at the referring institution until the experienced transport team arrives. The transport team should be capable of providing pediatric ALS at the referring hospital and maintaining that level of care during transport.[6]

The referring facility and the tertiary care unit are both responsible for the establishment of well-defined protocols for specific clinical situations. EMS protocols should include indications for direct transport of pediatric patients to hospitals and facilities equipped to handle their critical care needs. This should reduce the need for secondary transport. Transfer and transport agreements must be finalized in advance to prevent needless transport delays.

Once the patient has been resuscitated and postresuscitation stabilization has begun, the most appropriate method of interhospital transport must be determined. Decisions to be made include selection of the mode of transport and the transport team[7-14]; transport triage[11-16]; advance preparation for transport[17]; preparation by the transport team; communication[5]; and posttransport follow-up.

Mode of Transport

Interhospital transport can be accomplished by local ambulance, mobile ICU ambulance from the receiving hospital, helicopter, or fixed-wing aircraft. A child with significant respiratory or circulatory compromise requires constant medical supervision, which precludes transfer in the parents' car.

Ground ambulances are readily available, relatively inexpensive, and spacious (compared with most transport aircraft). They can travel in most weather conditions and can stop easily if a procedure must be performed. Disadvantages of ground ambulance transport include increased transport time over long distances and the risk of traffic-related delays.

Helicopter transport is fast, allows rapid arrival at the receiving hospital, and allows the referring hospital to turn over care quickly. Traffic congestion is avoided. However, it is extremely difficult to monitor or evaluate the pediatric patient during helicopter transport, and it is usually impossible to perform emergency procedures. Weather conditions prevent flying as often as 15% of the time, and the cost is high.

Fixed-wing aircraft are used only for long-distance transport. These aircraft are pressurized and land at controlled sites. Patient monitoring and interventions are performed more easily in fixed- than in rotor-wing aircraft. Disadvantages of this form of transport include long start-up times (usually offset by the speed of flight) and the need to transfer the patient from hospital to ambulance to aircraft, with a reverse transfer sequence on landing.

Transport Team

Members of the transport team may include local EMS personnel, medical personnel from the referring hospital, hospital-based critical care teams that transport patients of all ages, and dedicated pediatric and neonatal transport teams. Local EMS teams rarely have the training, experience, or equipment for long-distance transport of a critically ill or injured child following resuscitation.[18,19] In addition, use of local EMS personnel may deprive the region of service in the event of other emergencies.

Healthcare professionals from the referring hospital may be mobilized rapidly, but their travel may deprive the referring hospital of necessary personnel unless they are specifically scheduled for transport. Personnel with limited experience in pediatric prehospital and critical care will find patient management especially difficult in a moving vehicle with limited equipment (eg, portable monitors). Anticipated care during transfer should not exceed the level that the transport team is capable of providing.

Critical care transport teams that transport patients of all ages may or may not have appropriate training, experience, and equipment for optimal care of a critically ill or injured child.[20] The ability of transport teams in a given region to care for critically ill or injured children should be evaluated *before* this type of care is needed. The most qualified team (as measured by existing pediatric transport guidelines) should be used.[5]

Pediatric critical care transport teams provide optimal transport for critically ill children and often provide continuity of care from transport to pediatric ICU. However, such teams are not available in all areas and may not have access to all types of transport vehicles. If available, such a team should be used for transporting the most unstable children, even if that team takes longer to arrive or to stabilize the patient than would a less-skilled team. An exception to this "most-skilled" transport rule would be the child who requires immediate surgical intervention at the tertiary care center (eg, craniotomy for epidural hematoma).[6]

Transport Triage

No specific criteria are available to reliably determine the need for a pediatric critical care transport team,[15,21,22] although broad criteria include

- Patients expected to require pediatric ICU admission at the receiving hospital. Patients requiring that level of monitoring and care on arrival likely will need such care during transfer.
- Patients with a respiratory condition (eg, asthma or croup) with significant potential for deterioration during an hour-long ride.
- Patients who have recently experienced a life-threatening event (even if their condition is stable at the time of transfer), because the event may recur. These patients include neonates and infants with a history of apnea and any patient who has required aggressive stabilization (eg, following seizure with apnea or shock).

Advance Preparation (Table 3)

Every hospital should establish protocols that outline access to the various transport systems *before* a sick child actually requires care. The names and telephone numbers of facilities equipped to care for critically ill and injured children should be posted at the emergency department telephone, and a list of transport systems capable of transporting pediatric patients (if different from the receiving hospital's list) should be kept in the same location. If only one pediatric tertiary care center is located in the area, the nearest alternative hospital (even if in another state) should also be listed. Since bed capacity in pediatric ICUs usually is limited, a backup plan is essential.

Ambulance personnel who transport children should have specific training and ongoing experience in pediatric assessment, stabilization, and resuscitation. All EMTs should be encouraged to complete the pediatric ALS course and to maintain proficiency by assisting in the care of pediatric patients in the emergency department. Ambulance equipment should be evaluated periodically to ensure that it is appropriate for the entire range of ages and sizes of pediatric patients and to ensure that lost or missing equipment is immediately replaced.[18]

Transport nurses should have specific training and experience in pediatric evaluation, stabilization, and resuscitation. Written protocols must be available delineating management of potential crises during transport (eg, respiratory failure or arrest, seizure activity, and cardiac arrest). A list of necessary equipment should be prepared in advance, and a more extensive list of equipment should be available if a physician accompanies the patient. Ideally, pediatric transport packs, including equipment of the correct size and medication doses for particular emergency situations, should be prepared in advance.

In some areas of the country, transfer of uninsured patients may be restricted, especially if the nearest available pediatric center is across a state line. Advance preparation for transport must include such administrative matters as written, prearranged contracts between the referring and receiving hospitals and development of written protocols to initiate appropriate communication between hospital administrators. If payment for transport is separate from payment for hospitalization, arrangements for transport reimbursement should be negotiated in advance.

Table 3. Advance Preparation for Interhospital Transport

List of names and telephone numbers of pediatric tertiary care facilities

List of pediatric transport systems

List (or pack) of equipment and supplies for pediatric patients to be added to the standard EMS equipment

Personnel trained and experienced in pediatric care

Administrative protocols

Immediate Preparation (Table 4)

When a transport team from other than the referring or receiving hospital is used, the referring hospital still must assist in the efficient transfer of the patient. Some transport teams operate on the basis of implied consent and consider transport part of treatment for a life-threatening emergency, without the need for formal consent. If possible, written consent to transport should still be obtained from the patient's legal guardian. Many transport teams request that the parents remain at the referring hospital to give consent directly to the team.

If airway patency or ventilatory status is questionable, it is best to secure the airway with an endotracheal tube before transport. Intravascular lines and the endotracheal tube must be securely taped in place before transfer. Unfortunately, vascular catheters and endotracheal tubes frequently dislodge during transport, often because they were inadequately secured for a moving environment. The movement and vibrations occurring during transport make replacement of dislodged catheters or endotracheal tubes extremely difficult. The cervical spine and any fractured bones must be stabilized before transport.

Copies of the patient's chart and radiographs should be made before the transport team arrives. If blood products may be required during transport, a supply should be prepared in advance to be sent with the patient. Transfer generally will be more efficient if the referring hospital anticipates the requirements of the transport team and prepares to meet those requirements.

Table 4. Responsibilities of Referring Hospital Before Transport

Copy all patient records and radiographs

Obtain transport consent (many teams require that their own consent forms be signed)

Secure vascular access and endotracheal tube

Stabilize cervical spine and any fractures

Prepare blood products, if indicated

Provide laboratory telephone number for pending laboratory results

Communication

The initial call to transfer a patient should be made by one physician to another.[17] In fact, the transport system should not be activated until the referring physician has discussed the patient's case with the physician who will accept the patient in transfer. The referring physician should consult the patient's chart at the time of the call to give specific details about vital signs, fluids administered, timing of events, etc. In a crisis, a brief history of the illness/accident, interventions, and current clinical status should facilitate decisions about treatment and method of transport. The names of the receiving physician and hospital and advice from the receiving physician should be documented; transport team personnel may need additional specific information to select the proper equipment for transport. Any potential need for isolation should be addressed at this time so that appropriate bed arrangements can be made at the receiving hospital.

The referring physician should call the receiving hospital if the patient's condition changes at any time during the transfer. Nurses from both hospitals should request and provide updates on the patient's status. When the transport team arrives, the referring physician should provide a current report about the patient directly and personally to the transport team to formally relinquish care of the patient. If a method of transport is chosen that does not involve the receiving hospital's transport team, the referring physician should telephone the receiving physician immediately before the patient's departure and report the patient's most recent vital signs, current clinical status, and estimated time of arrival at the receiving hospital. Successful communication between the receiving and referring hospitals is essential for a successful transport, and both hospitals must ensure that this communication is successful. The tertiary care center that accepts the patient must be accessible and provide recommendations by telephone, and the transferring hospital must provide adequate information about the patient so that appropriate recommendations can be offered.

Copies of all records, laboratory results, and radiographs should be transferred with the patient. Laboratory results pending at the time of transport should be noted. The laboratory phone number should be provided with the patient record so that the receiving physician can obtain the outstanding results.

Posttransport Follow-up

Many transport teams provide an evaluation form for the referring hospital to complete. The referring physician should be contacted by the receiving physician after the transport is complete to identify any problems and to be advised of the patient's status. The tertiary care center is also responsible for providing personnel at the referring hospital with subsequent follow-up information on the patient's condition, including ultimate outcome. If such communication does not occur, the referring physician should contact the medical director of the transport system to express any concerns about the transport. Such a discussion can often clarify misunderstandings about matters such as the necessity for interventions or timing of the transport. This feedback is required to improve the performance of the transport team and the referring hospital.

References

1. Pollack MM, Alexander SR, Clarke N, Ruttimann UE, Tesselaar HM, Bachulis AC. Improved outcomes from tertiary center pediatric intensive care: a statewide comparison of tertiary and nontertiary care facilities. *Crit Care Med.* 1991;19:150-159.

2. Hunt RC, Bryan DM, Brinkley VS, Whitley TW, Benson NH. Inability to assess breath sounds during air medical transport by helicopter. *JAMA.* 1991;265:1982-1984.

3. Andersen KH, Hald A. Assessing the position of the tracheal tube: the reliability of different methods. *Anaesthesia.* 1989;44:984-985.

4. Fletcher SA, Henderson LT, Miner ME, Jones JM. The successful surgical removal of intracranial nasogastric tubes. *J Trauma.* 1987;27:948-952.

5. American Academy of Pediatrics Task Force on Interhospital Transport. *Guidelines for Air and Ground Transport of Neonatal and Pediatric Patients.* Elk Grove Village, Ill: American Academy of Pediatrics; 1993.

6. Aoki BY, McCloskey K, eds. *Evaluation, Stabilization, and Transport of the Critically Ill Child.* St. Louis, Mo: Mosby Year Book; 1992.

7. Baxt WG, Moody P. The impact of a physician as part of the aeromedical prehospital team in patients with blunt trauma. *JAMA.* 1987;257:3246-3250.

8. Kanter RK, Tompkins JM. Adverse events during interhospital transport: physiologic deterioration associated with pretransport severity of illness. *Pediatrics.* 1989;84:43-48.

9. Kanter RK, Boeing NM, Hannan WP, Kanter DL. Excess morbidity associated with interhospital transport. *Pediatrics.* 1992;90: 893-898.

10. McCloskey KA, King WD, Byron L. Pediatric critical care transport: is a physician always needed on the team? *Ann Emerg Med.* 1989;18:247-249.

11. McCloskey KA, Johnston C. Critical care interhospital transports: predictability of the need for a pediatrician. *Pediatr Emerg Care.* 1990;6:89-92.

12. McCloskey KA, Johnston C. Pediatric critical care transport survey: team composition and training, mobilization time, and mode of transportation. *Pediatr Emerg Care.* 1990;6:1-3.

13. Macnab AJ. Optimal escort for interhospital transport of pediatric emergencies. *J Trauma.* 1991;31:205-209.

14. Snow N, Hull C, Severns J. Physician presence on a helicopter emergency medical service: necessary or desirable? *Aviat Space Environ Med.* 1986;57:1176-1178.

15. Orr R, Venkataraman ST, Cinoman MI, Hogue BL, Singleton CA, McCloskey KA. Pretransport pediatric risk of mortality (PRISM) score underestimates the requirement for intensive care or major interventions during interhospital transport. *Crit Care Med.* 1994;22:101-107.

16. Rubenstein JS, Gomez MA, Rybicki L, Noah ZL. Can the need for a physician as part of the pediatric transport team be predicted? A prospective study. *Crit Care Med.* 1992;20:1657-1661.

17. American Academy of Pediatrics Committee on Pediatric Emergency Medicine; Singer J, Ludwig S, eds. *Emergency Medical Services for Children: The Role of the Primary Care Provider.* Elk Grove Village, Ill: American Academy of Pediatrics; 1992.

18. Seidel JS. Emergency medical services and the pediatric patient: are the needs being met? II: training and equipping emergency medical services providers for pediatric emergencies. *Pediatrics.* 1986;78:808-812.

19. Seidel JS, Hornbein M, Yoshiyama K, Kuznets D, Finklestein JZ, St Geme JW Jr. Emergency medical services and the pediatric patient: are the needs being met? *Pediatrics.* 1984;73:769-772.

20. McCloskey K, Orr R, Hardwick W. Pediatric transport by teams transporting patients of all ages. *Pediatr Emerg Care.* 1992;8:307. Abstract.

21. Kissoon N, Frewen TC, Kronick JB, Mohammed A. The child requiring transport: lessons and implications for the pediatric emergency physician. *Pediatr Emerg Care.* 1988;4:1-4.

22. Orr R, Venkataraman S, McCloskey K, King W, Cinoman M. Predicting the need for major interventions during pediatric interhospital transport using pretransport variables. *Pediatr Emerg Care.* 1992;8:371. Abstract.

Suggested Reading

McCloskey K, Orr R. Interhospital transport. In: Ludwig S, ed. *Emergency Medical Services for Children: What the Practitioner Needs to Know.* Elk Grove Village, Ill: American Academy of Pediatrics; 1992.

Barkin RM, ed. Pediatrics in the emergency medical services system. *Pediatr Emerg Care.* 1990;6:72-77.

Day S, McCloskey K, Orr R, Bolte R, Notterman D, Hackel A. Pediatric interhospital critical care transport: consensus of a national leadership conference. *Pediatrics.* 1991;88:696-704.

Ethical and Legal Aspects of CPR in Children

Chapter 11

External chest compression was introduced three decades ago.[1] Since that time CPR has gained acceptance as an effective emergency technique that can significantly reduce mortality and be mastered readily by healthcare professionals and laypersons. CPR has become a standard treatment modality with attendant legal and ethical issues.

The search for principles to guide the conduct of potential rescuers in these encounters with sudden death is part of the larger, continuing exploration of the impact of modern medical technology on the traditional patient-provider relationship. Of particular relevance is the continually evolving position of children in our society, their legal standing, and the legal predicates of the special relationships among provider, parent, and child in the pediatric healthcare setting.

This chapter presents some of the general principles underlying the ethical and legal rights and duties of pediatric patients, healthcare providers, and hospitals, and relates those principles specifically to CPR, highlighting aspects unique to the care of children.

The Child as Patient

Appreciation of the physical, physiologic, and psychosocial development of children is central to the recognition of pediatrics as a specialty discipline within medicine. Practitioners and hospitals who provide care for children are legally judged by widely accepted pediatric standards. It should be anticipated that these pediatric standards will be the reference point for identification of legal issues involving resuscitative care.

The Patient-Physician Relationship

Ethical Principles

Throughout much of medical history, physicians have been guided by principles derived from the Hippocratic oath. The dominant Hippocratic theme instructs physicians to use their knowledge and skills for the benefit of their patients and to protect their patients from harm. Contemporary writers have noted the absence of any explicit patient role in decision making and questioned whether this paternalistic stance is appropriate in an era in which highly invasive technology may blur the line between "benefit" and "harm."[2]

The modern view frames the patient-physician relationship as a collaborative process to which the physician contributes medical knowledge, skill, and judgment and

the patient contributes a personal valuation of the potential benefits and risks inherent in the proposed treatment, thus incorporating important moral principles of patient autonomy and right to self-determination.

Issues of patient autonomy, shared decision making, and the dilemma of balancing benefit and harm are particularly germane to CPR and the appropriate application of life-support technology. These issues are further complicated in cases involving minors because highly valued traditions of family privacy and parental authority may be challenged.

The Physician-Patient Relationship

Physicians generally enter into a legal relationship with a patient by two routes. Typically the physician agrees in advance to provide a specific course of treatment in exchange for compensation. Less typical but more applicable to the CPR context, however, are the legal obligations that arise when a physician must render care without prior agreement. Once a physician or other person performs an act that may be construed as rendering care, a legal duty generally follows to meet some "reasonable standard" (discussed more fully below) in the performance of that act and to continue the effort.[3] *Once treatment has been undertaken either in the hospital or in the prehospital setting, the provider may not unilaterally terminate the legal relationship unless care is no longer needed, the patient agrees to the termination, or appropriate procedures for the transfer of care have been carried out.*[4]

Informed Consent

Central to the patient-physician relationship is the notion of "consent," a traditional moral and legal concept that has evolved into a complex codification of patients' rights of self-determination. At first glance these considerations may seem irrelevant in emergency care situations, when consent to treatment is usually implied.[5] However, familiarity with this issue is needed in light of the increasing use of advanced patient directives prescribing preferred treatment in the event of cardiac arrest, the rising number of competent patients refusing consent for life support, and the frequency with which third parties serve as proxy decision makers for patients who are incompetent.

In his classic assertion that every person of sound mind and mature age has the right to determine what shall happen to his or her own body,[6] Cardozo defined patients' rights to grant *permission* for treatment, without which a physician may be guilty of committing an assault. Modern court decisions and state statutes have shaped this concept into the doctrine of "informed consent," which requires much more than mere acquiescence.

The essential operational elements of informed consent involve a careful assessment of the patient's decision-making capacity, a judgment as to the "voluntariness" of the decisions, and a determination of the nature and extent of the information to be disclosed. Decision-making capacity is reflected in the patient's ability to comprehend, communicate, and appreciate the consequences of available choices. "Voluntariness" refers to the absence of internal or extrinsic pressures that may coercively restrict patient options.[7] Considerable controversy and legal variability surround the required content of the information disclosure. Traditionally, and in many states by law, prevailing practice patterns have been accepted as the reference standard for required disclosure. The modern view, furthering patient autonomy, rejects this professional standard in favor of a lay, objective, "reasonable person" standard that requires physicians to disclose those material facts concerning treatment alternatives and risks that a reasonable person would need to make an informed decision.[8]

The law recognizes several exceptions to the informed consent doctrine that may apply in cases involving CPR and life support. Most significantly, in emergencies involving the risk of serious injury or death, consent may be implied if the need for treatment is immediate or the patient has lost decision-making capacity. If there is strong reason to believe that the disclosure involved may cause serious psychological harm, physicians may rely on "therapeutic privilege" and be excused for failing to obtain informed consent.[9] States vary considerably with respect to their statutory or common-law definition of informed consent.[10]

The Parent-Child-Professional Triad

The Rights of Parents and Children

An increased potential for conflict is introduced into the patient-professional relationship when the patient is a minor under parental guardianship. Parental decision making on behalf of children, particularly in the area of life support, can provoke questions regarding parental rights versus rights of children, parental rights versus the duty of the pediatric professional, and the interests of the decision makers versus those of the state.

As a rule, the law protects the natural rights of parents to raise children free from unwarranted state interference, presuming that parents will act in the best interests of their children.[11] Accordingly, parents are allowed considerable latitude for medical decisions on behalf of their children, even if the choices may not concur with the physician's recommendation.[12,13] These rights are conditional on parental fulfillment of the duty to provide neces-

sary care for minor children. If parents fail to provide their children with at least a minimum standard of medical care, the state may assert its interest in protecting the welfare of children by invoking child protection statutes to override parental wishes. Courts regularly uphold such interventions when parental refusals, even when genuinely motivated by strong family convictions, may be life-threatening.[14] However, when the consequences for the child are grave but not life-threatening, states have varied in their willingness to intervene, reflecting the continuing struggle to balance the rights of individual children and family privacy.[15] Thus, courts have overruled parental refusal to consent when cosmetic surgery is recommended for a severely deformed child[16] but upheld parental objections to a spinal fusion that would correct the child's paralytic scoliosis.[12]

The ambivalence of courts about medically inappropriate parental decisions is further exemplified in cases in which the treatment chosen is predictably ineffective but not immediately life-threatening. In one case the court ordered conventional chemotherapy for a child suffering from leukemia over the objections of the parents, who preferred metabolic and laetrile treatment.[17] Conversely, another court upheld a parental decision to treat the child with laetrile, reasoning that the parents fulfilled the legal requirement of providing minimum treatment necessary by demonstrating that some medical opinion exists supporting the use of laetrile.[18] Many state child-protection statutes include exemptions for parents who seek nontraditional forms of treatment based on religious convictions, although the American Academy of Pediatrics has urged states to repeal such provisions.[19]

"Baby Doe" Cases

The widely publicized "Baby Doe" cases involve decisions by parents and physicians to withhold life-sustaining treatment from severely handicapped or critically ill newborns. The general ethical and legal concepts of physician-patient relationships, informed consent, rights of the incompetent, and conflict between the family and the state are at issue in these situations.

The President's Commission for the Study of Ethical Problems in Medicine and Biomedical and Behavioral Research has identified significant problems in the decision-making process concerning neonates and offered an approach to a "best interest" analysis, including the use of ethics committees to advise in ambiguous cases.[20] Congress has established controversial guidelines suggesting that treatment may be withheld from neonates under the following conditions:

- The infant is chronically and irreversibly comatose.
- Treatment would merely prolong dying or would not be effective in ameliorating or correcting all of the infant's life-threatening conditions.
- Treatment would be virtually futile in terms of survival and therefore inhumane.

The Department of Health and Human Services has construed these provisions narrowly to specifically exclude any consideration of the potential "quality of life" of the affected infant.[21] While many neonatologists believe that these guidelines have led to excessive treatment of hopelessly ill infants,[22] others report that they have not affected their practice patterns.[23]

Difficult decisions about initiating CPR may arise unexpectedly in the delivery room with the birth of a very premature, critically ill neonate or a baby with multiple congenital malformations. Many hospitals follow a policy of initiating CPR attempts in the delivery room for all viable neonates pending thorough assessment and review of therapeutic options. There is accumulating evidence, however, that very low birthweight infants (<750 g) who require aggressive CPR during the first days of life have a very low likelihood of survival.[24-26] In most cases a well-documented review of the clinical data supported by appropriate clinical consultation and discussions with the family will result in a clear consensus concerning the appropriateness of continued life-support measures based on the child's best interest. Ethical dilemmas remain, however, in those complex cases in which the participants in the decision seek to balance the benefits of prolonging life through the use of multiple invasive medical and surgical procedures against the continuing burden on the child and family. Consultation with hospital ethics committees can provide a method to ensure careful consideration of the clinical and ethical issues in such cases.[20,27]

Consent by Minors

Historically the right of self-determination is recognized at the legal age of maturity, defined as 18 years. Many legislatures and courts have expanded minors' rights to consent to medical treatment, although great variability in this approach exists from state to state. A child may acquire status as an "emancipated minor" entitled to treatment as an adult through marriage, judicial decree, military service, parental consent, failure by the parents to meet legal responsibilities, living apart from and being financially independent of parents, and (in some circumstances) motherhood. In addition, statutory "mature minor" rules uphold the validity of consent given by minors if the treatment is appropriate and the minor is considered capable of comprehending the clinical circumstances and therapeutic options.[28] Many state statutes permit minors to consent to treatment for specified conditions, such as venereal disease and substance abuse. A "variable competence" approach to minors' consent may be used, which considers developmental aspects of cognitive and psychosocial maturation.[29] As a child's powers to interpret and integrate life's experiences evolve from a characteristically concrete, shortsighted perspective to an appreciation of abstract, future-oriented concepts, a concomitant expansion of decisional rights involving increasingly complex and risky alternatives may follow. Professionals have been encouraged to obtain "assent" for some treatments from children as young as 7 years and, in the interest of promoting children's rights, to consider persistent expressions of dissent by young children.[30]

Courts have recognized the rights of minors approaching the age of 18 years to participate in decision making, including choices involving life-and-death consequences.[31,32]

Essential Elements of Medical Malpractice

General Considerations

Medical malpractice actions are based on allegations of negligent conduct by the healthcare provider. To prevail, the patient must prove that the healthcare provider failed in his or her *duty* to provide the patient with the degree of knowledge, skill, and care usually exercised by a reasonable and prudent provider under similar circumstances, given the prevailing state of medical knowledge and available resources,[33] and that the *specific injury* was *caused* by that failure. Each emphasized element of this definition must be supported separately by sufficient evidence to make the allegation more likely than not. Poor results, complications of treatment, and errors in judgment are not necessarily evidence of malpractice.[33]

The provider's legal duty toward the patient begins with a mutual agreement to provide care for compensation or with any act that may represent an undertaking to provide care. To prevail in a malpractice action the patient must prove that the provider breached that duty by failing to provide care or by providing care that did not meet an acceptable standard. In addition, the patient must, in fact, have suffered an injury. Therefore, even if evidence demonstrates that the care provided was substandard, a claim of medical malpractice will fail if the patient escaped injury. Finally, the plaintiff must prove that the provider's failure to provide care of an acceptable standard caused the patient's injury. While these general elements apply to medical malpractice cases, specific criteria may vary considerably from state to state.

Standards of Care

General Standards

Key to the finding of medical malpractice is the *standard of care* by which the provider's conduct will be measured. Healthcare providers are required to exercise the degree of care and skill expected of a reasonably competent practitioner of the same class, acting in the same or similar circumstances. Courts vary, however, on the geographic limits from which the comparison practitioner may be drawn. The traditional "strict locality rule," which limited the comparison standard to the same geographic area as the defendant provider, has been abandoned in some courts (and some states) in favor of a regional or national standard.[34] Many courts, recognizing the widespread improvement in the standard of medical care, greater access to information and facilities, and standardized training programs for medical specialists, prefer to use nationally accepted standards of care. This wider geographic standard greatly expands the range of medical expert opinions available to parties in malpractice litigation.

Medical malpractice cases concerning CPR have been limited to in-hospital cases in which the risk of cardiac arrest could be anticipated. Successful action against laypersons who attempt out-of-hospital CPR seems unlikely.[35]

Standards and Guidelines for CPR

The key to medical malpractice litigation is often determination of the reference standard of care. A person at the scene of a cardiac arrest may be bound by a duty to provide care based on prior relations with the patient or by employment in an organized EMS system. The standard of care by which the rescuer's conduct may be measured in initiating, performing, or terminating CPR takes into account the class of the rescuer, the level of expertise that the rescuer may have or is expected to have, and the circumstances surrounding the event. Whether a person trained in CPR may be legally held to AHA guidelines is unclear. Some courts regard the AHA CPR guidelines as a national standard of care.[35,36]

Failure to Obtain Consent

Proof of negligence in malpractice cases may be based on failure to obtain informed consent. The plaintiff must prove that the provider failed to disclose all the material facts that a reasonable person would require to make an informed decision, that the patient's injury was caused by the provider's act (for which the patient granted uninformed permission), and that a reasonable person would have withheld consent had the material facts been disclosed.[8] These elements may vary according to the laws of individual states.

Consent for CPR may be implied in cardiac arrest cases, as it is in any emergency in which circumstances preclude an opportunity for prior discussion with the patient or guardian. However, problems may arise in emergency situations when documents on the victim's person or statements by family members purport to represent the victim's intended refusal of CPR. Authorities encourage the exercise of medical judgment in such cases.[5,37] It is extremely difficult to validate such information in an emergency setting, so the practice of initiating resuscitative efforts is generally accepted with the understanding that CPR may be discontinued based on subsequent authentication of the patient's previously expressed wishes.

Hospital Liability

The professional who provides CPR will often be functioning as part of an organization. Emergency department staff, hospital-based resuscitation teams, hospital medical staff, trained technicians in an EMS system, municipal firefighters, and police personnel deal with complex issues of accountability and legal liability.

A hospital may be held liable not only for the organized services it provides but also for the individual acts of its employees. A hospital that represents itself as operating an emergency department has a duty to accept and treat all patients coming through its doors and to provide a properly equipped facility.[38] A hospital has a positive duty to maintain sufficient personnel properly trained in CPR, to provide appropriate equipment for CPR, to implement an emergency alerting system within the hospital, and to monitor CPR performance. In many jurisdictions this legal duty of hospitals to ensure organization of CPR services and competence of their cardiac arrest teams has deprived hospital-based personnel of the legal immunity available to out-of-hospital rescuers.[39]

In recent years courts have expanded the notion of hospital liability beyond responsibility for the facility to include the duty to ensure that competent medical care is provided to each patient.[40,41] By this doctrine a hospital is considered an entity composed of both administrative and medical staff (paid and volunteer), each sharing joint responsibility for the development of standards and monitoring the quality of patient care. With the acceptance of national guidelines of pediatric CPR, the courts will likely recognize hospital corporate liability for the provision of appropriate CPR services for infants and children, including trained personnel, proper equipment, an organized system for response to pediatric cardiopulmonary arrests, and continuous monitoring of resuscitation performance.

Vicarious Liability

Customary CPR practices include prompt designation of a leader from among the responders to a cardiac arrest. This raises questions about potential special liability of the leader for the actions of others. Similar issues may arise in connection with the role of hospital-based medical personnel directing care via telecommunications with EMS personnel in the field.

The traditional legal view applied the "captain-of-the-ship doctrine" to such cases so that a leader would be held vicariously liable for the conduct of others in the group, depending on his or her level of control or right of control of group member actions. The modern legal trend, generally articulated with reference to surgical teams, recognizes the distinct areas of expertise contributed by each member and tends to hold each to a standard of his or her class and ultimately his or her employer rather than shift liability to the team leader.[42]

Duty to Rescue

Ethical and Legal Aspects of Duty to Rescue

The AHA stresses the crucial role the first responder plays before an organized resuscitation team arrives.[43-45]

Under the generally accepted moral principles of beneficence and nonmalfeasance, the fundamental proscription against actively harming others is complemented by an affirmative duty to benefit others when in a position to do so.[46] Traditional American law, however, does not enforce this moral obligation. Precedents in case law distinguish between an *affirmative act* that may give rise to liability in rescue situations if it is performed inappropriately and *failure to act*, which, however ignoble, may be above legal reproach.[3,47] This may result in a moral paradox in which a person making a well-intentioned but incompetent attempt to rescue another is held legally liable, whereas failure to act may not produce legal consequences.

Certain preexisting relations may create legal duties to rescue in emergency situations. These duties may stem from implied contracts, as in the case of emergency department healthcare providers, police, lifeguards, or emergency medical technicians. Special-status relationships, such as parent-child, captain-passenger, and employer-employee, may carry a general legal duty to rescue if the effort can be made without endangering the rescuer.[48] When not functioning in an official, obligatory capacity, healthcare providers are subject to similar disparate moral and legal standards. While the moral obligation of providers to assist in emergencies is asserted in the professional code of ethics,[49] no legal duty to act has been imposed simply because they are providers.[50]

It is interesting to note that statutes enacted in Vermont[51] and Minnesota[52] require persons to offer emergency assistance. These may indicate a movement toward recognition of a general duty to rescue.[52,53]

Despite reluctance to assign legal liability for failure to act, courts have ruled that once steps are initiated and termination would place the victim in a worse position or compromise the likelihood of assistance from others, the potential rescuer incurs a legal duty to perform appropriately. This element of the law of rescue, coupled with the dramatic growth in medical malpractice litigation, created well-grounded fear that professionals would be hesitant to offer assistance and ultimately led to Good Samaritan immunity statutes in all states.

Good Samaritan statutory language generally identifies a protected class, usually focusing on protection of health professionals to encourage response by trained persons. In some states, statutes protect any person offering emergency assistance. As a general rule, legal immunity is granted only to persons rendering aid without compensation or attempts to collect compensation. However, many state statutes creating organized EMS systems protect trained professionals in the course of their official duties.

The scope of immunity granted varies considerably among statutes. Common to all is the requirement that the rescuer show "good faith" belief that the situation called for the immediate action undertaken. Most statutes confer legal immunity for incompetent rescue attempts unless the actions were grossly negligent (conduct that would be considered reckless, offensive, and shocking to most people). The rescue settings covered by Good Samaritan statutes also vary. In some states only actions at the site of the emergency are covered; other states include events during transport to a medical facility.[54] Some states extend immunity to persons responding to an emergency within a hospital if they have no preexisting duty to offer assistance. In contrast, other states have denied protection to these same persons, reasoning that members of a hospital staff are presumed to have sufficient expertise in emergency medical care.[54]

Traditional legal concepts hold persons offering assistance in an emergency to a "reasonable care" standard, taking into account all of the circumstances surrounding the incident and the rescuer's level of skill. Thus, common-law formula considers the existence of an emergency in determining what degree of care is reasonable.[55]

The capability and willingness of first responders to perform CPR on pediatric victims are important, especially because respiratory arrest is more common than primary cardiac arrest, and pediatric ALS may prevent the progression of respiratory to cardiac arrest.[56] Prolonged hypoxemia prior to actual cardiac arrest is thought to contribute to the poor results of out-of-hospital resuscitation.[4,56] First responders should not be dissuaded by fear of possible litigation from making reasonable attempts at CPR, regardless of their level of experience or training. Whether under Good Samaritan statutes or traditional common-law principles, CPR attempts in emergencies are likely to be viewed as reasonable, even when provided by an inadequately trained rescuer, as long as there is a good-faith belief that the possible benefits of the attempt outweigh the risk from the rescuer's incompetence.[57]

Decisions to Initiate and Terminate CPR

First responders at the scene of a cardiac arrest are encouraged to initiate full CPR measures in virtually all instances without attempting to assess resuscitability. The absence of accepted criteria for immediate determination of death, with a few exceptions, supports the requirement that rescuers give the victim the benefit of the doubt and initiate attempts at resuscitation.[58,59] Unreliable or unverifiable information about prior illness of the victim or about wishes previously expressed by the victim against CPR should not influence the exercise of medical judgment in prehospital emergencies. In a hospital setting some children may have preexistent "do-not-resuscitate" orders (see below). If these are determined to be valid, CPR should not be initiated or may be discontinued. From both an ethical and legal standpoint, discontinuing or withholding CPR under such circumstances is permissible.[59]

A decision to terminate CPR based on nonresuscitability is equivalent to determining death and therefore must be made by a physician. Nonphysicians are required to continue CPR to the limits of their physical endurance or until the care of the victim is transferred to another qualified, responsible person. An increasing number of states are exploring ways to authorize nonphysician emergency medical personnel to withhold or discontinue resuscitative efforts in the field based on criteria for poor survival or recognition of patients' requests not to resuscitate.[60] Once CPR is initiated, physicians are required to continue CPR as necessary until the victim is transferred to the care of other properly trained personnel or until cardiac death (as defined by cardiovascular unresponsiveness to acceptable resuscitative techniques) is determined.[58]

Some investigators have proposed guidelines for cessation of CPR based on predictability of cardiac recovery after specified periods of apnea, pulselessness, and resuscitation efforts.[61] Empirical studies demonstrate considerable physician variability in interpreting clinical data to decide whether to terminate CPR.[62,63] This variability in clinical practice, together with the complex ethical and psychological factors involved in individual cases, has led some commentators to prefer that no specific criteria be promulgated for ceasing CPR in children.[64]

Orders Not to Resuscitate

In marked contrast to earlier times when most people died at home in the comfort of familiar surroundings, an estimated 80% of all deaths now occur in hospitals.[20] It is not surprising that a large proportion of hospitalized patients die after one or more attempts at CPR.[65] Recognizing that attempts at resuscitation may not always promote patient well-being, the National Conference Steering Committee stated, "The purpose of cardiopulmonary resuscitation is the prevention of sudden, unexpected death." CPR may not be indicated when death is expected and prolonged cardiac arrest would render resuscitative efforts virtually futile.[66] Resuscitation in these circumstances may represent a violation of an individual's right to die with dignity. Contraindications to CPR must be noted in the patient's chart by the attending physician.[67] "Do-not-resuscitate" orders and chart notes legitimize decisions not to resuscitate hospitalized patients when CPR is not indicated. Under certain circumstances, do-not-resuscitate orders may apply to prehospital care of terminally ill patients when appropriate documentation is provided to the local EMS service.[68,69]

However, many state laws still make it illegal for prehospital personnel to honor a hospital DNR order.

Competent Patients

Consistent with the principle of self-determination, a competent patient's right to refuse CPR is virtually absolute.[70,71] Courts have limited the right of the competent patient to refuse lifesaving treatment in only a few narrowly defined circumstances, such as the protection of dependent children.[72]

In everyday legal contexts, such as the assignment of property rights, the definition of "competence" is straightforward. Determination of competence in terms of decision-making capacity in the healthcare process is considerably more complex yet critical to an analysis of resuscitation decisions. Patients may have decisional capacity for some medical alternatives but not for others. The degree to which a patient's decision-making capacity may be temporarily or permanently affected by pain, drugs, or mental state also must be assessed.[73,74] Once competence has been established, the patient, under the consent doctrine, has the right to refuse treatment, including lifesaving measures, even if the decision seems foolish or irrational to others.

Unfortunately studies suggest wide disparities in physician practices with respect to discussing resuscitation with competent patients.[75,76] Legal considerations aside, communication among practitioners, patients, and families on the subject of resuscitation appears to be influenced significantly by social and ethical values held by staff members and by differing views concerning the propriety of including competent patients in such discussions.[77-82]

Minors may express the wish to have life support withheld.[31] Caregivers may tend to underestimate the capacity of some adolescent patients to deal with concepts of death, terminal illness, and consequences.[30,83] In several recent cases courts have authorized caregivers to recognize decisions by older adolescents to withhold resuscitative attempts.[32,84] How courts respond to situations in which there is disagreement between parents and the adolescent patient is unclear.

Incompetent Patients

Promotion of the autonomy of hopelessly ill and incompetent patients can be very difficult.[85] Some general themes emerge from a review of court rulings.

The American Medical Association has stated that physicians have no obligation to provide futile or useless treatment. Thus, do-not-resuscitate orders are often appropriate for patients who are irreversibly and terminally ill when resuscitation would merely prolong the dying process.[86] The recognition that physicians have no ethical or legal duty to provide futile therapy has led to considerable controversy about the meaning of the term *futile* and its implications for unilateral decision making by physicians.[87] Current AHA guidelines suggest strictly defined circumstances for consideration of decisions to stop or withhold CPR efforts on the grounds of futility. The guidelines caution against unilateral decision making by physicians when value judgments are made about important goals of therapy from the patient's point of view.[67] Nevertheless, the subjective value judgments inherent in terms such as *hopeless, irreversible,* and *terminal* should be recognized, and open discussion among participants in the decision should be encouraged.[88]

Court decisions have also emphasized the same right of self-determination for incompetent patients that is granted competent patients.[89] Therefore, surrogate decision makers who are engaged in decisions about life-sustaining treatment (including CPR) for incompetent patients are required to ascertain and represent (to the extent possible) the wishes expressed by the patient while the patient was still competent (eg, "substituted judgment"). In other words, the surrogate decision maker attempts to reach the decision that the incapacitated person would make if able. Previous statements or indirect evidence of the patient's views regarding life-sustaining treatment or resuscitation provide legal ground for substituted judgment by the surrogate decision maker.[90] If it is impossible to ascertain the patient's prior wishes or if the patient was never competent, as in the case of minors, physicians and surrogate decision makers may decide the resuscitation status based on their assessment of the patient's "best interests."[91]

Designations of treatment as "ordinary" or "extraordinary" have been used to distinguish obligatory from optional care. Recent cases recognize the ambiguity of those terms and suggest that analysis should be shifted from the type of treatment to the condition of the patient, highlighting the potential benefit to the patient and the burden of the proposed treatment.[91] CPR, for example, might be considered disproportionately burdensome if it offers no reasonable possibility beyond very short-term survival.

Because previously expressed wishes may have little practical application to minors, parental decisions to withhold CPR or other life-sustaining treatment from children will be measured by the "best interest" test. Nevertheless, the surrogate decision makers are expected to exercise their judgment as to the child's best interest from the point of view of the child—what the child might choose if he or she were competent.[92] The conflicts that may arise between legitimate parental rights of family privacy and the state's interest in protecting the welfare of children will center on whether life-sustaining treatment serves the best interest of an individual child. When decisions must be made on behalf of never-competent patients, some urge that the autonomy of the family unit be upheld by deference to a guardian's or family's reasonable interpretation of a patient's best interest from the perspective of their own beliefs and values.[93]

Policies and Guidelines

To ensure protection of patients' rights in circumstances in which the healthcare provider must act rapidly with limited personal knowledge of the patient, many hospitals have adopted formal policies governing orders not to resuscitate. Explicit policies encourage prior deliberation, ensure adherence to informed consent requirements, and promote the assignment of decision-making responsibilities to appropriate persons. Such policies should include the following:

- Requirements that do-not-resuscitate orders be written on the order sheet, accompanied by progress notes that explain the rationale for the decision and identify the participants in the decision-making process
- Guidelines for prior judicial review in specifically enumerated circumstances.[94]

Orders not to resuscitate refer exclusively to the initiation of resuscitative measures in the event of cardiac or respiratory arrest and are entirely compatible with administration of all other diagnostic and therapeutic modalities.

Frequently physicians write orders for "partial codes," which limit the extent of resuscitation to be offered a patient.[95] Although rationalized as serving the patient's presumed best interest, partial code orders may create ethical and legal problems if they are not carefully considered and written. Do-not-resuscitate policies and forms used at some institutions provide opportunities to list specific associated life-support interventions that may or may not be incorporated into the limitation-of-treatment plan during the *prearrest* phase.

Ethics Committees

Legal scholars, professional organizations, and government agencies have recommended that hospitals establish ethics committees to encourage more systematic and disciplined approaches to medical decision making. The major functions envisioned for ethics committees are education, consultation, development of hospital policies and guidelines, and case review. Creation of a forum for discussion of ethical dilemmas, review of policies and guidelines related to medical ethics issues, and nonbinding case consultation may enhance the protection of patients' rights with little need for recourse to judicial intervention.[96] Experience to date suggests that a multidisciplinary ethics committee serves as an effective institutional resource, particularly in cases in which ambiguity, communication breakdown, disagreement, or apparent conflict of interest have complicated life-and-death decisions for incompetent patients.

A major impetus for the development of hospital-based ethics committees is the controversy surrounding the care of critically ill or seriously handicapped neonates. Many hospitals now have infant care review committees or subcommittees. Although many of the administrative and legal aspects of hospital ethics committees are still being developed, such groups appear to be playing an increasing role in life-support decisions.[97,98]

Emergency Medical Services

The establishment of EMS systems has significantly enhanced on-scene delivery of emergency care to cardiac arrest victims. These are complex, integrated systems of care with multidimensional responsibilities, including appropriate maintenance of equipment, delineation of standards of care at various levels of training, on-site decisions to initiate or terminate CPR, shared clinical and legal responsibility between the emergency medical technician and central medical control, and application of immunity statutes to professional EMTs. All of these areas are subjects of potential litigation.

Specially trained technicians (EMTs, paramedics) working within such systems will generally be held to a standard of care commensurate with their level of training or certification. Most states require paramedics to pass the Department of Transportation course reflecting criteria established by the Task Force on EMTs of the National Academy of Sciences–National Research Council. Because EMTs engage in a quasi-medical practice outside the hospital, their scope of practice relies on standing order protocols and offline medical direction.[99] System organization varies widely from place to place. In some states and some EMS sysems, EMTs are required to initiate resuscitation attempts in virtually all instances without attempting to determine viability[100] and to resolve any doubts as to patient viability in favor of the patient. CPR may be terminated only by order of a physician.[101,102]

As a rule, the EMT may not disregard or countermand an order given by a physician.[103] Conflicts may arise at the scene when an EMT and a physician who may be less skilled in prehospital emergency care respond to a cardiac arrest. Most EMS systems have specific policies dealing with this issue. The procedure used varies widely from system to system.

Training programs and transport protocols for the prehospital system of emergency care are primarily designed to respond to adult cardiac arrest victims. Evidence suggests that some systems fall short of providing optimal care for children.[104] Promotion of guidelines for pediatric emergency care, including CPR, should improve the quality and consistency of care provided to children.

Brain Death

Current technology may maintain cardiorespiratory function in patients with minimal or no brain function and no possibility for recovery. These developments challenge traditional legal, cultural, and religious concepts of death and highlight the need for reliable policy for deter-

mination of death when cardiorespiratory activity is maintained through technology.[105] A determination that death of the whole brain has occurred has become well established as a legal standard of death in the United States. Brain death statutes generally conform to the Model Uniform Determination of Death Act[106,107] and state that a person is legally dead when (1) irreversible cessation of circulation and respiratory function or (2) irreversible cessation of all functions of the entire brain including the brain stem has been determined according to accepted medical standards.[106,107] The brain death statute in New Jersey includes a controversial "conscience clause" that provides that in situations in which the physician is aware that the patient's or family's religious convictions would be violated by a declaration of brain death, only cardiorespiratory death criteria may be applied.[108]

The diagnosis of brain death in children may be difficult. Specific criteria for brain death developed for adults have not been validated for children. Authoritative statements that may serve as useful working guidelines have been issued for adults and children of various age groups.[109,110] Diagnosis of death based on neurologic criteria should be approached with particular caution in circumstances in which neurologic function may be altered by hypothermia, use of neuromuscular blocking agents or barbiturates, or unknown cause of brain insult.[111,112]

Cardiopulmonary support systems may be withdrawn from brain-dead patients without judicial review or fear of legal repercussions. In homicide cases courts have consistently rejected the alleged assailant's defense that the discontinuation of cardiorespiratory support of the brain-dead victim caused death.[113] Similarly, courts have authorized the discontinuance of cardiorespiratory support systems for brain-dead victims of child abuse without affecting the criminal charges against the alleged abuser.[114]

Extraordinary situations have occurred in which CPR or life support of brain-dead pregnant women was continued for the protection of a viable fetus.[115-117] Rapid advances in perinatology have brought into focus the potential conflicts between maternal and fetal rights. These conflicts of interest are expected to occasionally include the pregnant woman's right to refuse life-sustaining treatment.[118]

Advance Directives

The Patient Self-determination Act, passed by Congress in 1990, requires hospitals and other healthcare facilities and agencies that participate in Medicare and Medicaid to establish written policies and procedures to inform all adult patients of their right to prescribe binding limits to CPR and life-sustaining measures in the event of future decisional incapacity.[119,120] Advance directives may serve to provide surrogate decision makers with important evidence of an incompetent patient's wishes, even in states without living will statutes.[86] The Patient Self-determination Act was further revised in 1991 to require hospitals and healthcare agencies to establish written policies and procedures to inform all adult patients of their rights to make decisions concerning medical care, including the right to accept or refuse medical or surgical treatment and the right to formulate an advance directive.[121]

It is now accepted that competent adult patients have the right to decide their treatment with a living will. However, the usefulness of these living wills may be limited by the inability to foresee all possible situations that may arise. The addition of a durable power of attorney gives the appointed person the ability to make a decision based on the patient's beliefs.[122]

Application of advance directives is difficult in pediatric practice. The previously discussed issues of consent by minors and competence must be considered. Despite these limitations, the use of advance directives in pediatric patients is increasing.[123]

The Delivery Room

The standard of care in the delivery room has improved dramatically in recent years. Professional organizations have promulgated national guidelines for the appropriate organization of skilled personnel and equipment to ensure delivery of acceptable resuscitation services to high-risk neonates,[124,125] which may have important implications for the legal liability of physicians and nurses in delivery rooms.

The prediction of the need for neonatal resuscitation has been improved through widespread use of fetal monitoring, increased sophistication in neonatal resuscitation, and the general availability of regional referral centers. These improvements provide potential for professional liability. Birth-related problems are the largest single source of malpractice suits against pediatricians.[126]

Organ and Tissue Donation

Successful CPR does not guarantee successful cerebral resuscitation, and brain death may follow. Patients who are pronounced "brain dead" may become vascular organ donors. Cadaveric tissue donation is also possible after circulatory function ceases, and this form of donation does not require brain death. Permission from next of kin or prior consent must be obtained for any tissue or organ donation, and the patient's wishes, if expressed before resuscitation, should be considered.

The shortage of suitable organs has led to the enactment of "required request" laws that require documentation that families of potential donors are offered the option of organ donation and that the local organ procurement organization is notified of potential donors.[127] A controversial proposal has been made for "presumed consent," which would permit the body of every deceased person to be used as a potential organ donor unless that person had declared an objection to being a donor before death or the next of kin declares such an objection immediately upon notification of death.[128] Such measures have been adopted in several countries but not in the United States.

Ethics of Practicing Intubation Skills

Many healthcare providers lack sufficient clinical experience in management of the pediatric and infant airway. Under certain circumstances, intubation of newly deceased infants and children may be performed to improve the healthcare providers' skills. This practice, although controversial, is brief and beneficial to others and is an effective teaching technique. However, the sensibilities of family and staff should be respected and consent obtained.

Conclusions

Advanced life support providers should explore the ethical and legal obligations that attend pediatric lifesaving skills.

- Children are different from adults, and appropriate management regimens cannot safely be derived simply by scaling down adult versions.
- Performance of pediatric ALS trainees in pediatric resuscitation will be judged against the content of the pediatric BLS and pediatric ALS courses.
- Providers should develop an appreciation of the unique rights of parents and children, the limits of parental authority, and the role of the state in protecting the welfare of children.
- The professional should recognize when the rights of parents and children may conflict, especially when making decisions to withhold CPR. Available institutional and judicial resources should be consulted to ensure that the best interests of the child are protected.
- When there is doubt about the authority or reasonableness of guardian requests to withhold CPR, a presumption that resuscitation is indicated should govern professional conduct until the conflict can be resolved.
- Even if potential rescuers lack confidence in their pediatric skills, they should undertake good-faith efforts at resuscitation to the limits of their ability, relying on legal protection based on common-law doctrines or Good Samaritan statutes.
- The importance of postresuscitation care must be recognized even when resuscitation is unsuccessful in restoring cerebral and cardiopulmonary function. Respect and sensitivity in dealing with organ donation, postmortem examinations, and bereavement will ultimately benefit the child's family.

References

1. Kouwenhoven WB, Jude JR, Knickerbocker GG. Closed-chest cardiac massage. *JAMA.* 1960;173:1064-1067.
2. Veatch RM. *A Theory of Medical Ethics.* New York, NY: Basic Books; 1981:25.
3. *Prosser and Keeton on the Law of Torts.* 5th ed. St Paul, Minn: West; 1984:186, 341, 375, 378, 382.
4. Wadlington W, Waltz JR, Dworkin RB. *Cases and Materials on Law and Medicine.* Mineola, NY: Foundation Press; 1980:470.
5. Rozovsky FA. *Consent to Treatment: A Practical Guide.* Boston, Mass: Little Brown & Co; 1984:31,439.
6. *Scholendorff v Society of New York Hospital,* 211 NY 125, 105 NE 92 (1914).
7. President's Commission for the Study of Ethical Problems in Medicine and Biomedical and Behavioral Research. *Making Health Care Decisions: A Report on the Ethical and Legal Implications of Informed Consent in the Patient-Practitioner Relationship.* Washington, DC: US Government Printing Office; 1982:55.
8. *Canterbury v Spence,* 464 F2d 772, 787 (1972).
9. Capron AM. Informed Consent in Catastrophic Disease Treatment and Research. 123 U PA L R 340, 387 (1974).
10. Andrews LB. Informed consent statutes and the decisionmaking process. *J Leg Med.* 1984;5:163-217.
11. *Wisconsin v Yoder,* 406 US 205 (1972).
12. *In Re Green,* 307 A2d 279 (1973).
13. *In Re Seiferth,* 127 NE2d 820 (1955).
14. *Prince v Commonwealth of Massachusetts,* 321 US 158 (1944).
15. Rothman DJ, Rothman SM. The conflict over children's rights. *Hastings Cent Rep.* 1980;10:7-10.
16. *In Re Sampson,* 278 NE2d 918 (1972).
17. *Custody of a Minor,* 393 NE2d 836 (1979).
18. *Matter of Hofbauer,* 393 NE2d 1009 (1979).
19. American Academy of Pediatrics Committee on Bioethics. Religious exemptions from child abuse statutes. *Pediatrics.* 1988;81:169-171.
20. President's Commission for the Study of Ethical Problems in Medicine and Biomedical and Behavioral Research. *Deciding to Forego Life-Sustaining Treatment.* Washington, DC: US Government Printing Office; 1983:16, 227, 251, n58, 142, 443.
21. Pub L 98-457; Fed Reg 45CFR part 1340; April 15, 1985, p 14878.
22. Kopelman LM, Irons TG, Kopelman AE. Neonatologists judge the 'Baby Doe' regulations. *N Engl J Med.* 1988;318:677-683.
23. Carter BS. Neonatologists and bioethics after Baby Doe. *J Perinatol.* 1993;13:144-150.
24. Lantos JD, Meadow W, Miles SH, et al. Providing and forgoing resuscitative therapy for babies of very low birth weight. *J Clin Ethics.* 1992;3;283-287.
25. Allen MC, Donohue PK, Dusman AE. The limit of viability—neonatal outcome of infants born at 22 to 25 weeks' gestation. *N Engl J Med.* 1993;329:1597-1601.
26. Davis DJ. How aggressive should delivery room cardiopulmonary resuscitation be for extremely low birth weight neonates? *Pediatrics.* 1993;92:447-450.
27. Weir R. *Selective Nontreatment of Handicapped Newborns: Moral Dilemmas in Neonatal Medicine.* New York, NY: Oxford University Press; 1984.
28. Capron AM. The competence of children as self-deciders in biomedical intervention. In: Gaylin W, Macklin R, eds. *Who Speaks for the Child.* New York, NY: Plenum Publishing Corp; 1982:57.
29. Gaylin W. Competence, no longer all or nothing. In: Gaylin W, Macklin R, eds. *Who Speaks for the Child.* New York, NY: Plenum Publishing Corp; 1982:57.
30. Leikin SL. Minors' assent or dissent to medical treatment. *J Pediatr.* 1983;102:169-176.
31. Schowalter JE, Ferholt JB, Mann NM. The adolescent patient's decision to die. *Pediatrics.* 1973;51:97-103.
32. *In Re EG,* 549 NE2d 322 (1989).
33. American College of Legal Medicine. *Legal Medicine: Legal Dynamics of Medical Encounters.* 2nd ed. St Louis, Mo: Mosby Year Book; 1991.
34. *Shilkret v The Annapolis Emergency Hospital Association,* 349 A2d 245 (1975).
35. *Proceedings of the National Conference on the Medicolegal Implications of Emergency Medical Care.* Dallas, Tex: American Heart Association; 1975:133, 155.
36. Dalen JE, Howe JP III, Membrino GE. Sounding board: CPR training for physicians. *N Engl J Med.* 1980;303:455-457.
37. Quimby CW Jr, Spies FK. Liability of the hospital cardiac team. *Ark L R.* 1972;26:17, 24.
38. *Guerrero v Copper Queen Hospital,* 537 P2d 1329 (1975).
39. Mancini MR, Gale AT. *Emergency Care and the Law.* Rockville, MD: Aspen Systems Corp; 1981:99.
40. *Darling v Charleston Community Memorial Hospital,* 211 NE2d 253 (1965).
41. Smith WB. Hospital liability for physician negligence. *JAMA.* 1984;251:447-448.
42. *Sparger v Worley Hospital, Inc,* 547 SW2d 582 (1977).
43. *Textbook of Advanced Cardiac Life Support.* Dallas, Tex: American Heart Association; 1983:4, 241.
44. Cummins RO, Eisenberg MS. Prehospital cardiopulmonary resuscitation: is it effective? *JAMA.* 1985;253:2408-2412.
45. Anderson AM, Haag B, Michelback AP. Help when needed: lay public confident of CPR skills. *J Kans Med Soc.* 1980;81:572-573.
46. Beauchamp TL, Childress JF, eds. *Principles of Biomedical Ethics.* 2nd ed. New York, NY: Oxford University Press Inc; 1983:148.
47. Weinrub EJ. The case for a duty to rescue. *Yale L J.* 1980; 90:247, 250.
48. Lipkin RJ. Beyond Good Samaritans and moral monsters: an individualistic justification of the general legal duty to rescue. *UCLA L R.* 1983;31:252-253, 262.
49. *Current Opinion of the Judicial Council of the American Medical Association.* 1984: IX.
50. Helminski FJ. Good Samaritan statutes: time for uniformity. *Wayne L R.* 1980;27:217, 221, 231.
51. Vt Stat Ann tit 12, §519 (1973).
52. Minn Stat Ann, §605.05 (West 1983).
53. Feuerhelm KW. Taking notice of Good Samaritan and Duty to Rescue laws. *J Contemp Law.* 1984;11:219.
54. Mapel FB III, Weigel CJ II. Good Samaritan laws — who needs them: the current state of Good Samaritan protection in the United States. *S Tex L J.* 1981;21:327, 351.
55. Restatement of Torts, 2d 289, 296, 298 (1965).
56. Zaritsky A, Nadkarn V, Getson P, Kuehl K. CPR in children. *Ann Emerg Med.* 1987;16:1107-1111.
57. Sullivan B. Some thoughts on the constitutionality of Good Samaritan statutes. *Am J Law Med.* 1982;8:27.
58. Standards and guidelines for cardiopulmonary resuscitation (CPR) and emergency cardiac care (ECC). *JAMA.* 1986;255:2905-2989.
59. Emergency Cardiac Care Committee and Subcommittees, American Heart Association. Guidelines for cardiopulmonary resuscitation and emergency cardiac care. *JAMA.* 1992;268: 2171-2302.
60. Kellermann AL. Criteria for dead-on-arrivals, prehospital termination of CPR, and do-not-resuscitate orders. *Ann Emerg Med.* 1993;22:47-51.
61. Eliastam M, Duralde T, Martinez F, Schwartz D. Cardiac arrest in the emergency medical service system: guidelines for resuscitation. *J Am Coll Emerg Phys.* 1977;6:525-529.
62. Eliastam M. When to stop cardiopulmonary resuscitation. *Top Emerg Med.* 1979;1:109.
63. O'Marcaigh AS, Koenig WJ, Rosekrans JA, Berseth CL. Cessation of unsuccessful pediatric resuscitation: how long is too long? *Mayo Clin Proc.* 1993;68:332-336.
64. Chipman C, Adelman R, Sexton G. Criteria for cessation of CPR in the emergency department. *Ann Emerg Med.* 1981;10:11-17.
65. DeBard ML. Cardiopulmonary resuscitation: analysis of six years' experience and review of the literature. *Ann Emerg Med.* 1981;10:408-416.
66. Lantos JD, Berger AC, Zucker AR. Do-not-resuscitate orders in a children's hospital. *Crit Care Med.* 1993;21:52-55.
67. Emergency Cardiac Care Committee, American Heart Association: Guidelines for cardiopulmonary resuscitation and emergency cardiac care, VIII: ethical considerations in resuscitation. *JAMA.* 1992;268:2282-2288.

68. American College of Emergency Physicians. Guidelines for 'do not resuscitate orders' in the prehospital setting. *Ann Emerg Med.* 1988;17:1106-1108.

69. Miles SH, Crimmins TJ. Orders to limit emergency treatment for an ambulance service. *JAMA.* 1985;254:525-527.

70. *Satz v Perlmutter,* 362 So2d 160 (1978).

71. *Lane v Candura,* 376 NE2d 1232 (1978).

72. *Belchertown State School v Saikewicz,* 370 NE2d 417, 425 (1977).

73. Drane JF. The many faces of competency. *Hastings Cent Rep.* 1985;15:17-21.

74. Jackson DL, Youngner S. Patient autonomy and 'death with dignity': some clinical caveats. *N Engl J Med.* 1979;301:404-408.

75. Bedell SE, Delbanco TL. Choices about cardiopulmonary resuscitation in the hospital: when do physicians talk with patients? *N Engl J Med.* 1984; 310:1089-1093.

76. Evans AL, Brody BA. The do-not-resuscitate order in teaching hospitals. *JAMA.* 1985;253:2236-2239.

77. Eisenberg JM. Sociologic influences on decision-making by clinicians. *Ann Intern Med.* 1979;90:957-964.

78. Youngner S, Jackson DL, Allen M. Staff attitudes towards the care of the critically ill in the medical intensive care unit. *Crit Care Med.* 1979;7:35-40.

79. Spencer SS. Sounding board: 'code or no code': a nonlegal opinion. *N Engl J Med.* 1979;300:138-140.

80. McPhail A, Moore S, O'Connor J, Woodward C. One hospital's experience with a 'do not resuscitate' policy. *Can Med Assoc J.* 1981;125:830-836.

81. Robertson JA. *The Rights of the Critically Ill: The Basic ACLU Guide to the Rights of Critically Ill and Dying Patients.* Cambridge, Mass: Ballinger; 1983:77, 79, 100.

82. Farber NJ, Bowman SM, Major DA, Green WP. Cardiopulmonary resuscitation (CPR): patient factors and decision making. *Arch Intern Med.* 1984;144:2229-2232.

83. Hashimoto DM. A structural analysis of the physician-patient relationship in no-code decision making. *Yale L R.* 1983;93:363, 381.

84. *In Re Swan,* 569 A2d 1202 (1990).

85. Wanzer SH, Federmann DD, Adelstein SJ, et al. The physician's responsibility toward hopelessly ill patients: a second look. *N Engl J Med.* 1984;310:955-959.

86. *In Re Dinnerstein,* 380 NE2d 134 (1978).

87. Jecker NS, Schneiderman LJ. An ethical analysis of the use of 'futility' in the 1992 American Heart Association Guidelines for Cardiopulmonary Resuscitation and Emergency Cardiac Care. *Arch Intern Med.* 1993;153:2195-2198.

88. Lo B, Steinbrook RL. Deciding whether to resuscitate. *Arch Intern Med.* 1983;143:1561-1563.

89. *Matter of Quinlan,* 355 A2d 647 (1976).

90. *Matter of Conroy,* 486 A2d 1209 (1985).

91. *Barber v Superior Court.* 195 Cal Rptr 484 (1983).

92. *Custody of a Minor,* 434 NE2d 601 (1982).

93. Veatch RM. Limits of guardian treatment refusal: a reasonableness standard. *Am J Law Med.* 1984;9:427-468.

94. *In Re Storar,* 52 NY2d 363 (1981).

95. Youngner SJ, Lewandowski W, McClish DK, Juknialis BW, Coulton C, Bartlett ET. 'Do not resuscitate' orders: incidence and implications in a medical-intensive care unit. *JAMA.* 1985; 253:54-57.

96. Cranford RE, Doudera AE, eds. *Institutional Ethics Committees and Health Care Decision Making.* Ann Arbor, Mich: Health Administration Press; 1984.

97. Fost N, Cranford RE. Hospital ethics committees: administrative aspects. *JAMA.* 1985;253:2687-2692.

98. AMA Judicial Council. Guidelines for ethics committees in health care institutions. *JAMA.* 1985;253:2698-2699.

99. Smith JP, Bodai BI. The urban paramedic's scope of practice. *JAMA.* 1985;253:544-548.

100. 5 *EMT Legal Bull* 4. 1981.

101. 7 *EMT Legal Bull* 7. 1983.

102. 5 *EMT Legal Bull* 3. 1981.

103. Caroline NL. *Emergency Care in the Streets.* 2nd ed. Boston, Mass: Little Brown & Co; 1983:7.

104. Seidel JS, Hornbein M, Yoshiyama K, Kuznets D, Finklestein JZ, St Geme JW Jr. Emergency medical services and the pediatric patient: are the needs being met? *Pediatrics.* 1984;73:769-772.

105. President's Commission for the Study of Ethical Problems in Medicine and Biomedical and Behavioral Research. *Defining Death: A Report on the Medical, Legal, and Ethical Issues in the Determination of Death.* Washington, DC: US Government Printing Office; 1983:13.

106. Guidelines for the determination of death: report of the medical consultants on the diagnosis of death to the President's Commission for the Study of Ethical Problems in Medicine and Biomedical and Behavioral Research. *JAMA.* 1981; 246:2184-2186.

107. Uniform Determination of Death Act. 1990 (West Supp.). Uniform Laws Annotated. Title 12, pp. 320-323.

108. Olick RS. Brain death, religious freedom and public policy: New Jersey's landmark legislation initiative. *Kennedy Institute of Ethics Journal.* 1991;1:275-282.

109. The Hastings Center. *Guidelines on the Termination of Life-Sustaining Treatment and the Care of the Dying: A Report.* Briarcliff Manor, NY: The Center; 1987:85.

110. American Academy of Pediatrics Task Force on Brain Death in Children. Report of a special task force: guidelines for the determination of brain death in children. *Pediatrics.* 1987;80:298-300.

111. Freeman JM, Rogers MC. On death, dying and decisions. *Pediatrics.* 1980;66:637-638.

112. Robinson RO. Brain death in children. *Arch Dis Child.* 1981;56:657-658.

113. Eisner JM, Randell LL, Tilson JQ. Judicial decisions concerning brain death. *Conn Med.* 1982;46:193-194.

114. Cook JW, Hirsch L. *I: Medicine and Law.* New York, NY: Springer International; 1982;1:135, 140.

115. Dillon WP, Lee RV, Tronolone MJ, Buckwald S, Foote RJ. Life support and maternal brain death during pregnancy. *JAMA.* 1982;248:1089-1091.

116. Siegler M, Wikler D. Brain death and live birth. *JAMA.* 1982;248:1101-1102. Editorial.

117. Veatch RM. Maternal brain death: an ethicist's thoughts. *JAMA.* 1982;248:1102-1103. Editorial.

118. Bowes WA Jr, Selgestad B. Fetal versus maternal rights: medical and legal perspectives. *Obstet Gynecol.* 1981;58:209-214.

119. Society for the Right to Die. September 1990.

120. Omnibus Reconciliation Act of 1990, Public L. No 101-508 Sec 4206, 4751.

121. Wolf SM, Boyle P, Callahan D, et al. Sources of concern about the Patient Self-determination Act. *N Engl J Med.* 1991; 325:1666-1671.

122. Silverman HJ, Vinicky JK, Gasner MR. Advance directives: implications for critical care. *Crit Care Med.* 1992;20:1027-1031.

123. Jefferson LS, White BC, Louis PT, Brody BA, King DD, Roberts CE. Use of the Natural Death Act in pediatric patients. *Crit Care Med.* 1991;19:901-905.

124. American Academy of Pediatrics, American College of Obstetricians and Gynecologists. *Guidelines for Perinatal Care.* 3rd ed. Evanston, Ill/Washington, DC; 1992.

125. Neonatal Resuscitation Program. American Academy of Pediatrics/American Heart Association.

126. *American Academy of Pediatrics News.* February 1985.

127. Omnibus Budget Reconciliation Act of 1986 (OBRA), Public Law 99-509, October 21, 1986.

128. Moskop JC. Organ transplantation in children: ethical issues. *J Pediatr.* 1987;110:175-180.

Index

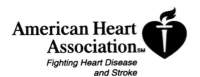

National Center
7272 Greenville Avenue
Dallas, Texas 75231-4596
Tel 214 373 6300
Fax 214 706 1341

Dear Colleague:

Every five to seven years the American Heart Association hosts a major conference to revise the *Guidelines for Cardiopulmonary Resuscitation (CPR) and Emergency Cardiac Care (ECC)*, published in the *Journal of the American Medical Association*. These guidelines are the scientific foundation on which our programs in basic life support, advanced cardiac life support, and pediatric advanced life support are based.

Because important medical advances in the field of cardiopulmonary resuscitation and emergency cardiac care occur in the years between major conferences, the Committee on Emergency Cardiac Care and its subcommittees have created a means through which new recommendations can be made and the algorithms revised when necessary. *Currents in Emergency Cardiac Care* is the official newsletter of the AHA and the Citizens CPR Foundation. This quarterly publication allows us to communicate with instructors and providers of CPR and ECC throughout the world. For as little as $1 a month, *Currents* subscribers receive

- Reports from the ECC Committee and its subcommittees

- Changes in the scientific guidelines and algorithms

- Reports from the Citizen CPR Foundation

- Highlights from other ECC publications from the United States and around the world.

In addition, *Currents* features

- A readers' forum to facilitate two-way communication between local and national ECC volunteers and staff

- An instructors' column on educational issues

- And much, much more.

As chairman of the ECC Committee, I urge you to subscribe to *Currents in Emergency Cardiac Care*. To place your order, mail or fax the subscription card in this book or call 1-800-AHA-1793, ext. 1310.

Best personal wishes,

Joseph P. Ornato, MD
Chairman, Committee on Emergency Cardiac Care

For immediate response, take advantage of our customer services. We provide prompt and courteous service for:

- Change of address

- Missing issues

- Free catalog of Scientific Councils and Journals

- Special trainee and emeritus rates

- Scientific Council Membership information

Please call Scientific Publishing Customer Service at (214) 706-1310 Fax (214) 691-6342

Advance payment is required on all orders.

We accept MasterCard, Visa, American Express, and checks for:

- Renewals
- New orders
- Single copies

Make checks payable to the American Heart Association in US dollars drawn on a US bank.

Information you need from the authority you trust

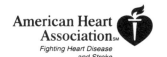

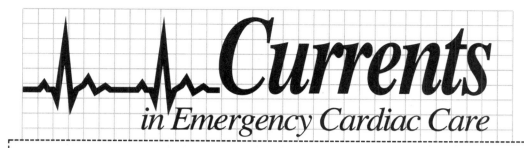

Get to the heart of cardiac care.

In this age of information overload, you need a resource that keeps you professionally current. CURRENTS IN EMERGENCY CARDIAC CARE saves you valuable time by getting to "the heart of the matter." It provides the most vital, up-to-date, and authoritative data on CPR and ECC procedures, treatments, and guidelines in a style that's clear and concise. Each issue includes timely reports from the American Heart Association's Committee on Emergency Cardiac Care and its Basic, Advanced, Pediatric and Program Administration Subcommittees as well as news on trends, developments, and innovations in emergency cardiac care from around the world.

The American Heart Association invites you to become a scientific council member. Membership allows you to contribute your knowledge and expertise to the advancement of pulmonary, critical care, and resuscitation science within the AHA as well as to receive important information regarding research findings and patient education materials.

This offer expires March 31, 1997.

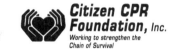

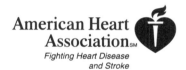

Fold on the line below and tape - DO NOT STAPLE

☐ **YES,** I want to subscribe to Currents in Emergency Cardiac Care!
___ US Individual......................................$12
___ Non-US Individual..............................$16

☐ **YES,** I want to become a Scientific Council Member!

___ Cardiopulmonary and Critical Care......$25

___ Cardiovascular Nursing.........................$25

___ Cardiovascular Disease in the Young....$30

Please start my subscription with the issue indicated (check one):

___ March ___ June ___Sept. ___ Dec.
      Year ____ or ___next issue

Advanced payment required
__ Check enclosed, in US dollars, drawn on a US bank
__ MasterCard __ Visa __ American Express
Account number

_____

Expiration date: Month____ Year_____
Signature as it appears on card
_____

Total order $ _____

Name_____

Address_____

_____

State_____Zip _____

Country_____

Phone_____ Fax_____

E-Mail _____

Month/year of birth __/__

___Male ___ Female

Race/Ethnicity: ___American Indian ___Asian
                        ___Black ___Hispanic
                        ___White

% of time spent: ___Administrative ___ Research
                        ___Patient Care ___Teaching
                        ___Other

My Specialty is: (check one)

___ Physician   ___ Anesthesiology
___ Nurse   ___ Critical Care
___ EMS personnel   ___ Cardiology
___ CPR/ACLS instructor   ___ Other (specify)

5ECC01/2

SCIENTIFIC PUBLISHING
AMERICAN HEART ASSOCIATION
PO BOX 843543
DALLAS TX 75284-3543